ROBOTIC AND NAVIGATED SPINE SURGERY

Surgical Techniques and Advancements

ROBOTIC AND NAVIGATED SPINE SURGERY

Surgical Techniques and Advancements

ANAND VEERAVAGU, MD, FAANS
Assistant Professor of Neurosurgery
Director of Minimally Invasive NeuroSpine Surgery
Stanford University School of Medicine
Stanford, California
United States

MICHAEL Y. WANG, MD, FAANS
Professor of Neurological Surgery and Rehabilitation Medicine
Neurosurgery
University of Miami Miller School of Medicine;
Chief of Neurosurgery and Director, Neurosurgical Spine Fellowship
University of Miami Hospital,
Miami, Florida
United States

ELSEVIER

Elsevier
1600 John F. Kennedy Blvd.
Ste 1800
Philadelphia, PA 19103-2899

ROBOTIC AND NAVIGATED SPINE SURGERY
Surgical Techniques and Advancements

ISBN: 978-0-323-71160-9

Content Development Manager: Somodatta Roy Choudhury
Content Strategist: Humayra R. Khan
Senior Content Development Specialist: Priyadarshini Pandey
Publishing Services Manager: Shereen Jameel
Project Manager: Vishnu T. Jiji
Design Direction: Renee Duenow

Printed in India

Last digit is the print number: 9 8 7 6 5 4 3 2 1

This book is dedicated to my incredible family
who has supported me every step of the way,
and to the entire healthcare community who stood steadfast
in the face of the worldwide COVID-19 pandemic.

Anand Veeravagu, MD, FAANS

To Amy, Patrick, Evan, and Sarah.
Thank you for all of your support.

Michael Y. Wang, MD, FAANS

CONTRIBUTORS

A. Karim Ahmed, MD
Resident
Department of Neurosurgery
Johns Hopkins School of Medicine
Baltimore, Maryland
United States

Adriel Barrios-Anderson, BSc
Medical Student
Neurosurgery
The Warren Alpert Medical School of Brown University
Providence, Rhode Island
United States

Phillip Behrens, MD
Orthopedic Surgery
Cedars-Sinai Medical Center
Los Angeles, California
United States

Atiq Ur Rehman Bhatti, MD
Research Fellow
Neurologic Surgery
Mayo Clinic
Rochester, Minnesota
United States

Mohamad Bydon, MD
Professor
Neurologic Surgery
Mayo Clinic
Rochester, Minnesota
United States

Joaquin Q. Camara, MD
Assistant Professor
Neurosurgery
Brown University
Providence, Rhode Island
United States

Dean Chou, MD
Professor
Neurosurgery
University of California, San Francisco
San Francisco, California
United States

Richard Danilkowicz, MAT, MD
Orthopedic Surgery
Duke University Hospital
Durham, North Carolina
United States

Nader Delavari, MD
Chief Resident
Neurosurgery
New York University
New York City, New York
United States

Brian Dial, MD
Surgeon
Orthopedic Surgery
Duke University
Durham, North Carolina
United States

Doniel Drazin, MD, MA
Neurosurgeon
Pacific Northwest University of Health Sciences
Yakima, WA, USA,
Providence Regional Medical Center
Everett, Washington
United States

Jeff Ehresman, MD
Resident
Neurosurgery
Barrow Neurological Institute in Phoenix Arizona
Johns Hopkins University School of Medicine
Baltimore, Maryland
United States

Cyrus Elahi MS, MD
Resident Neurosurgery
Barrow Neurological Institute
Phoenix, Arizona
United States

Melissa Erickson, MD
Associate Professor of Orthopedic Surgery & Neurosurgery
Duke University School of Medicine
Durham, North Carolina
United States

S. Harrison Farber, MD
Resident
Neurosurgery
Barrow Neurological Institute
Phoenix, Arizona
United States

Parastou Fatemi, MD
Resident Physician
Neurological Surgery
Stanford University
Stanford, California
United States

Anthony K. Frempong-Boadu, MD
Associate Professor
Neurosurgery and Orthopedic Surgery
New York University Langone Health
Director of Spinal Surgery
New York University
New York City, New York
United States

Anshit Goyal, MBBS, MS
Resident
Department of Neurosurgery
Mayo Clinic
Jacksonville, Florida
United States

Joseph Hsieh, MD, MBA, MPH, MS
Assistant Professor
UT Health Neurosciences
UT Houston
Houston, Texas
United States

Jeremy Huang, BS
Clinical Research Coordinator
Department of Neurological Surgery
University of California, San Francisco
San Francisco, California
United States

Ibrahim Hussain, MD
Clinical Instructor
Neurological Surgery
University of Miami
Miami, Florida
United States

Bowen Jiang, MD
Neurosurgery
Providence St. Jude Medical Center
Fullerton, California
United States

Michael Jin, BS
Medical Student
School of Medicine
Stanford University
Stanford, California
United States

J. Patrick Johnson, MS, MD, FACS, FAANS
Director
Spine Center
Cedars Sinai
President and CEO
Neurosurgery
Spine Institute Foundation
Los Angeles, California
United States

Isaac Karikari, MD
Assistant Professor
Neurosurgery and Orthopedic Surgery
Duke University Medical Center
Durham, North Carolina
United States

Jayanidhi Kedda, BS
Medical Student Researcher
Department of Neurosurgery
Johns Hopkins Hospital
Baltimore, Maryland
United States

Terrence T. Kim, MD
Director of Education and Fellowship
Orthopedic Surgery
Cedars-Sinai Medical Center
Los Angeles, California
United States

Jason I. Liounakos, MD
Resident
Neurological Surgery
University of Miami
Miami, Florida
United States

Ann Liu, MD
Resident Physician
Neurosurgery
Johns Hopkins Hospital
Baltimore, Maryland
United States

Sheng-Fu Larry Lo, MD, MHS
Assistant Professor of Neurosurgery
Neurosurgery
Johns Hopkins University
School of Medicine
Baltimore, Maryland
United States

Victor Lo, MD, MPH
Neurosurgery
Kaiser Permanente—Southern
California Permanente Medical Group
San Diego, California
United States

Nicolai Maldaner, MD
Junior Consultant
Department of Neurosurgery
University Hospital Zürich
Zürich
Switzerland

Rory R. Mayer, MD
Clinical Instructor
Neurosurgery
University of California, San Francisco
San Francisco, California
United States

Praveen V. Mummaneni, MD, MBA
Joan O'Reilly Endowed Professor
Vice Chairman
Department of Neurological Surgery
Director Minimally Invasive Spine Fellowship
University of California, San Francisco
San Francisco, California
United States

Adetokunbo 'Toki' Oyelese, MD, PhD
Professor
Department of Neurosurgery
Brown University Medical School
Director Division of Spine Surgery
Department of Neurosurgery
Rhode Island Hospital
Providence, Rhode Island
United States

Mark A. Pacult, MD
Resident
Neurosurgery
Barrow Neurological Institute
Phoenix, Arizona
United States

Zach Pennington, MD
Resident
Department of Neurosurgery
Mayo Clinic
Rochester, Minnesota
United States

Robert C. Ryu, MD
Adjunct Assistant Professor
Department of Orthopaedics
The Ohio State University Wexner Medical Center
Columbus, Ohio
United States

Ethan Schonfeld
Masters Student
Biomedical Informatics
Stanford University
Stanford, California
United States

Marc Schroder, MD, PhD
Chairman
Department of Neurosurgery
Bergman Clinics
Amsterdam
The Netherlands

Daniel M. Sciubba, MD
Professor and Chair
Department of Neurosurgery
Hofstra University/Northwell
Manhasset, New York
United States

Victor E. Staartjes, MD
Resident, Research Group Leader
Machine Intelligence in Clinical Neuroscience (MICN)
Laboratory
Department of Neurosurgery
University Hospital Zürich
Zürich
Switzerland

Martin Nikolaus Stienen, MD, FEBNS
Senior Attending, Department of Neurosurgery
Deputy Chair, Spine Center of Eastern Switzerland
Kantonsspital St. Gallen
St. Gallen
Switzerland

Nicholas Theodore, MD
Professor of Neurosurgery
Orthopedic Surgery, Pediatrics and Biomedical Engineering
Johns Hopkins University School of Medicine
Director, Neurosurgical Spine Center
Co-Director, Carnegie Center for Surgical Innovation
Johns Hopkins University
Baltimore, Maryland
United States

Juan S. Uribe, MD
Chief, Division of Spinal Disorders
Professor and Vice Chair
Volker K. H. Sonntag Chair of Spine Research
Neurological Surgery
Barrow Neurological Institute
Phoenix, Arizona
United States

Anand Veeravagu, MD, FAANS
Assistant Professor of Neurosurgery
Director of Minimally Invasive NeuroSpine Surgery
Stanford University School of Medicine
Stanford, California
United States

Harsh Wadhwa, BS
Medical Student
Neurosurgery
Stanford School of Medicine
Stanford, California
United States

Michael Y. Wang, MD, FAANS
Professor of Neurological Surgery and
Rehabilitation Medicine
Neurosurgery
University of Miami Miller School of Medicine
Chief of Neurosurgery and Director
Neurosurgical Spine Fellowship
University of Miami Hospital
Miami, Florida
United States

Ketan Yerneni, BA
Department of Neurosurgery
Stanford University
Stanford, California
United States

Corinna Clio Zygourakis, MD
Assistant Professor
Neurosurgery
Stanford University
Palo Alto, California
United States

ACKNOWLEDGMENT

The editors wish to thank the Elsevier publishing team including Humayra Khan, Laura Klein and Priyadarshini Pandey, whose invaluable assistance made the publication of this text possible. The editors would also like to thank Ethan Schonfeld whose contribution to content, organization, and management was vital to the publication of this book.

Anand Veeravagu and Michael Y. Wang

PREFACE

The rapid acceleration of robotic and computer technology has expanded the application of intelligent tools during routine and complex spine surgery. From image guidance to endoscopic techniques, the utilization of advanced technology in spine surgery has improved accuracy, decreased postoperative complications, and lowered radiation exposure. Notably, the integration of computer technology into clinical decision making has shown promise in predicting not only postoperative outcomes but also cage selections, rod bending angles, and surgical construct planning.

Data is the driving force of many of these advancements. For years, medicine has been slow to develop intelligent systems largely hindered by the difficulties in collecting and sharing data. Now, robotic systems reduce the need for surgeon directed data collection, with the systems themselves able to collect, share, and learn from this data directly. Yet, the need for collaboration and cooperation has only been accentuated.

As these technologies continue to grow in both their complexity and their outcomes, it is imperative for surgeons to stand at the forefront of their innovation. This book addresses both the foundational technologies (i.e., shared control robots, telesurgical robots, machine learning, and augmented reality) and clinical case reports demonstrating their utilization as well as the respective considerations involved in their current clinical practice. Through this dichotomy, it is evident that these technologies, from the most obvious to the most esoteric, can directly improve patient outcomes.

Anand Veeravagu and Michael Y. Wang

CONTENTS

1

Computer-Assisted Spine Surgery—A New Era of Innovation

Anand Veeravagu, MD, FAANS, Ethan Schonfeld, and Michael Y. Wang, MD, FAANS

The idea of surgical intelligence is finally coming to fruition. The use of both computer and robotic assistance, and increasing use of the two together, has already demonstrated the promise of surgical intelligence to transform spine surgery. Offering potential improvements in surgical accuracy, reductions in postoperative complications, and decreased revision surgeries, computer assistance provides the novel ability to base decision-making support on hundreds of thousands of prior cases. Poor measures of predictive power have been found for the surgeon's ability to predict risk and benefit of surgery.[1] The use of patient demographic and operative characteristics when creating complex analytical models allowed for the development of frailty scores that can better predict risks and benefits for a patient.[1] Coupling such decision-making support for surgical uses, such as rod bending angles, with the precise ability of robotics to carry out the task, continues to improve patient outcomes. To date, the use of robotics in surgery has resulted in improved screw placements and improved navigation and reduced radiation dose, length of stay, and need for revision surgeries.[2–6] However, as with many novel applications of technology, an array of challenges exists. These include reliance on single-centered retrospective data and limited data sharing, limited data for rare diseases and uncommon procedures, straight line trajectories of robotic movements, high costs of computer and robotic assistance (infeasible for small centers), high learning curves, a limited set of procedures for the use of such technologies (currently mainly used for screw placements), and legal issues regarding who is at fault in case of adverse events.

Recently, robotic uses for spine surgery are expanding from screw placements to include tissue-focused uses such as tumor resections, spurred by developments in haptic feedback systems, 3D printing, and mechanical advances.[7] Further expansion of procedure types arose for microscopic-based surgeries with augmented reality support, visualizing tool orientation with respect to the anatomy of interest with no disruptions to the surgical view.[8] Similar technological improvements, catalyzed by 5G, gave rise to huge advances in telesurgical robotics, with the successful demonstration of the first 12 cases in 2020.[9] With these advances, four dominant uses for computers and robotics in spine surgery have become apparent: telesurgical robotic surgery, shared-control robots with computer navigation, augmented reality systems, and machine learning decision-making support.

TELESURGICAL ROBOTIC SURGERY

While previously limited by bandwidth and speed of networks, the implementation of 5G eliminates such concerns with its high speed, high bandwidth, and low latency. Demonstrations of telesurgical spine procedures, using a one-to-many workflow, open the door for the possibility of state-of-the-art surgeons being able to reach populations otherwise unable to present to the hospital. The workflow for the first 12 cases of successful spinal robotic telesurgery is presented below.[9]

The telesurgery (demonstrated for pedicle screw implantation on patients with fracture, spondylolisthesis, or stenosis) involved a local operative team responsible for the peripheral tasks. First, the patients were anesthetized and the robotic system registered and positioned. A motorized C-arm took 3D images that were then transmitted to a control room (in a different city) over a 5G system. The surgeon using the robotic software chose the entry point, screw orientation, and surgical path under navigational guidance. However, the K-wire and screw placement was done by surgeons on the patient side along with all image acquisitions, positioning of tools, equipment and patient preparation, and patient tracker installation. Furthermore, any bone resection and nerve decompressions would be done on the patient side. In this way, for full telesurgical uses, further innovations to technology, including advanced robotic movement capabilities, are necessary.

Necessary future innovations to telesurgery for spine surgeries include better control, increased dependence on the master surgeon, and expansion of procedure types. Haptic feedback presents the potential for improvements to master surgeon control of the robot by mimicking hand movements.[10] Soft tissue surgery appears to be accomplishable by the current telesurgical systems, although data does not conclusively support this; soft tissue procedural safety, however, is supported by case reports using the da Vinci Surgical System.[11]

SHARED-CONTROL ROBOTS AND COMPUTER NAVIGATION

Most of the current uses of robotics for spine surgery involve shared-control robots, including the Mazor X, ExcelsiusGPS, and ROSA One. Allowing both the surgeon and robot to control instruments and motions, these technologies improve placement, bending, and cutting. With the ability to position the robotic arms along pre-planned trajectories, the surgeon is able to preoperatively plan procedures, thereby reducing complex movements and decision-making during the operation for the surgeon. The five main steps involved in most shared-control procedures include the surgeon marking the trajectory on preoperative CT scans in the robotic system, a mounting frame being attached to the patient for image registration, fluoroscopic imaging being performed to facilitate synchronization with the preoperative imaging, robotic attachment to the mounting frame, and screw placement with guide wires.

Shared-control screw fixation surgical procedures have been shown to result in improved screw placement and navigation, and reduced radiation dose, length of stay, and need for revision surgeries.[2–6] Furthermore, robotic use during surgery allows for data collection that does not require the surgeon to be involved. Such intraoperative data is already being collected and shared to develop better decision-making support for cage fitting and rod bending based on the patient outcomes of prior cases.[12]

However, such workflows suffer from limitations. One such limitation is that minor patient movements during surgery can desynchronize the robotic path from the pre-planned trajectories; to address this, a reliance on intraoperative imaging is needed. Such reliance poses significant radiation concerns to both the patient and surgeon. Furthermore, the linear restrictions of the robot allow for limited paths with the inability to perform some tissue procedures. However, advances in current state-of-the-art shared-control robots include mechanical advantages such as movement stabilization (no-fly zones, restriction of movements based on pre-planning, tremor filtering) as well as significant reductions to radiation exposure. The latter is accomplished through the use of computer navigation.

With robotics relying on minimally invasive procedures to prevent excess tissue damage, surgeons lost the ability to visualize the key anatomical landmarks as was possible in open surgery. Thus, a reliance on intraoperative repetitive fluoroscopy was created. To eliminate this, computer navigation began to make use of advances in machine learning. Machine learning is the ability for the computer to make predictions based on its knowledge of past data. In the lens of spine surgery, with the input of a camera-captured (no radiation) image of a patient's spine, the desired outcome may be to locate a specific landmark and synchronize it to a similarly located landmark in the preoperative CT image. To predict this desired outcome, a computer may be trained by repeated exposure to past cases where the desired output is known. Thus, with every case, a computer may learn how to predict better. Using such technology, advances in computer navigation have reduced radiation exposure by 80%; this method takes low-quality, low-dose intraoperative imaging and predicts how best to construct a higher quality image from this.[13] Similar computer vision advances have used non-radiation-based photography to capture patient landmark features and predict synchronization to preoperative imaging, thereby addressing patient movement desynchronization during the course of surgery.[14] While further research is required to develop synchronization and navigation based on optic cameras, such technology suggests a radiation-free intraoperative future workflow and thus illustrates the benefits computer navigation brings to shared-control and minimally invasive surgery.

AUGMENTED REALITY SYSTEMS

All the above procedures involve intraoperative imaging being displayed on a screen. This requires continuous disruption of the surgeon's workflow to match the orientation of their surgical equipment and tools with the anatomy displayed on the nearby screen. Such separation in the display increases surgical time, decreases the surgeon's understanding of the orientation of tools to anatomy, and requires more radiation exposure for continued intraoperative imaging. Augmented reality systems such as XVision, which is already cleared by the FDA, can superimpose the position of surgical tools on the CT imaging in real time and display the resulting augmented reality on a surgical headpiece that is worn by the surgeon.[8] A similar use of augmented reality involves projecting the pre-planned surgical path onto the patient in a surgical headpiece to guide navigation better. Furthermore, segmentations of vertebrae have been combined with augmented reality visualizations of screw orientations to guide placement accuracy. By superimposing O-arm imaging with the live view from the microscope, superimposed videos can guide surgeons during the course of tumor surgeries and degenerative spine disease procedures.[15]

Augmented reality uses are not limited to screw planning. Augmented reality can be used to project necessary anatomical landmarks into a surgeon's microscopic view during minimally invasive anterior cervical discectomy and fusion, posterior cervical laminotomy, and foraminotomy. Furthermore, augmented reality display of resection planes has been used in combination with microscopic eyepieces during osteotomy for deformity.[16]

Leveraging augmented reality systems for spine surgery may also serve as an educational tool. Allowing complex surgical procedures to be recreated in augmented reality environments can aid in the training of surgeons. Advanced future uses could expand such recreation to include simulation of a pre-planned technique and allow the surgeon to revise their plan based on the patient's anatomy and visualization with the augmented reality system before the surgery itself.

MACHINE LEARNING AND DECISION-MAKING SUPPORT

We have already discussed the applications of machine learning for spine surgery including lower-dose imaging, anatomic landmark synchronization to preoperative imaging during patient movements, cage selection, and rod bending. All these technologies rely on a shared infrastructure: they take input information relevant to the patient (demographic variables, operative characteristics, preoperative imaging, and intraoperative imaging) and output a prediction (best cage shape, best rod angle, simulated high-dose imaging, anatomical orientation and synchronization). This infrastructure is built upon each machine learning-driven system being trained on thousands of cases from past surgeries.

However, the use of machine learning in spine surgery extends to include the conversion of imaging information (MRI to CT), algorithmic decision-making support for path planning, and risk prediction.[17–19] Systems have already been developed that help with trajectory planning, avoiding at-risk tissue, and aiding the surgeon in obstacle avoidance during complex navigation. However, it is risk prediction that poses an immediate potential benefit to the current operating workflows. Using the available demographic and operative characteristics (including comorbidity status, procedural history, preoperative imaging, and operative plan), it is difficult for the surgeon to predict, based on their medical experience, the success of the planned surgery and risk of complication to the patient. With high-risk and high-cost procedures, high predictive capabilities in this domain hold incredible value. Machine learning allows for increased predictive power by learning from similar patients' outcomes. A surgeon is unable to compare the current patient to hundreds of thousands of others and consider how similar the patient is; however, the current algorithms allow for such techniques. Recent systems aimed to support surgical decision-making, rather than simply being a black box to output a prediction, resulted in the surgeon seeing the 5 or 10 past cases most similar to the current patient along with their respective outcomes. Such similarity determination is based on complex information including personality type and genetic information in the most recent work.[1] Such algorithms to be used for risk prediction have been instrumental in identifying risk factors. One such study found risk factors for sustained postoperative opioid use by leveraging a machine learning workflow.[20]

To train better and more predictive machine learning algorithms requires high amounts of data. This poses a problem in rare and more specialized cases; however, an increasing effort is resulting in better methods and availability of such data. Robotics allows continuous data collection without surgeon assistance being necessary. Companies have developed data sharing technology to be coupled with robotic systems for the simulation of surgical plans.[21]

CONCLUSION

Computer and robotic technologies are presenting clinically significant improvements to surgery, allowing them to make their way into state-of-the-art practice. However, there exists a need for formal cost-benefit analysis of the integration of these spine robotic systems into practice. There are potential high costs associated with the technology itself, high setup time, training curve, and increased surgical times as users are not familiar with the system; these may be offset by improved outcomes leading to decreased revision surgeries, readmission, and length of stay.

Further remaining to be studied is the potential for dissimilar distributions used for machine learning training. As data is scarce for many spine surgery tasks, such data may be taken from only one clinical center. For example, a machine learning system to segment the vertebrae may use the training data of CT scans from only one hospital. The CT scans of other hospitals may not closely resemble those from the first hospital, either in their distribution of anatomical abnormalities or even their imaging format. Such distribution shifts may pose a threat to the successful application of machine learning systems across varied users in spine surgery. As the field progresses, it will become necessary to use data for training that is obtained across a multitude of centers, capturing a wide range of types of conditions, imaging, and formats. We may soon begin to see the possibility for semi-, and even full, automation of surgical subroutines by robotics. As decision-making shifts toward increased reliance on the robotic and computer system predictions, standardized and regularized development of the deployment of such algorithms to patient care is imperative.

Computers and robotics offer, and have already partially achieved, a revolution in geographical reach, surgical precision, decision-making support, and decreased radiation in spine surgery.

REFERENCES

1. UCSF. Neurosurgery. How Big Data Is Changing Practice in Adult Deformity. YouTube. https://www.youtube.com/watch?v=TfgWilYXuJs. Accessed 10/15/2021. November 17, 2020.
2. Benech CA, Perez R, Benech F, Greeley SL, Crawford N, Ledonio C. Navigated robotic assistance results in improved screw accuracy and positive clinical outcomes: an evaluation of the first 54 cases. *J Robot Surg*. 2020;14(3):431–437. https://doi.org/10.1007/s11701-019-01007-z.
3. Fan M, Liu Y, He D, et al. Improved accuracy of cervical spinal surgery with robot-assisted screw insertion: a prospective, randomized, controlled study. *Spine*. 2020;45(5):285–291. https://doi.org/10.1097/BRS.0000000000003258.
4. Zhang Q, Han XG, Xu YF, et al. Robotic navigation during spine surgery. *Expert Rev Med Devices*. 2020;17(1):27–32. https://doi.org/10.1080/17434440.2020.1699405.
5. D'Souza M, Gendreau J, Feng A, Kim LH, Ho AL, Veeravagu A. Robotic-assisted spine surgery: history, efficacy, cost, and future trends. *Robot Surg*. 2019;6:9–23. https://doi.org/10.2147/RSRR.S190720.
6. Staub BN, Sadrameli SS. The use of robotics in minimally invasive spine surgery. *J Spine Surg*. 2019;5(suppl 1):S31–S40. https://doi.org/10.21037/jss.2019.04.16.
7. Sayari AJ, Pardo C, Basques BA, Colman MW. Review of robotic-assisted surgery: what the future looks like through a spine oncology lens. *Ann Transl Med*. 2019;7(10):224. https://doi.org/10.21037/atm.2019.04.69.
8. Dibble CF, Molina CA. Device profile of the XVision-spine (XVS) augmented-reality surgical navigation system: overview of its safety and efficacy. *Expert Rev Med Devices*. 2021;18(1):1–8. https://doi.org/10.1080/17434440.2021.1865795.
9. Tian W, Fan M, Zeng C, Liu Y, He D, Zhang Q. Telerobotic spinal surgery based on 5G network: the first 12 cases. *Neurospine*. 2020;17(1):114–120. https://doi.org/10.14245/ns.1938454.227.
10. Mohan A, Wara UU, Arshad Shaikh MT, Rahman RM, Zaidi ZA. Telesurgery and robotics: an improved and efficient era. *Cureus*. 2021;13(3):e14124. https://doi.org/10.7759/cureus.14124.
11. Trybula SJ, Oyon DE, Wolinsky JP. Robotic tissue manipulation and resection in spine surgery. *Neurosurg Clin N Am*. 2020;31(1):121–129. https://doi.org/10.1016/j.nec.2019.08.014.
12. Eisner W. FDA clearance completes Medicrea's AI spine platform. *Orthop This Week*. https://ryortho.com/breaking/fda-clearance-completes-medicreas-ai-spine-platform/. Accessed 10/15/2021. August 15, 2019.
13. Isaacs RE, Karikari IO, Anderson DG. Reducing radiation an order of magnitude during x-ray intensive spine procedures using a standard fluoroscope. *Spine J*. 2014;14(11). https://doi.org/10.1016/j.spinee.2014.08.206.
14. Burström G, Nachabe R, Persson O, Edström E, Elmi Terander A. Augmented and virtual reality instrument tracking for minimally invasive spine surgery: a feasibility

and accuracy study. *Spine*. 2019;44(15):1097–1104. https://doi.org/10.1097/BRS.0000000000003006.
15. Carl B, Bopp M, Saß B, Voellger B, Nimsky C. Implementation of augmented reality support in spine surgery. *Eur Spine J*. 2019;28(7):1697–1711. https://doi.org/10.1007/s00586-019-05969-4.
16. Yoo JS, Patel DS, Hrynewycz NM, Brundage TS, Singh K. The utility of virtual reality and augmented reality in spine surgery. *Ann Transl Med*. 2019;7(suppl 5):S171 https://doi.org/10.21037/atm.2019.06.38.
17. Goyal A, Ngufor C, Kerezoudis P, McCutcheon B, Storlie C, Bydon M. Can machine learning algorithms accurately predict discharge to nonhome facility and early unplanned readmissions following spinal fusion? Analysis of a national surgical registry. *J Neurosurg Spine*. 2019;31(4):1–11. https://doi.org/10.3171/2019.3.SPINE181367.
18. Staartjes VE, Seevinck PR, Vandertop WP, van Stralen M, Schröder ML. Magnetic resonance imaging–based synthetic computed tomography of the lumbar spine for surgical planning: a clinical proof-of-concept. *Neurosurg Focus*. 2021;50(1):E13. https://doi.org/10.3171/2020.10.FOCUS20801.
19. Zhang Q, Li M, Qi X, Hu Y, Sun Y, Yu G. 3D Path planning for anterior spinal surgery based on CT images and reinforcement learning. *IEEE International Conference on Cyborg and Bionic Systems (CBS)*. 2018. https://doi.org/10.1109/cbs.2018.8612190.
20. Karhade AV, Ogink PT, Thio QCBS, et al. Machine learning for prediction of sustained opioid prescription after anterior cervical discectomy and fusion. *Spine J*. 2019;19(6):976–983. https://doi.org/10.1016/j.spinee.2019.01.009.
21. Surgimap. *Overview*. https://www.surgimap.com/overview/.

2

Navigation in Occipital and Cervical Spine Surgery

Robert C. Ryu, MD, Phillip Behrens, MD, Doniel Drazin, MD, MA, Victor Lo, MD, MPH, Joseph Hsieh, MD, MBA, MPH, MS, Terrence T. Kim, MD, and J. Patrick Johnson, MS, MD, FACS, FAANS

INTRODUCTION OF TECHNOLOGY

In the occipital and cervical spine, posterior cervical instrumentation is a commonly selected procedure for stabilization in trauma, neoplasia, deformity, and spondylosis. The earliest techniques described wiring between the spinous processes to achieve bony arthrodesis.[1] Several types of instrumentation systems and screws were subsequently developed, including compression clamps, hook-rod systems, and eventually pedicle screws.[2–7] Roy-Camille et al. initially proposed the lateral mass screw in 1979, and the trajectory along with the technique was later modified by Anderson et al., An et al., and Jeanneret et al.[6–10]

The use of lateral mass screws in the dorsal cervical spine has since increased for multiple reasons.[8,11,12] The advantages include the relative safety of the anatomy around the lateral mass, the ability to place instrumentation post-laminectomy, ease of instrumenting multiple levels, ability to extend the construct, and biomechanical strength.[8,13–15] The disadvantages of the lateral mass screw include possible injury to the vertebral artery and/or nerve root, junctional facet violation, and lateral mass fracture.[16] Several studies have implicated misjudging screw length and trajectory as possible contributing factors to many of the aforementioned complications.[17–20]

The introduction of CT image-guided neuronavigation has changed the landscape of modern spine surgery, with improved accuracy, increased visualization of deep spine anatomy and reduction of radiation exposure. Current generation CT image-guidance placement of instrumentation has been well demonstrated in thoracic and lumbar spine, as well as the pelvis.[21–24] In the cervical spine, several studies have been conducted to determine the accuracy and complication rates in instrumentation placement with navigation.[25–27] In addition, there have been more limited reports on the use of navigation in difficult-to-image areas of the cervical spine including the craniocervical junction, cervical-thoracic junction, and cervical pedicles.[27–32] In this chapter, we present our technique for the safe and efficient placement of posterior cervical instrumentation from the occiput to the subaxial cervical spine under modern CT image-guided neuronavigation.

SURGICAL TREATMENT FOR SPINAL PATHOLOGY

Clinical Studies

Clinical Presentation

- There is no absolute contraindication for posterior cervical navigation. The indications for posterior cervical instrumentation include instability from traumatic, neoplastic, infectious, iatrogenic, or congenital etiologies, as well as multilevel cervical spinal stenosis with degenerative instability, deformity, or kyphosis. The use of CT image-guided navigation in the cervical spine is typically indicated in regions where visualization of the deep bony anatomy is extremely beneficial. At the occipitocervical junction, identifying the location of the occipital protuberance, spinal canal, and vertebral artery are necessary in order to safely introduce spinal instrumentation. In the subaxial and cervicothoracic junctions, the overlying soft tissue and bony structures of the shoulder girdles often obstruct conventional fluoroscopy, making navigation a superior alternative.[33] Aside from improving accuracy and safety of cervical instrumentation, image-guided neuronavigation has the added benefit of smaller incisions and less soft tissue mobilization.[34]

Preoperative Imaging

- Carefully reviewing all available preoperative advanced imaging including CT, MRI, and radiographs of the cervical spine, may reveal anomalous anatomy such as presence of a ponticulus posticus. With a prevalence of 16.7% (range, 4.3%–52.9%),[35] a ponticulus posticus can easily be mistaken for a thickened posterior arch, leading to a potentially devastating vertebral artery injury during C1 screw fixation. C2 and subaxial dorsal anatomy can also be highly variable. Atretic or congenitally abnormal bony C2 pedicles, abnormal subaxial cervical landmarks and variable anatomy of the intervertebral foramen[36,37] can be identified with preoperative imaging review. The potential hazards associated with these anomalies can be carefully and safely avoided intraoperatively with neuronavigation systems.

Surgical Plan and Workflow

- Room layout: We use the Medtronic mobile CT scanner O-arm® Surgical Imaging with StealthStation® Navigation System (Medtronic, Inc., Minneapolis, MN). The StealthStation® Navigation System and optical tracking camera are typically placed at the head or foot of the bed for optimal visualization of the surgical field. We use either a Skytron 3100 with gel pads or the Mizuho OSI® Jackson table with the arms tucked at the sides. The patients are positioned prone and the cranium is secured with a radiolucent Mayfield® head-holder. Care is taken not to use any table extenders that drop below the table as this may block the entry, closure, and imaging of the mobile CT scanner.
- Reference frame: The selection of an ideal optical dynamic reference frame (DRF) is dependent on the type of cervical surgery and exposure that is warranted. The two main options for reference frames are a spinous process clamp affixed to any of the C2–T1 spinous processes and a Mayfield extension arm that allows positioning of the DRF near the occiput (Figs. 2.1 and 2.2). The DRF is typically affixed between the StealthStation optical tracking camera and the working surgical level to provide the best uninterrupted line of sight to both the DRF and navigated spinal instruments. The DRF should be placed out of the surgical working area with the camera positioned at either the patient's head or the foot of the bed. The motor-evoked and somatosensory potentials are routinely monitored, and electromyographic monitoring is performed in all patients.

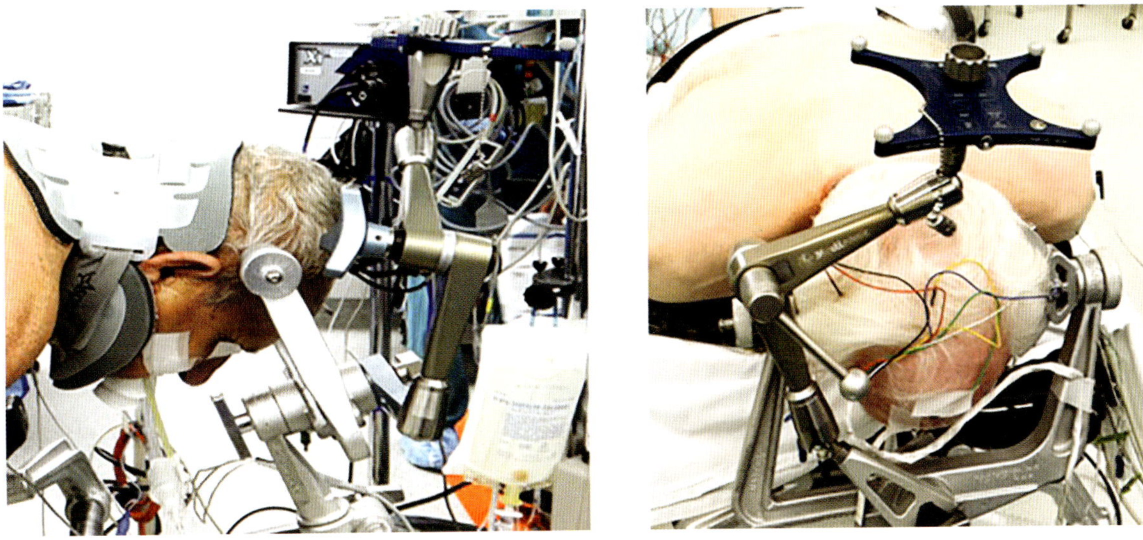

FIG. 2.1 Optical Dynamic Reference Frame attached to the Mayfield extension arm.

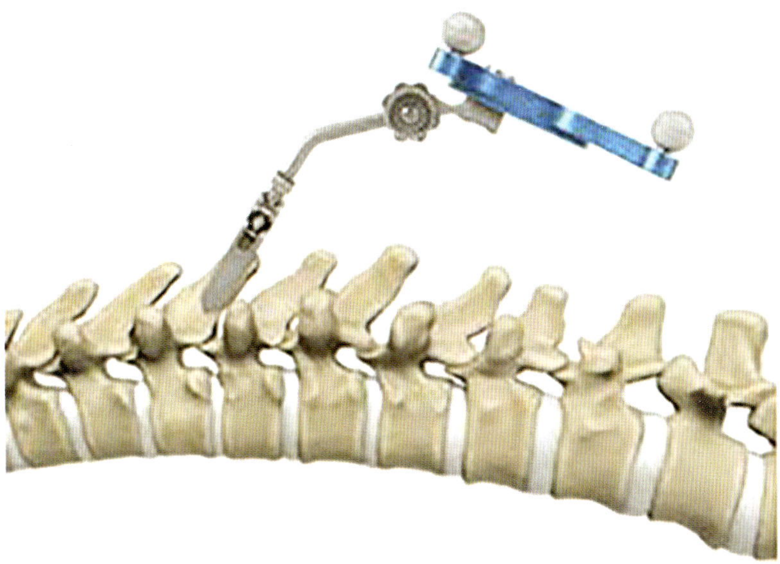

FIG. 2.2 Optical Dynamic Reference Frame attached with a spinous process clamp.

Intraoperative Imaging

- A straight midline incision is made to expose the levels of interest. After complete exposure, retractors are placed and left in during the O-arm image acquisition so as not to be adjusted after the O-arm spin and instrument registration. The O-arm is then brought into the protected field for image acquisition (Fig. 2.3). The anesthesiologist is asked to hold ventilation throughout the entire scan and resume respiration after image

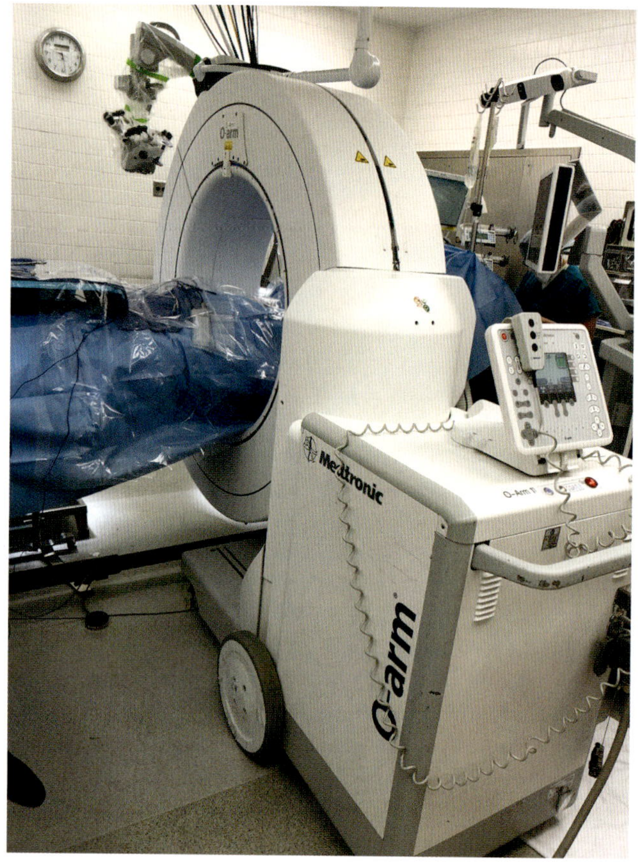

FIG. 2.3 Medtronic mobile CT scanner O-arm® Surgical Imaging.

acquisition is completed. If possible, the tidal volumes are reduced to at least 30% of the baseline to reduce chest wall excursion during the navigated instrumentation portion of the surgery. All neuronavigation instruments are then registered and utilized for intraoperative planning of screw placement including choice of screw diameter, length, and trajectory based upon the relevant anatomy (Fig. 2.4).

- The insertion of posterior cervical screws with navigation can be achieved according to several different methods. In general, in our practice, a high-speed drill is used initially to identify the ideal starting points on the bony surface anatomy. This starting point is confirmed with navigation and the deep bony anatomy analyzed to determine the ideal screw trajectory. In all cases, navigation is used as a confirmatory tool and as an adjunct to the direct visual and tactile information available from the surgical field.
- With minor adjustments made with navigation, the anatomic entry points and trajectories for the various screws are as follows: C1 lateral mass screws are initially determined by palpation of the medial and lateral edges of the C1–C2 facet joint. The starting point is selected directly beneath the edge of the posterior arch in the center of the C1 lateral mass, with a sagittal trajectory parallel to the posterior arch of C1, angled approximately 10 degrees medially (Fig. 2.5). Care is taken to identify and protect the C2 nerve

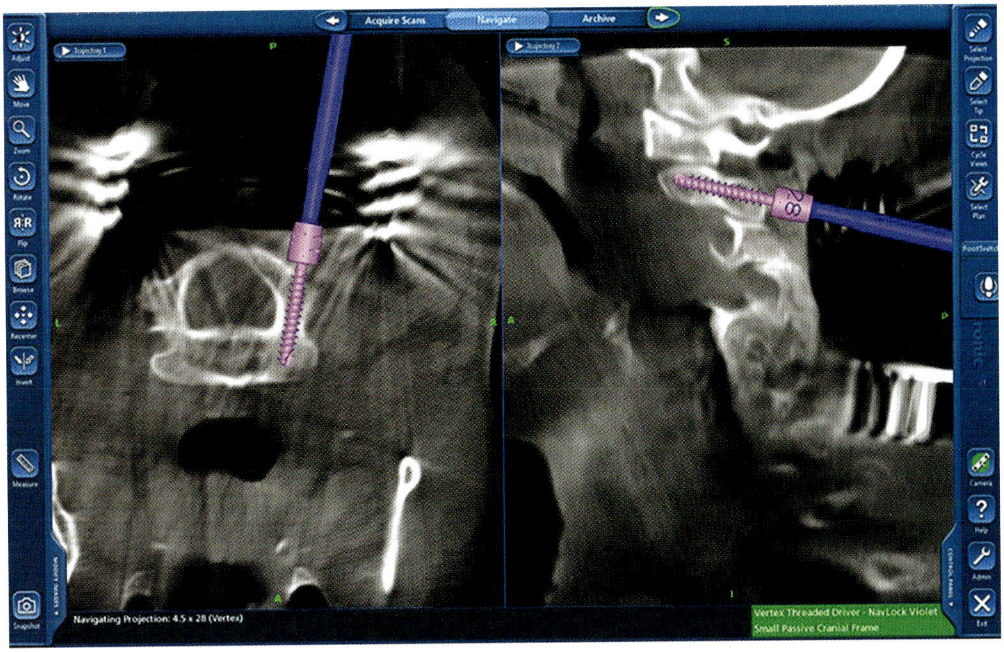

FIG. 2.4 StealthStation® Navigation System (Medtronic, Inc.) display.

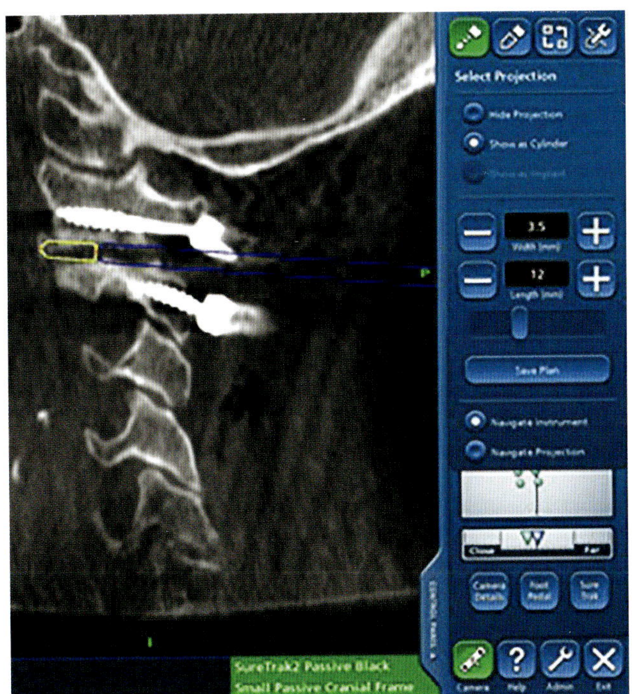

FIG. 2.5 Placement of C1 lateral mass screws using StealthStation® Navigation System.

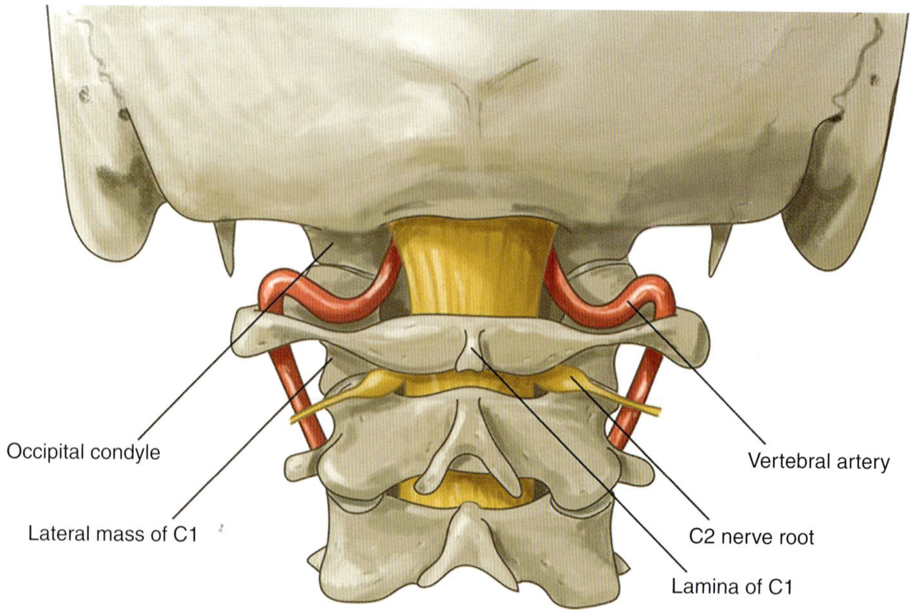

FIG. 2.6 Posterior atlantoaxial anatomy showing C1 lateral mass screw start point just above the C2 nerve. *(From Pittman JL, Bransford RJ. Cervical Spine Surgery: Standard and Advanced Techniques. 2019:201–206.)*

running just below the C1 start point (Fig. 2.6). A pilot hole is drilled with a 2.4-mm or 2.9-mm drill bit, and the trajectory is confirmed with navigation. The software on the StealthStation workstation allows users to "save" the drilled trajectory as a projection and provides the ability to measure screw length and width. Finally, the screw tract is palpated with a ball probe to confirm the absence of a bony wall breach, and a final screw is inserted into its ideal trajectory, as determined by CT-guided navigation (Fig. 2.7).

- The C2 pedicle screw starting point is at the midpoint of the C2 pars with the drill bit guide directed into the central cancellous channel of the C2 pedicle by navigation. Generally, C2 pedicle screw placement begins 3 to 4 mm above the C2–C3 facet, angled 20 to 30 degrees medial and 20 to 30 degrees cephalad. The exposure of the medial and superior aspect of the C2 pedicle within the spinal canal allows the direct visualization of any medial bony wall breach with instrumentation. Due to gross variations in pedicle orientation, size, and vertebral artery anatomy, the C2 pedicle screw length and trajectory can be highly variable (Fig. 2.8). Care is always taken to review the preoperative advanced imaging at the occipitocervical junction in order to anticipate any anatomic variations.
- Other non-pedicle trajectories for the instrumentation of the C2 can be easily achieved with navigation guidance. The C2 pars screws begin 3 mm above the C2–C3 facet and 3 mm lateral to the lamina-lateral mass junction, angled 10 to 15 degrees medial and 35 degrees cephalad (Fig. 2.9). The C2 transarticular screws start 2 to 3 mm superior to the facet and 3 mm lateral to the lamina-lateral mass junction, aimed 10 to 15 degrees medial to the anterior tubercle of C1. The C2 translaminar screws have an offset starting point with a trajectory slightly less than the slope of the lamina in relation to the

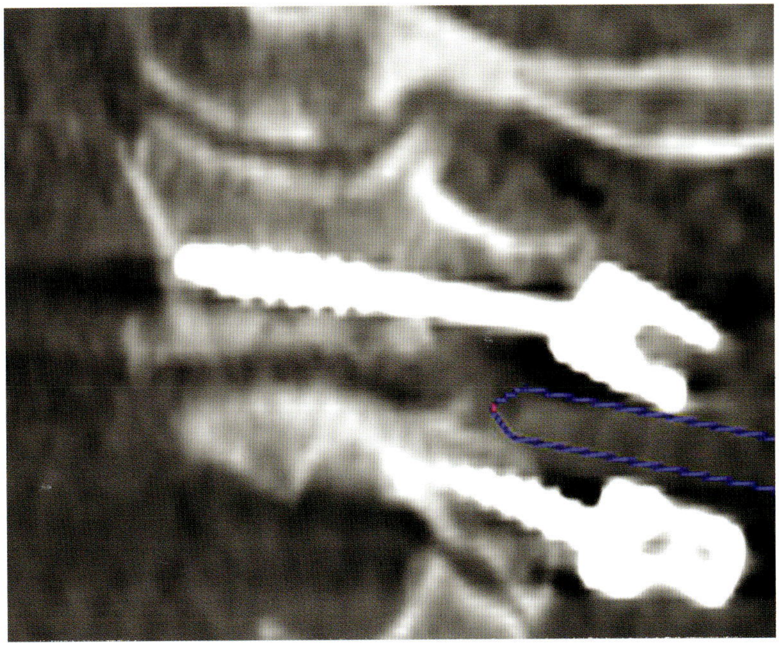

FIG. 2.7 Placement of C1 lateral mass screws using StealthStation® Navigation System.

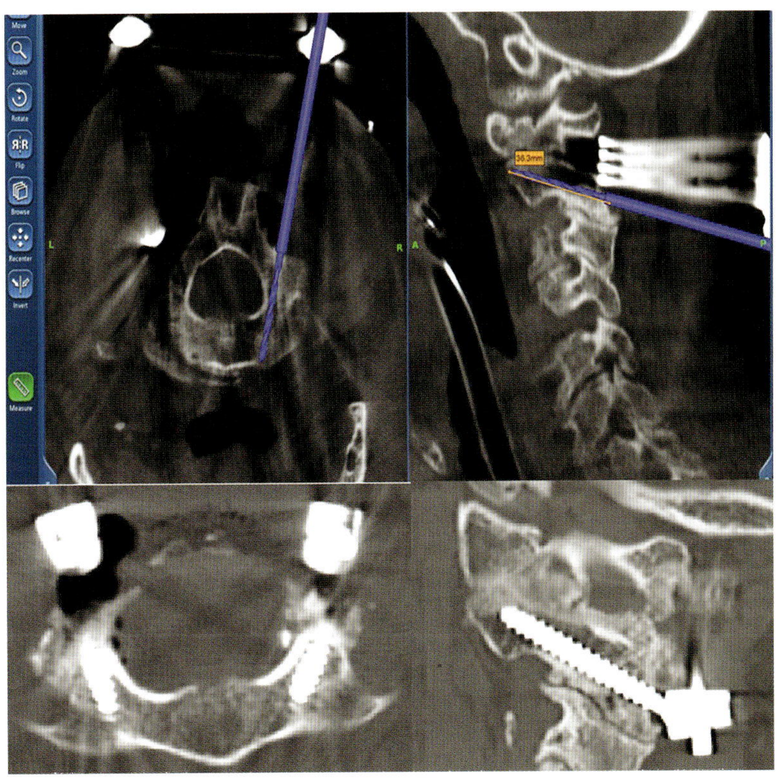

FIG. 2.8 Placement of C2 pedicle screws using StealthStation® Navigation System.

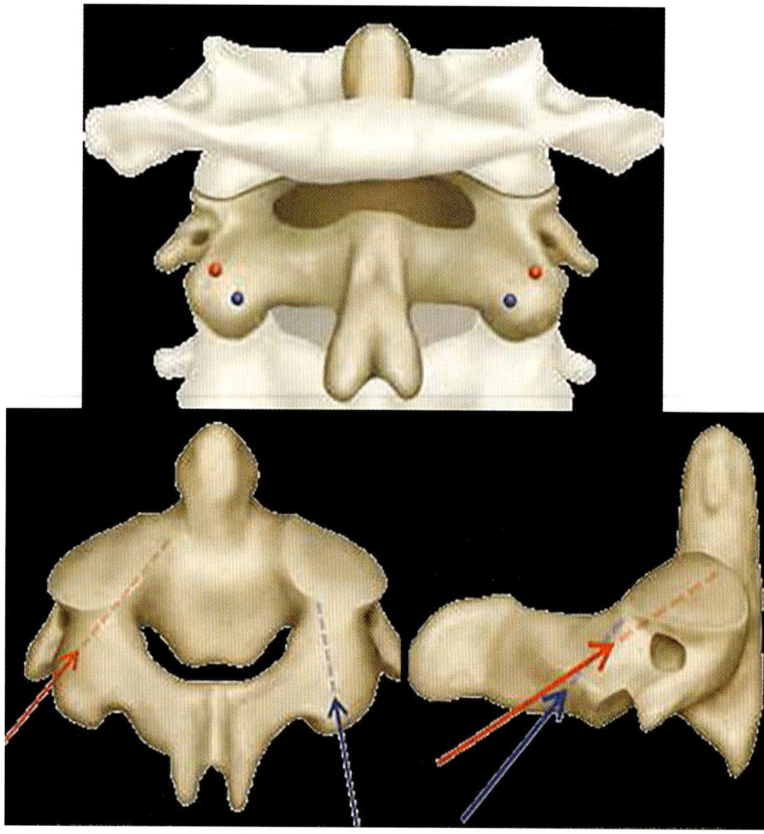

FIG. 2.9 Starting point and trajectory for C2 pars screws.

vertebral body. With the ability to visualize the deep bony anatomy, all of the non-pedicle C2 screw trajectories can be determined confidently, and screw head alignment for rod insertion can be planned better.

- The subaxial lateral mass screws from C3 to C7 follow the modified Anderson technique, with a starting point approximately 1 mm medial to the center of the lateral mass, a trajectory parallel to the facet joint, and approximately 30 degrees of lateral angulation in the parasagittal plane[8] (Fig. 2.10). Although free-hand and fluoroscopic techniques are well described, navigation is particularly helpful in preventing adjacent segment degeneration by avoiding screw violation of the proximal and distal facet joints. Additionally, navigation allows the easy alignment of all the lateral mass screw starting points to help facilitate eventual rod placement.
- The traditional subaxial C3–C7 pedicle screws *without* navigation have not been considered as a first-line instrumentation choice. With image-guided navigation, subaxial C3–C7 pedicle screws have been gaining popularity, especially in the revision setting in patients with permissible anatomy.[26] In addition, C7 pedicle screws have been increasingly utilized for instrumentation of the cervicothoracic junction. The trajectory of the pedicle screws can be variable, from 25 to 45 degrees medial as one progresses from C3 to C7. Ultimately, the ideal axial and sagittal trajectories are best determined with navigation.

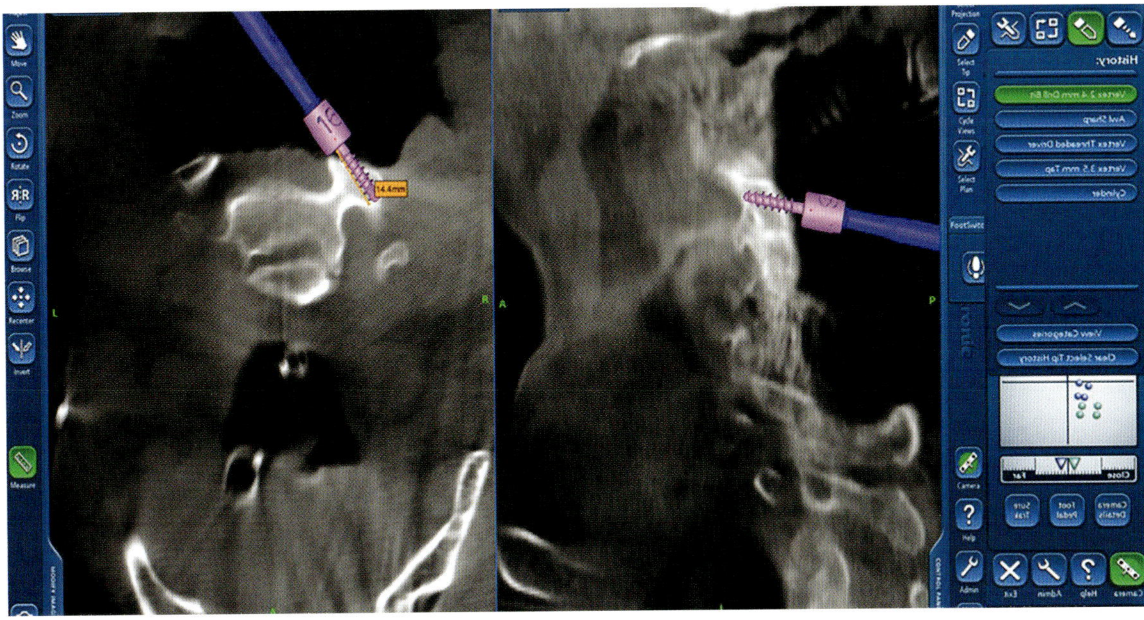

FIG. 2.10 Placement of subaxial lateral mass screws using StealthStation® Navigation System.

- CT image-guided navigation is also utilized with occipital plate placement. There is great variability of the posterior skull and bony anatomy. The location of the external occipital protuberance can be identified visually with direct dissection. However, the identification of the internal bony anatomy of the occipital cranium is the critical portion for instrumentation purposes. With navigation, the visualization and localization of the internal occipital protuberance, midline inferior keel, and inferior nuchal line are extremely straightforward. Understanding the depth of screws and selecting the thickest portion of the occiput allows for maximal bony purchase of the occipital screws and plate. In addition, knowing the thinnest regions of the posterior occipital bone (particularly in the occipital squamous bone laterally) helps with avoiding injury to internal structures such as the transverse sinus, cerebellar vasculature, or cerebellum itself.
- In general, for all screw instrumentation in the occipitocervical spine, all instruments including the probe, high-speed drill, awl, pedicle finder probes, screw tap, and screw are calibrated for navigation purposes. In our hands, specifically, a navigation probe is initially placed on the appropriate starting entry point based on the standard anatomic surface landmarks. Reformatted CT images centered on the corresponding point in the image data set will be displayed, allowing the selection of the appropriate entry point and screw trajectory in the axial, sagittal, and coronal planes. The navigated probe can be placed in different positions and angles, to check the ideal trajectory in real time. The cortical entry site is prepared with a navigated high-speed drill, while the appropriate trajectory in both the sagittal and axial planes is checked. The entry hole is then pre-drilled with a navigated drill/awl and then probed for sidewall breach and to determine depth. A navigated tap is used, followed by final screws that are inserted with the navigated screwdriver into their ideal trajectories.

Postoperative Imaging

- In order to reduce the radiation burden on the patient, we do not routinely perform confirmatory intraoperative CT scans for navigated placed screws. However, upright plain radiographs are obtained postoperatively in the hospital and again at 3 and 12 months after surgery. In the case of intraoperative breach, navigation inaccuracy, surgeon request, or intraoperative neuromonitoring changes there is a low threshold to repeat a CT scan for confirmation of instrumentation placement.

Postoperative Recovery and Follow-Up

- The patients are evaluated immediately postoperatively for any signs of neurologic deficit or clinical symptoms associated with the remote possibility of a malpositioned screw during the inpatient hospitalization and outpatient settings. Except for patients with osteoporosis, or those in whom poor bone quality is identified intraoperatively, those with stable instrumentation do not require postoperative immobilization with a cervical collar. Drains are routinely placed during surgery and ultimately removed after the output reaches a threshold minimum. All sutures are buried under the subcutaneous skin, dressings are applied, and the first follow-up is scheduled within the first 2 weeks.

Procedural Concerns in Detail

System accuracy is checked following the insertion of each screw by placing the navigated probe onto a known anatomic landmark and visually confirming accuracy with the image guidance system. Often times, the hex-shaped metal fixation screwhead to the spinous process reference clamp is used as a known landmark to determine inaccuracies of navigation. If the accuracy deviates by more than 1 mm, an intraoperative scan is performed on the same region.

Treatment Side Effects

Although navigation systems are a useful adjunct in spine surgery and have markedly reduced radiation exposure to surgeons and surgical staff, the radiation exposure to the patient has increased. Urbanski et al. reported that patients undergoing navigated pedicle screw placement received a greater mean radiation dose than did those whose screws were placed with traditional fluoroscopic guidance (1071 ± 447 mGy-cm vs. 391 ± 53 mGy-cm; $P < .001$).[38] It is our opinion that certain cervical spinal cases that require multiple fluoroscopic images for bony visualization may in fact expose the patient to more radiation than does navigation. The literature is still not clear as to this comparison, and it is best left to the decision of the surgeon to practice as low as reasonably achievable (ALARA) techniques.

Workflow Disruptions

- Workflow disruptions of navigated cervical spine cases can lead to various negative outcomes including surgeon dissatisfaction, increased operative time, increased blood loss, and even inaccurate instrumentation placement. The implementation of this new technology in the operating room requires careful attention to avoiding disruptions that can negatively impact the efficiency of a surgeon's workflow. The most common ones are described here.
- Displacement of the reference frame in relation to the spine can alter the accuracy of neuronavigation significantly. This can occur from leaning on the patient, accidental movement of the reference frame, or adjustment of the soft tissue retractors. The inability

of neuronavigation to adjust for dynamic changes of the spine after intraoperative CT image acquisition is a major issue in spinal navigation.

- Obstruction of the reference frame line of sight to the LED-camera detector can create a major issue in navigation accuracy and time delay. Whether the block of visualization arises from an individual in the operative field or from blood/tissue on the reflective spheres, these flow disruptions can negatively impact the progression of the surgery and lead to inaccuracies.
- Proficiency and familiarity of the surgical team with spinal navigated cases are key to a successful cervical navigation case. Understanding that each individual from the scrub technician to the imaging technician to the navigation technician has full competency with the imaging modality, instruments, and software is critical to avoiding workflow disruptions. In addition, coordination of the OR personnel and navigation team is critical in the successful implementation of spinal navigation. Prolonged wait times for team members and inexperienced navigation technologists can lead to delayed surgical time, surgeon fatigue, and abandonment of this technology during a cervical case.

Management of Complications

- Ensure that the reference frame is securely fastened to a stable structure (i.e., uninjured spinous process or the Mayfield clamp) and that it exists outside of the working field so as not to be bumped accidentally or obstruct any instruments including the probe, pneumatic drill, awl, pedicle finder probes, screw tap, and screw holder, each of which may displace the reference frame.
- Minimize activity that will cause the reference frame to displace in relation to the spine such as leaning on the patient, adjusting or moving retractors, or altering the height or position of the OR bed. To minimize chest wall excursion during respiration, we also ask the anesthesiologist to decrease the respiratory tidal volumes during the screw instrumentation steps.
- Clear the reflective spheres on the DRF and on all handheld navigated tools from blood and other tissue that would obstruct the ability of the camera to detect the reflective surfaces.
- Check the accuracy of the navigation with placement of the handheld navigation probe on the known visualized anatomic landmarks (i.e., the spinous process or facet joint), ensuring that they correspond with the displayed image dataset. If any discrepancy of the navigated position from the true anatomic position is sensed, recalibrate the navigated instrument, analyze the fiduciary for movement or displacement, and have a low threshold to repeat CT image capture.
- Start with placement of those screws that are most distal to the reference frame or are the most navigation-intensive, as accuracy degrades with time and distance away from the reference frame. Progress toward the reference frame if possible. Moreover, as the case progresses, due to the high mobility of the cervical spine, activities such as drilling and screw placement may cause the reference frame to displace in relation to the spine, causing inaccurate projections. Frequent check of accuracy and re-registering handheld equipment is recommended.
- To optimize workflow efficiency, the surgeon should try to remain in the operating room at all times. Assisting with O-arm positioning and removal, coordinating all individuals as needed, and scrubbing back into the case will minimize delay and maximize overall workflow efficiency.

Case Examples

- Case example #1 is a 67-year-old male with a history of metastatic renal cell carcinoma with a lesion to the right C1 lateral mass (Fig. 2.11). He presented with a complaint of severe axial neck pain and the inability to sit or stand upright due to a pathologic fracture through the C1 lateral mass and subsequent cervical instability (Fig. 2.12). He failed an extensive course of nonoperative medical management and elected to proceed with

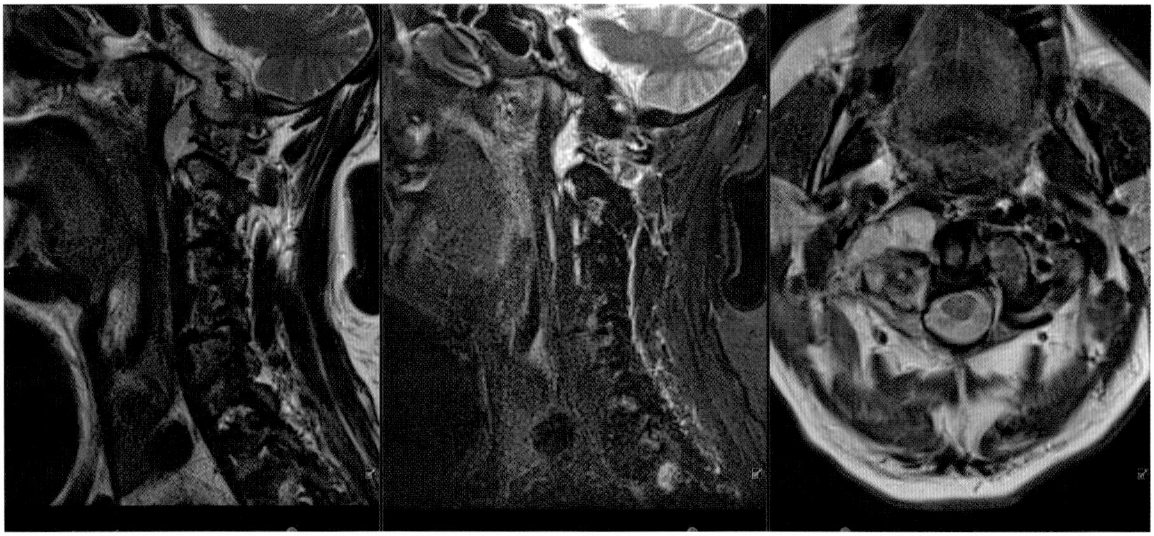

FIG. 2.11 MRI cervical spine revealing an unstable pathologic fracture through the C1 lateral mass from metastatic renal cell carcinoma.

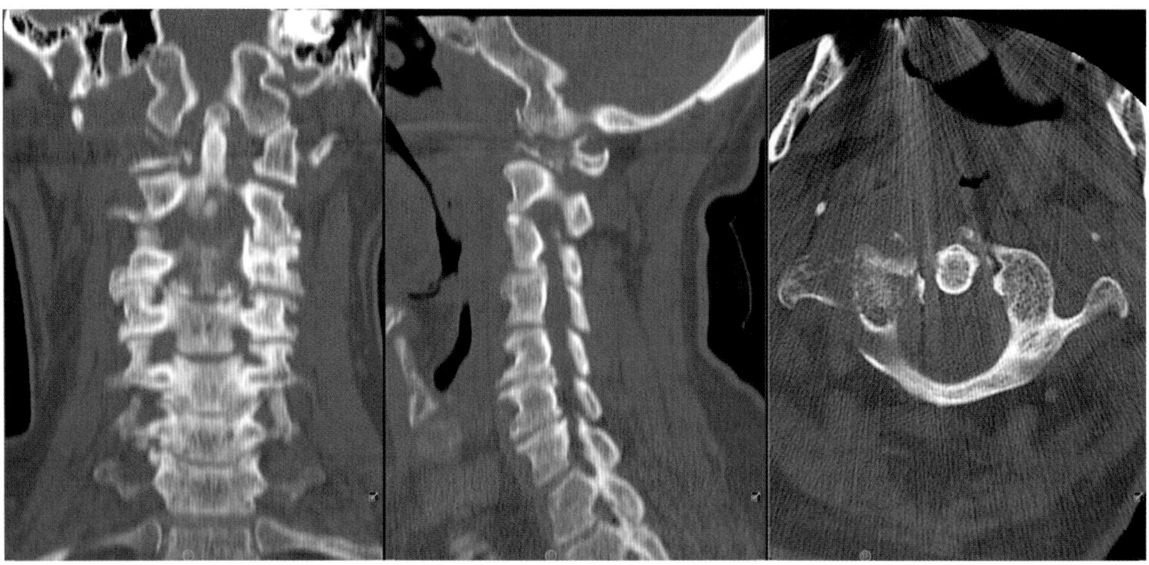

FIG. 2.12 CT cervical spine revealing an unstable pathologic fracture through the C1 lateral mass from metastatic renal cell carcinoma.

surgical intervention. He underwent an occiput to C2 posterior spinal instrumented fusion with O-arm CT-guided navigation (Figs. 2.13 and 2.14). His postoperative course was uneventful and he recovered well, denying significant neck or arm pain.

- Case example #2 is an 89-year-old male who sustained a C1–C2 fracture dislocation after a fall. Subsequent imaging revealed a C1 anterior arch fracture, a C2 type 2 dens fracture, and progressive instability with a C1–C2 rotatory facet dislocation (Fig. 2.15). He underwent a closed reduction of the C1–C2 dislocation with manipulation of the cervical spine, followed by an occiput to C2 posterior spinal instrumented fusion with O-arm CT-guided navigation (Fig. 2.16). His postoperative course was uneventful and he recovered well.
- Case example #3 is a 64-year-old male with a complex history including prior radiation therapy for tonsillar cancer, who subsequently developed rare, episodic, and spasmodic seizure-like disorder consistent with stiff person syndrome. He developed a severe cervicothoracic kyphotic deformity resulting in a chin-on-chest deformity (Fig. 2.17). Given his severe, chronic neck pain and inability to maintain a functional, horizontal gaze, refractory to nonoperative management, he elected to proceed with surgical intervention. He underwent an occiput to T6 posterior spinal instrumented fusion with O-arm CT-guided navigation and correction of his sagittal plane kyphotic deformity (Figs. 2.18 and 2.19). Postoperatively, he did well with significant improvement in both pain and horizontal gaze.
- Case example #4 is a 56-year-old female with a complex surgical history including previous C2–C7 anterior spinal fusion that subsequently went on to develop subjunctional degenerative changes, screw pullout, and fracture dislocation, with consequent cervicothoracic kyphosis and instability resulting in a severe chin-on-chest deformity (Fig. 2.20). Her deformity was exacerbated by left-sided torticollis that also caused a coronal deformity. She underwent multiple, staged surgical interventions which included halo placement, traction, and posterior cervical laminectomy decompression osteotomy

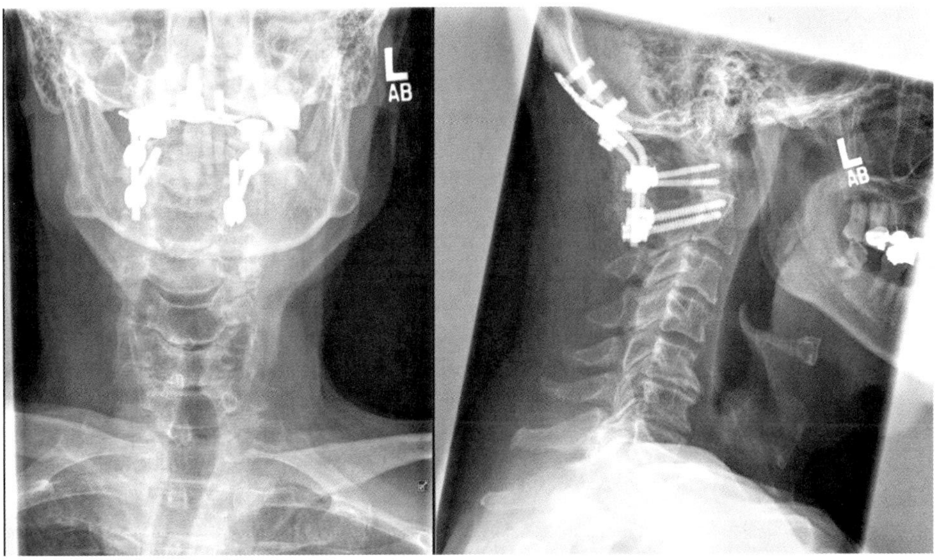

FIG. 2.13 Postoperative radiographs revealing occiput to C2 posterior instrumented fusion.

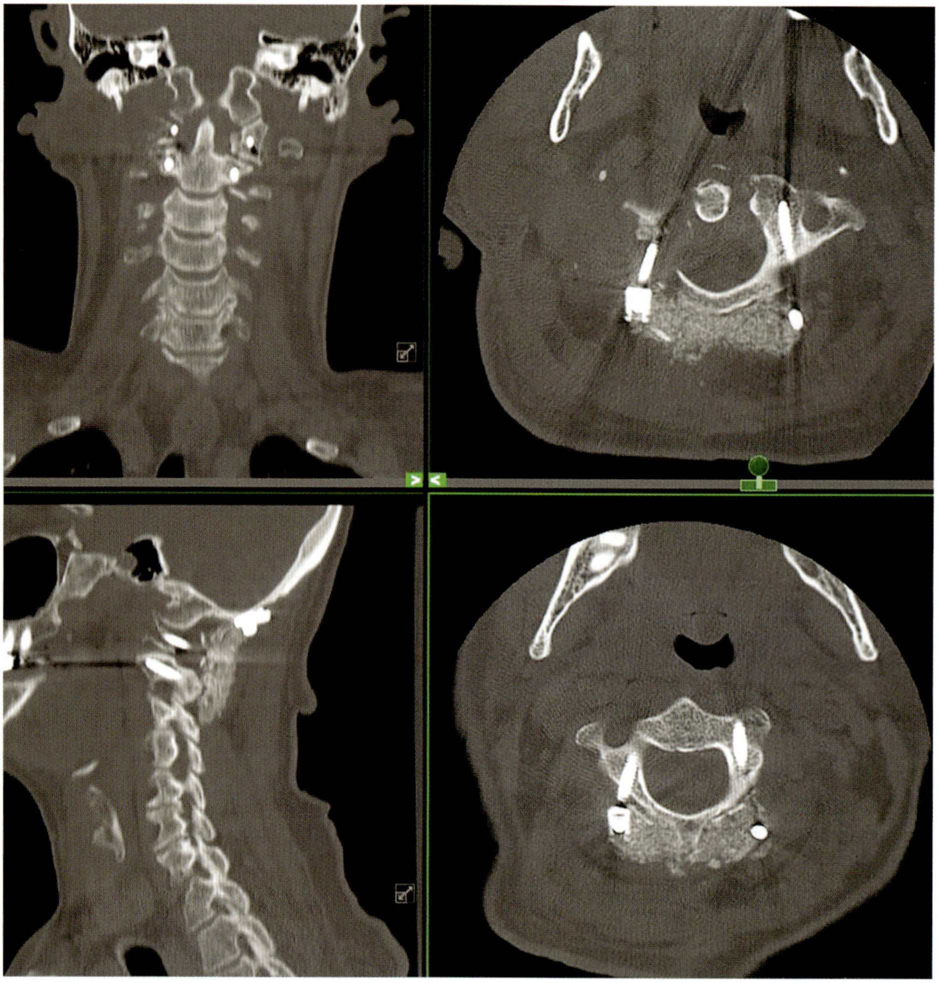

FIG. 2.14 Postoperative CT cervical spine revealing occiput to C2 posterior instrumented fusion with well-positioned screws.

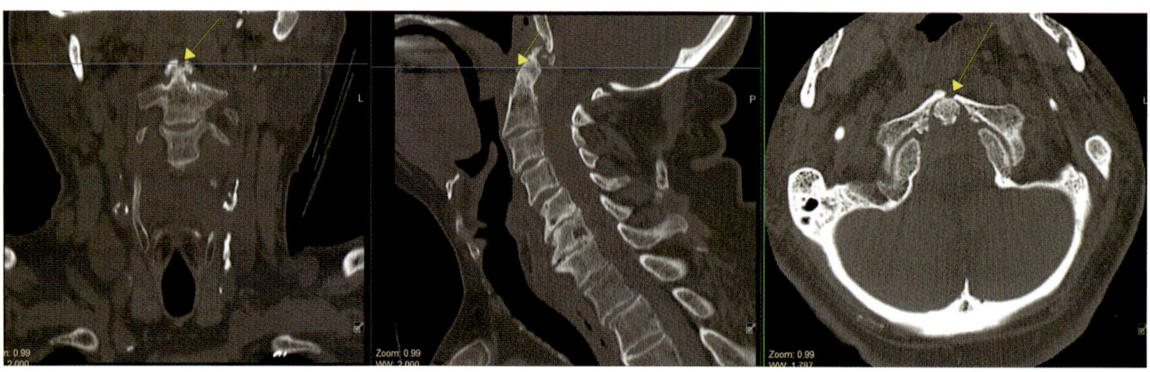

FIG. 2.15 CT cervical spine revealing C1–C2 fracture dislocation with C1 anterior arch fracture, and C2 type 2 dens fracture, and progressive instability with C1–C2 rotatory facet dislocation.

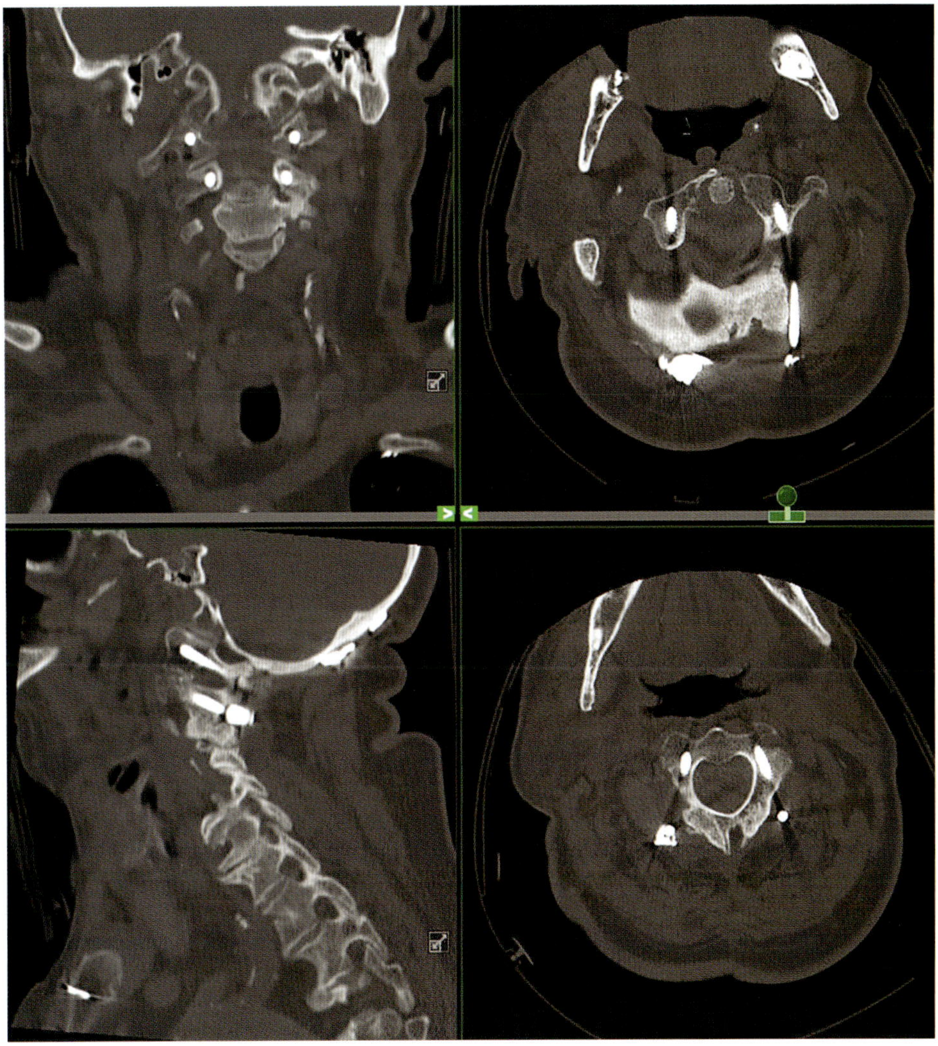

FIG. 2.16 Postoperative CT cervical spine revealing of interval reduction and C1–C2 posterior instrumented fusion with well-positioned screws.

with instrumentation and anterior C7–T1 corpectomy. The final stage of the treatment included a revision C2–T3 posterior spinal fusion with O-arm CT-guided navigation (Figs. 2.21 and 2.22). Her postoperative course was uneventful and she recovered well with significant improvement in pain and posture.

RESULTS

In a retrospective review, we discuss our experience and present our findings regarding lateral mass screw placement accuracy and complications with the Medtronic O-arm® Surgical Imaging with StealthStation® Navigation compared to C-arm fluoroscopic-guided placement. We evaluated 83 consecutive patients (ages 24–93 years) undergoing new or

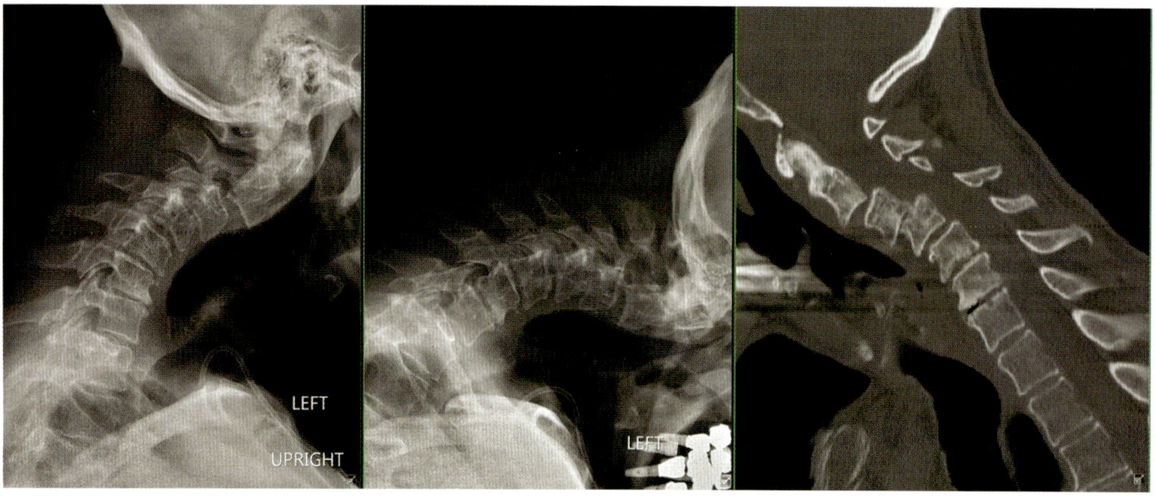

FIG. 2.17 Preoperative cervical radiographs and CT scan revealing severe cervicothoracic kyphosis from multilevel cervical anterolisthesis, worse at C2–C3, with motion on flexion-extension views.

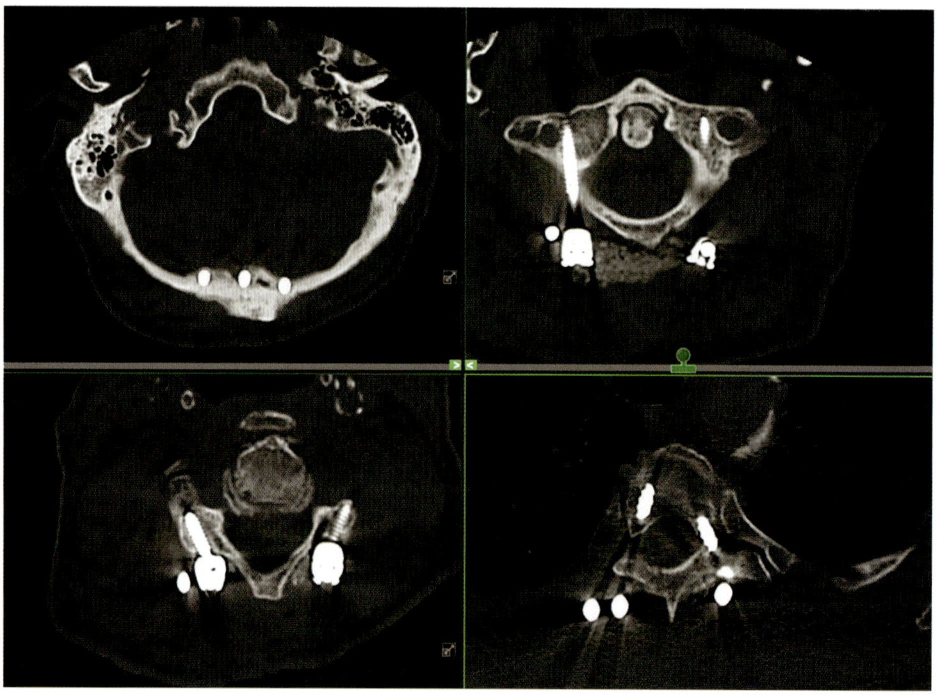

FIG. 2.18 Postoperative CT cervical-thoracic spine revealing well-positioned occipital screws, C1 lateral mass screws, subaxial lateral mass screws, and upper thoracic pedicle screws.

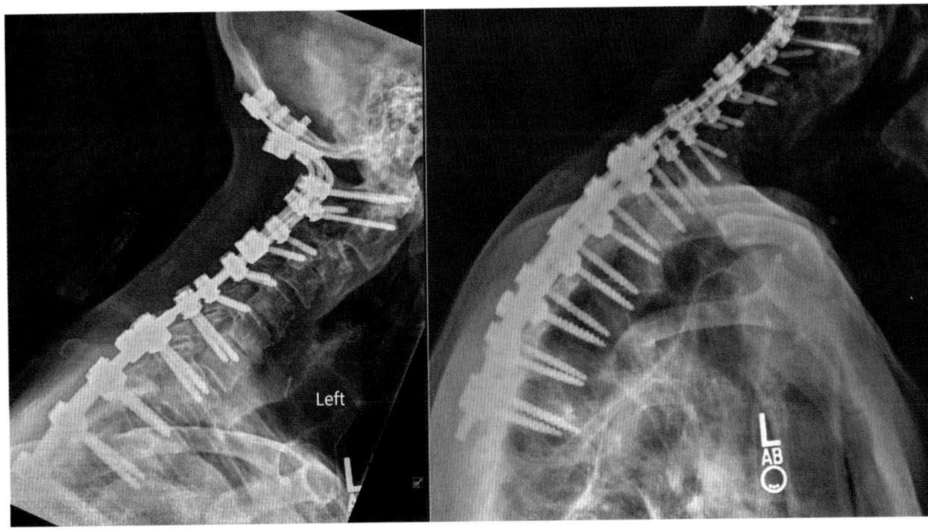

FIG. 2.19 Postoperative cervical radiographs revealing well-positioned occiput to T6 posterior instrumented fusion and correction of cervicothoracic kyphosis.

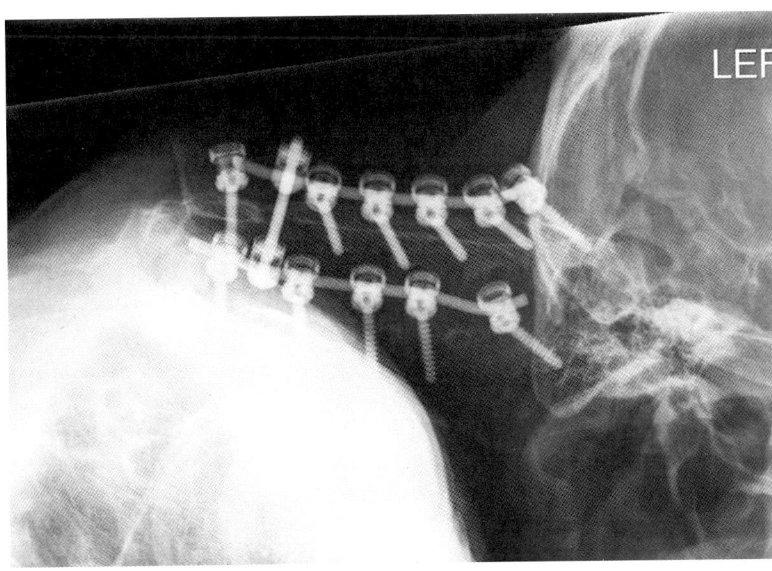

FIG. 2.20 Preoperative cervical radiograph revealing severe cervicothoracic kyphosis.

revision C1 lateral mass, C2 pars/pedicle, and C3–C7 lateral mass instrumentation and undergoing postoperative CT imaging from 2008 to 2014 (Table 2.1). In comparing screw lengths, designated as unicortical, bicortical, or breached (>2 mm past the second cortex), the O-arm group had 69.6% unicortical, 28.2% bicortical, and 1.8% breached screws. The fluoroscopy group had 24.2% unicortical, 69.7% bicortical, and 6.1% breached screws. The screw trajectories were assessed by theoretic violation of critical anatomic structures. There were significantly higher theoretic violations in the transverse foramen (11.0% vs. 2.5%;

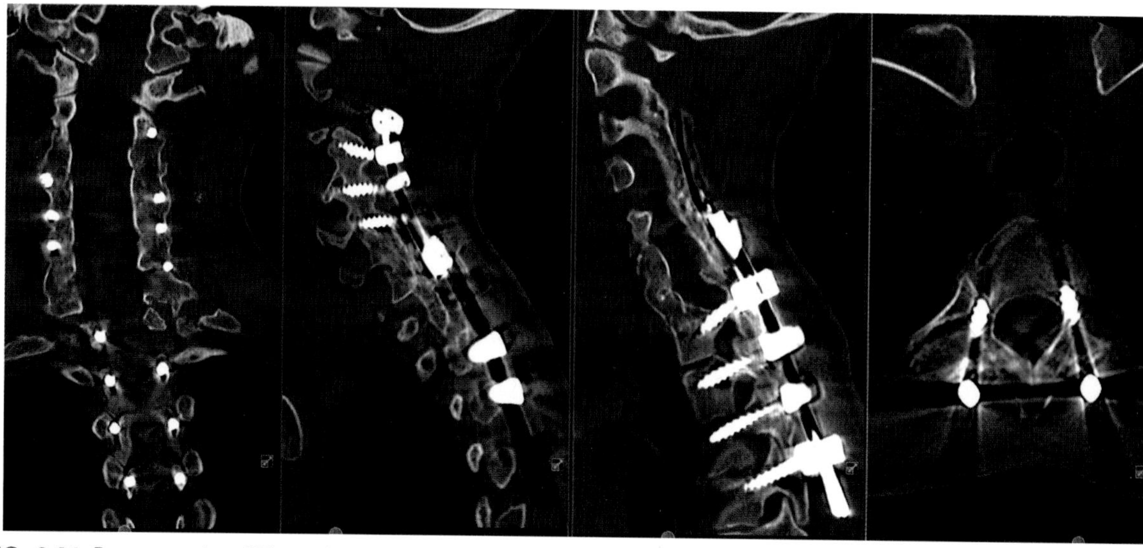

FIG. 2.21 Postoperative CT cervical spine revealing C2–T3 posterior instrumented fusion with well-positioned screws.

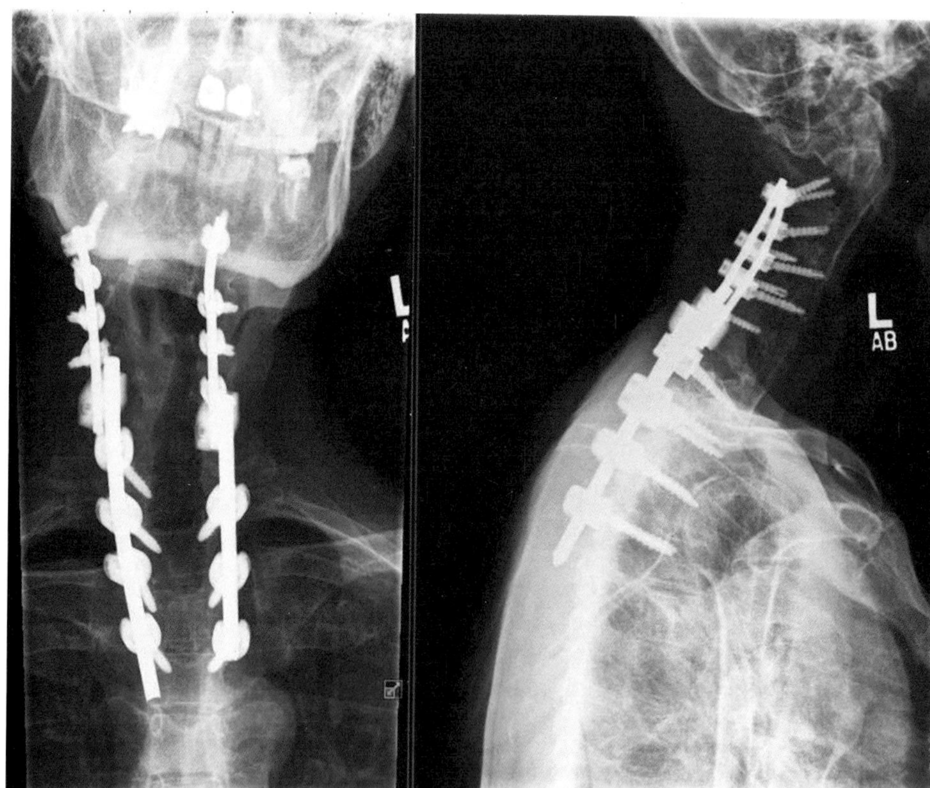

FIG. 2.22 Postoperative cervical radiograph C2–T3 posterior instrumented fusion and correction of cervicothoracic kyphosis.

TABLE 2.1 Patient demographics and diagnoses

	Fluoroscopic Guided	**O-Arm Navigated**
Patient Demographics		
Number of Patients	43	40
Age Range	24-93	48-92
Mean Age ± Std Dev	60±17.6	67.3±10.4
Male	39.5%	60%
Diagnosis	**Number of cases (%)**	**Number of cases (%)**
C1-2 Subluxation	3 (7.0)	2 (5)
Osteomyelitis	1 (2.3)	2 (5)
DDD/Stenosis	10 (23.2)	24 (60)
Epidural abscess	2 (4.7)	0
Fracture	8 (18.6)	2 (5)
Os odontoideum	3 (7.0)	0
Pseudoarthrosis	12 (27.9)	8 (20)
Segmental instability	2 (4.7)	2 (5)
Adjacent level disease	1 (2.3)	0
Odontoid pannus	1 (2.3)	0

$P = .0003$) and facet joint (14.0% vs. 3.6%; $P = .001$) for fluoroscopy compared to O-arm. The overall aggregated theoretic violation rate was significantly higher in the fluoroscopic group (28.8%) compared to the navigation group (7.1%). In evaluating the biomechanically optimal placement of lateral mass screws, purchase within bone was determined as placement of the screw into one of three lateral mass zones defined by Heller et al.[18] The navigation group had a statistically significant more screws placed in the biomechanically favored zone 2 compared to the fluoroscopic-guided screws (81.5% vs. 65.2%; $P = .0002$). The fluoroscopy group had greater rates of biomechanically suboptimal screws placed in zone 3 (i.e., within the facet joint itself), than the O-arm group (27.3% vs. 6.8%; $P < .0001$). Within the 40-patient O-arm group, one patient required reoperation for radicular pain, which was not clearly related to screw placement. Within the 43-patient anatomic C-arm group, there was 1 death in a critically ill patient and 5 reoperations for screw pullout, pseudarthrosis, adjacent segment degeneration, and wound washout.

DISCUSSION

Dorsal cervical fixation has advanced significantly since Gallie's initial description of spinous process wiring.[1] Advances in technology and material in instrumentation have increased our treatment options for cervical pathologies. Lateral mass screw insertion is a prevalent procedure for dorsal cervical fixation and is considered a safe option to transpedicular screws.[39,40] Despite its relative safety, lateral mass screw insertion still runs the potential risk of damage to the vertebral artery or nerve root, facet violation, and lateral mass fracture.[16] Punyarat et al. found that, even in experienced hands, up to 23% of C2 pedicle screws and 11% of C2 pars screws placed using a free-hand technique without navigation may be malpositioned.[41] Ludwig et al. found that navigation is more accurate than topographic landmarks in accurate cervical pedicle screw placement.[42] Three systematic reviews of the literature have demonstrated the various applications of neuronavigation in the cervical spine with improved accuracy and safety.[25,43,44] The application of neuronavigation has the added benefit of improved accuracy, increased visualization of spine anatomy, and reduction of radiation exposure to the surgeon.

Wang et al. compared the radiation exposure from CT-based navigation versus conventional C-arm fluoroscopy, finding that CT-based navigation led to a statistically significant reduction of overall radiation exposure of 91.8% ($P < .0001$).[45] Although navigation systems are a useful adjunct in spine surgery that have markedly reduced radiation exposure to surgeons and surgical staff, they have led to increased exposure to the patient. Urbanski et al. reported that patients undergoing navigated pedicle screw placement received a greater mean radiation dose than did those whose screws were placed with traditional fluoroscopic guidance (1071 ± 447 mGy-cm vs. 391 ± 53 mGy-cm; $P < .001$).[38]

Harel et al. retrospectively evaluated patients treated with the Harm procedure for C1–C2 screw fixation under either fluoroscopic guidance or navigation.[27] Although they found that the accuracy rate of C1 and C2 screw placement was higher for the navigated group, this was not a statistically significant difference. Of note, the mean surgical duration was 27 minutes longer in the O-arm than in the fluoroscopy group ($P = .03$).

Kraus et al. performed an analysis of lateral mass screw placement, comparing the accuracy of navigation-assisted (Arcadis Orbic 3D, Siemens, Erlangen, Germany) with fluoroscopic-guided procedures in patients requiring fusion for the treatment of a fracture.[46] Accuracy was determined with a reference distance to the cortical bone and the position of the tip of the screw. Their study noted that the accuracy of navigation-assisted lateral mass screws was significantly higher than that of fluoroscopic guidance in terms of the percentage of screws perforating the cortex and contacting critical structures.[46]

We also evaluated lateral mass screw placement with respect to the cortical bone, designated at unicortical, bicortical, and long (>2 mm beyond the cortex). Interestingly, there was a significantly greater number of bicortical lateral mass screws in the fluoroscopic-guided group compared to the O-arm navigated group. This is likely due to variation in screw insertion techniques. With the fluoroscopic-guided lateral mass screws, each hole is made with a hand drill set starting at 10 mm and is checked with a ball probe for bony breach. In order to maximize bony purchase, the hand drill guide is then advanced 2 mm in length, the hole drilled, and probed for bony breach. In holes where the ball probe detected a breach, a screw of the same length as the drill guide is inserted. The addition of navigation provides real-time trajectories in three dimensions during the drilling, tapping, and screw placement, which allows the surgeon to monitor the screw placement in greater detail than that provided by fluoroscopy. Therefore, the screw length is determined by what is seen on the navigation system. This could explain the observation that the majority of navigated lateral mass screws were unicortical. The surgeon could visualize the precise maximal length of the screw without breach of the distal cortex. Lateral mass screws that are too long have the increased potential of injury or complication. In reviewing the lateral mass screws that were deemed long (i.e., >2 mm beyond the cortex), the fluoroscopically guided screws had a significantly greater number of long screws compared with the navigated group.

Screw trajectory has been cited as an important factor contributing to potential complications.[17–20] Thus, our analysis of breach violations allows us to quantify optimal versus suboptimal trajectories. Our data reveals that there was a significantly lower rate of violation of the transverse foramen and facet with the lateral mass screws placed with navigation. The types of violations that did not have a significant difference between navigation and fluoroscopy were of the spinal canal and neuroforamen. This is likely attributable more to the general lateral mass placement technique in both the fluoroscopic and navigation groups of directing the screws rostral and lateral to avoid neural elements. Overall, there was a statistically significant lower rate of breach violation in the O-arm navigated group compared with that in the fluoroscopic-guided group. Given the importance of trajectory and its contribution to potential complications, we consider this finding a useful marker of optimal screw placement. This trajectory may be even more important in revision cases, as often the anatomy may be distorted.

The desired target zone for the lateral mass screw is the superior articular process (zone 1) or main lateral mass body (zone 2). These were considered biomechanically optimal as they allowed for the maximal amount of screw length and purchase.[18] The screws placed in the inferior portion of the lateral mass (zone 3) are considered suboptimal due to the least amount of bony purchase. Our findings also demonstrated a statistically significant decrease in suboptimally placed lateral mass screws in those placed with navigation. There was also a significantly greater proportion of screws in the navigation group in zone 2. There was no statistical significance noted in zone 1 between the groups, but there was a trend toward statistical significance. Along the same lines as the improved trajectory, this decrease in biomechanically suboptimal placement is due to the better anatomical visualization during screw placement with navigation technology.

Revision cases have traditionally been more challenging than the index procedure due to scar tissue and distorted anatomy. In the analysis of revision cases, it was found that in the O-arm navigated placement of lateral mass screws, a significantly greater percentage were of a favorable length (i.e., unicortical and bicortical). A significantly greater percentage of screws also had no theoretic violation (i.e., spinal canal, nerve, transverse foramen, and facet joint) and were in the biomechanically favored zones (i.e., zones 1 and 2). Our findings suggest that the application of navigation would be beneficial in the setting of revision surgery, where there is often distortion of the normal anatomic landmarks both on direct visualization and fluoroscopy.

Since the initial collection of our data, we have continued to use navigation routinely for subaxial cervical lateral mass screw placement as well as C1 and C2 screw placement. Based on our experience, accuracy and efficiency comes with consistent use of the technology. Lack of familiarity with the navigation system, setup, and instruments for use in the cervical spine can potentially lead to a false sense of accuracy. For surgeons deciding to adopt navigation technology for cervical spine instrumentation, we recommend initial use in all consecutive cases with intraoperative confirmation of anatomical landmarks until comfort and efficient workflow are achieved. The initial learning curve must be passed in order to achieve greatest accuracy and superior clinical outcomes.

SUMMARY

Navigation in the occipital and cervical spine is a safe, accurate, and effective technological advancement. The consistent use of navigation assistance has enabled spine surgeons to direct ideal instrumentation trajectories accurately, thereby decreasing the potential rate of damage to the neural or vascular structures. In addition, in our findings, there was an additional increase in biomechanically optimal screw placement with navigation. The superior imaging quality and three-dimensional views of the deep bone anatomy over conventional fluoroscopic modalities make its use ideal in primary and revision procedures. We recommend the advanced use of spinal navigation before addressing the occipitocervical spine, but, once employed, this serves as an excellent adjunct to anatomic visualization, and facilitates safe clinical outcomes for the patient and spine surgeon.

REFERENCES

1. Gallie WE. Skeletal traction in the treatment of fractures and dislocations of the cervical spine. *Ann Surg*. 1937;106(4): 770–776.https://doi.org/10.1097/00000658-193710000-00026.
2. Aldrich EF, Crow WN, Weber PB, Spagnolia TN. Use of MR imaging-compatible Halifax interlaminar clamps for posterior cervical fusion. *J Neurol Surg*. 1991;74(2):185–189. https://doi.org/10.3171/jns.1991.74.2.0185.
3. Statham P, O'Sullivan M, Russell T. The Halifax interlaminar clamp for posterior cervical fusion: initial experience in the United Kingdom. *Neurosurgery*. 1993;32(3):396–398. discussion 398. https://doi.org/10.1227/00006123-199303000-00009.
4. Abumi K, Itoh H, Taneichi H, Kaneda K. Transpedicular screw fixation for traumatic lesions of the middle and lower cervical spine: description of the techniques and preliminary report. *J Spinal Disord*. 1994;7(1):19–28. https://doi.org/10.1097/00002517-199407010-00003.
5. Abumi K, Kaneda K. Pedicle screw fixation for nontraumatic lesions of the cervical spine. *Spine*. 1997;22(16):1853–1863. https://doi.org/10.1097/00007632-199708150-00010.
6. Roy-Camille R, Gaillant G, Bertreaux D. Early management of spinal injuries. In: McKibben B, ed. *Recent Advances in Orthopedics*. Edinburgh: Churchill Livingstone; 1979:57–87.
7. Roy-Camille R, Sailant G, Mazel C, eds Internal fixation of the unstable cervical spine by a posterior osteosynthesis with plates and screws. In: Sherk H, Dunn H, Eismont F, et al., eds. *The Cervical Spine*. 2nd ed. Philadelphia: JB Lippincott Publishers; 1989:390–404.
8. Anderson PA, Henley MB, Grady MS, Montesano PX, Winn HR. Posterior cervical arthrodesis with AO reconstruction plates and bone graft. *Spine*. 1991;16(3 suppl):S72–S79. https://doi.org/10.1097/00007632-199103001-00012.
9. An HS, Gordin R, Renner K. Anatomic considerations for plate-screw fixation of the cervical spine. *Spine*. 1991; 16(10 suppl):S548–S551. https://doi.org/10.1097/00007632-199110001-00019.
10. Jeanneret B, Magerl F, Ward EH, Ward JC. Posterior stabilization of the cervical spine with hook plates. *Spine*. 1991;16(3 suppl):S56–S63. https://doi.org/10.1097/00007632-199103001-00010.
11. Cooper PR, Cohen A, Rosiello A, Koslow M. Posterior stabilization of cervical spine fractures and subluxations using plates and screws. *Neurosurgery*. 1988;23(3):300–306. https://doi.org/10.1227/00006123-198809000-00003.
12. Swank ML, Sutterlin CE, Bossons CR, Dials BE. Rigid internal fixation with lateral mass plates in multilevel anterior and posterior reconstruction of the cervical spine. *Spine*. 1997;22(3):274–282. https://doi.org/10.1097/00007632-199702010-00009.
13. Errico T, Uhl R, Cooper P, Casar R, McHenry T. Pullout strength comparison of two methods of orienting screw insertion in the lateral masses of the bovine cervical spine. *J Spinal Disord*. 1992;5(4):459–463. https://doi.org/10.1097/00002517-199212000-00011.
14. Shapiro S, Snyder W, Kaufman K, Abel T. Outcome of 51 cases of unilateral locked cervical facets: interspinous braided cable for lateral mass plate fusion compared with interspinous wire and facet wiring with iliac crest. *J Neurol Surg*. 1999;91(1 suppl):19–24. https://doi.org/10.3171/spi.1999.91.1.0019.
15. Ulrich C, Arand M, Nothwang J. Internal fixation on the lower cervical spine—biomechanics and clinical practice of procedures and implants. *Eur Spine J*. 2001;10(2):88–100. https://doi.org/10.1007/s005860000233.
16. Heller JG, Silcox DH, Sutterlin CE. Complications of posterior cervical plating. *Spine*. 1995;20(22):2442–2448. https://doi.org/10.1097/00007632-199511001-00013.
17. Ebraheim NA, Klausner T, Xu R, Yeasting RA. Safe lateral-mass screw lengths in the Roy-Camille and Magerl techniques. An anatomic study. *Spine*. 1998;23(16):1739–1742. https://doi.org/10.1097/00007632-199808150-00006.
18. Heller JG, Carlson GD, Abitbol JJ, Garfin SR. Anatomic comparison of the Roy-Camille and Magerl techniques for screw placement in the lower cervical spine. *Spine*. 1991;16(10 suppl):S552–S557. https://doi.org/10.1097/00007632-199110001-00020.
19. Barrey C, Mertens P, Jund J, Cotton F, Perrin G. Quantitative anatomic evaluation of cervical lateral mass fixation with a comparison of the Roy-Camille and the Magerl screw techniques. *Spine*. 2005;30(6):E140–E147. https://doi.org/10.1097/01.brs.0000155416.35234.a3.
20. Seybold EA, Baker JA, Criscitiello AA, Ordway NR, Park CK, Connolly PJ. Characteristics of unicortical and bicortical lateral mass screws in the cervical spine. *Spine*. 1999;24(22):2397–2403. https://doi.org/10.1097/00007632-199911150-00018.
21. Yson SC, Sembrano JN, Sanders PC, Santos ER, Ledonio CG, Polly DW. Comparison of cranial facet joint violation rates between open and percutaneous pedicle screw placement using intraoperative 3-D CT (O-arm) computer navigation. *Spine*. 2013;38(4):E251–E258. https://doi.org/10.1097/BRS.0b013e31827ecbf1.

22. Jeswani S, Drazin D, Hsieh JC, et al. Instrumenting the small thoracic pedicle: the role of intraoperative computed tomography image-guided surgery. *Neurosurg Focus*. 2014;36(3):E6. https://doi.org/10.3171/2014.1.FOCUS13527.
23. Hsieh JC, Drazin D, Firempong AO, Pashman R, Johnson JP, Kim TT. Accuracy of intraoperative computed tomography image-guided surgery in placing pedicle and pelvic screws for primary versus revision spine surgery. *Neurosurg Focus*. 2014;36(3):E2. https://doi.org/10.3171/2014.1.FOCUS13525.
24. Kim TT, Drazin D, Shweikeh F, Pashman R, Johnson JP. Clinical and radiographic outcomes of minimally invasive percutaneous pedicle screw placement with intraoperative CT (O-arm) image guidance navigation. *Neurosurg Focus*. 2014;36(3):E1. https://doi.org/10.3171/2014.1.FOCUS13531.
25. Tjardes T, Shafizadeh S, Rixen D, et al. Image-guided spine surgery: state of the art and future directions. *Eur Spine J*. 2010;19(1):25–45. https://doi.org/10.1007/s00586-009-1091-9.
26. Chachan S, Bin Abd Razak HR, Loo WL, Allen JC, Shree Kumar D. Cervical pedicle screw instrumentation is more reliable with O-arm-based 3D navigation: analysis of cervical pedicle screw placement accuracy with O-arm-based 3D navigation. *Eur Spine J*. 2018;27(11):2729–2736. https://doi.org/10.1007/s00586-018-5585-1.
27. Harel R, Nulman M, Knoller N. Intraoperative imaging and navigation for C1–C2 posterior fusion. *Surg Neurol Int*. 2019;10:149. https://doi.org/10.25259/SNI_340_2019.
28. Guppy KH, Chakrabarti I, Banerjee A. The use of intraoperative navigation for complex upper cervical spine surgery. *Neurosurg Focus*. 2014;36(3):E5. https://doi.org/10.3171/2014.1.FOCUS13514.
29. Richter M, Mattes T, Cakir B. Computer-assisted posterior instrumentation of the cervical and cervico-thoracic spine. *Eur Spine J*. 2004;13(1):50–59. https://doi.org/10.1007/s00586-003-0604-1.
30. Rajasekaran S, Kanna PR, Shetty TA. Intra-operative computer navigation guided cervical pedicle screw insertion in thirty-three complex cervical spine deformities. *J Craniovertebr Junction Spine*. 2010;1(1):38–43. https://doi.org/10.4103/0974-8237.65480.
31. Theologis AA, Burch S. Safety and efficacy of reconstruction of complex cervical spine pathology using pedicle screws inserted with stealth navigation and 3D image-guided (O-Arm) technology. *Spine (Phila Pa 1976)*. 2015;40(18):1397–1406. https://doi.org/10.1097/BRS.0000000000001026.
32. Verma R, Krishan S, Haendlmayer K, Mohsen A. Functional outcome of computer-assisted spinal pedicle screw placement: a systematic review and meta-analysis of 23 studies including 5,992 pedicle screws. *Eur Spine J*. 2010;19(3):370–375. https://doi.org/10.1007/s00586-009-1258-4.
33. Djurasovic M, Dimar JR, Glassman SD, Edmonds HL, Carreon LY. A prospective analysis of intraoperative electromyographic monitoring of posterior cervical screw fixation. *J Spinal Disord Tech*. 2005;18(6):515–518. https://doi.org/10.1097/01.bsd.0000173315.06025.c6.
34. Schlenzka D, Laine T, Lund T. Computer-assisted spine surgery. *Eur Spine J*. 2000;9(suppl 1):S57–S64. https://doi.org/10.1007/pl00010023.
35. Zhang XL, Huang DG, Wang XD, et al. The feasibility of inserting a C1 pedicle screw in patients with ponticulus posticus: a retrospective analysis of eleven patients. *Eur Spine J*. 2017;26(4):1058–1063. https://doi.org/10.1007/s00586-016-4589-y.
36. Sioutas G, Kapetanakis S. Clinical anatomy and clinical significance of the cervical intervertebral foramen: a review. *Folia Morphol*. 2016;75(2):143–148. https://doi.org/10.5603/FM.a2015.0096.
37. Karaikovic EE, Daubs MD, Madsen RW, Gaines RW Jr. Morphologic characteristics of human cervical pedicles. *Spine*. 1997;22(5):493–500. https://doi.org/10.1097/00007632-199703010-00005.
39. Katonis P, Papadakis SA, Galanakos S, et al. Lateral mass screw complications: analysis of 1662 screws. *J Spinal Disord Tech*. 2011;24(7):415–420. https://doi.org/10.1097/BSD.0b013e3182024c06.
40. Sekhon LH. Posterior cervical lateral mass screw fixation: analysis of 1026 consecutive screws in 143 patients. *J Spinal Disord Tech*. 2005;18(4):297–303. https://doi.org/10.1097/01.bsd.0000166640.23448.09.
41. Punyarat P, Buchowski JM, Klawson BT, Peters C, Lertudomphonwanit T, Riew KD. Freehand technique for C2 pedicle and pars screw placement: is it safe? *Spine J*. 2018;18(7):1197–1203. https://doi.org/10.1016/j.spinee.2017.11.010.
42. Ludwig SC, Kramer DL, Balderston RA, Vaccaro AR, Foley KF, Albert TJ. Placement of pedicle screws in the human cadaveric cervical spine: comparative accuracy of three techniques. *Spine*. 2000;25(13):1655–1667. https://doi.org/10.1097/00007632-200007010-00009.
43. Tian NF, Huang QS, Zhou P, et al. Pedicle screw insertion accuracy with different assisted methods: a systematic review and meta-analysis of comparative studies. *Eur Spine J*. 2011;20(6):846–859. https://doi.org/10.1007/s00586-010-1577-5.
44. Mason A, Paulsen R, Babuska JM, et al. The accuracy of pedicle screw placement using intraoperative image guidance systems. *J Neurosurg Spine*. 2014;20(2):196–203. https://doi.org/10.3171/2013.11.SPINE13413.
45. Wang TY, Hamouda F, Sankey EW, Mehta VA, Yarbrough CK, Abd-El-Barr MM. Computer-assisted instrument navigation versus conventional C-arm fluoroscopy for surgical instrumentation: accuracy, radiation time, and radiation exposure. *AJR Am J Roentgenol*. 2019;213(3):651–658. https://doi.org/10.2214/AJR.18.20788.
38. Urbanski W, Jurasz W, Wolanczyk M, et al. Increased radiation but no benefits in pedicle screw accuracy with navigation versus a freehand technique in scoliosis surgery. *Clin Orthop Relat Res*. 2018;476(5):1020–1027. https://doi.org/10.1007/s11999.0000000000000204.
46. Kraus M, von dem Berge S, Perl M, Krischak G, Weckbach S. Accuracy of screw placement and radiation dose in navigated dorsal instrumentation of the cervical spine: a prospective cohort study. *Int J Med Robot Comput Assist Surg*. 2014;10(2):223–229. https://doi.org/10.1002/rcs.1555.

3

Navigation in Spine Trauma

Joaquin Q. Camara, MD, and Adetokunbo 'Toki' Oyelese, MD, PhD

INTRODUCTION OF TECHNOLOGY

Practice and Standard of Care

We are in a technological era where advancements in image-guided systems, robotics, machine learning/neuromodulation, and state-of-the-art image-guided operating suites are creating new possibilities in operative neurosurgery. This is resulting in numerous changes and improvements with respect to patient experience, care, and outcomes. Spine surgery is uniquely affected given its heavy reliance on intraoperative devices, biologics, and imaging. Novel tools are allowing us to perform surgeries with smaller incisions, as is the case with video-assisted endoscopy, with others fully relying on computer assisted navigation (CAN), as in cases of minimally invasive spine surgery (MISS). The integration of these, and similar technologies, is pushing the boundaries of spine tumor surgery, degenerative spine surgery, deformity surgery, MISS, and spine trauma surgery.

While traditional intraoperative imaging tools (i.e., radiography, C-arm fluoroscopy, biplanar fluoroscopy) remain a mainstay of most spine practices, newer technologies like 3D fluoroscopy, cone-beam CT, real-time flash registration, and intraoperative CT/MRI are allowing a new generation of spine surgeons safer, more accurate placement of hardware and better localization of difficult anatomy in real time. These modalities offer the added benefit of less radiation exposure to the surgeon, operative staff, and patient. Naturally, there are limitations to these technologies that have kept them from replacing the aforementioned mainstays. Among the challenges posed by novel technology is a steep learning curve for the appropriate implementation and effective use of such tools and techniques. As with all new developments, the upfront costs associated with the technology demands there be critical analysis of patient outcomes and long-term cost-effectiveness, prior to embracing them fully. Spine trauma surgery specifically has benefited from these advances as we continue to learn from its limitations to help make these technologies better for surgeon use.

Outcomes

The management of spine trauma patients has evolved rapidly over the last decade, from the imaging modalities used to diagnose them to the treatment of spinal cord injury. CAN is among the most revolutionary additions to spine surgery, allowing real-time feedback based on intraoperative radiography (3D x-ray, CT, and/or MRI) or registration points. It has been well established in the literature that, for pedicle screw placement, CAN demonstrates superior accuracy over that of a free-hand technique in the placement of pedicle screws.[1] A case report by Kakarla et al. showed the use of navigated percutaneous thoracic pedicle screw fixation in six spine trauma patients with unstable spine fractures.[2] In this study, a total of 37 pedicle screws were placed, with 16% of screws having a breach less than 2 mm and 3% with a breach beyond 2 mm. Additionally, the study noted no neurological complications detected and no revisions. Studies in both elective and trauma spine surgery repeatedly demonstrate the accuracy of pedicle screw placement with CAN, as well as the safety and decreased need for revision surgery for malpositioned screws.

Other modalities for spinal trauma, like percutaneous MISS techniques, are believed to improve outcomes by limiting soft tissue disruption and avoiding the risks of conventional open approaches. These result in shorter recovery periods and hospital stays.[3] The application of this technique additionally limits blood loss, which, importantly, can be substantial in open trauma cases, and is not infrequently complicated by patients with multisystem issues. Percutaneous CAN options offer an important alternative in such cases. Furthermore, for trauma cases where the anatomy is completely distorted from injury and/or prior intervention, navigation can be useful for real-time feedback in instrumentation and assessing the corrected deformity. Although the literature is starting to support the application of MISS in degenerative surgery, the level of evidence supporting its use in the trauma population is lacking compared to its use in those with degenerative disease.[4]

While intraoperative time was originally felt to be a likely disadvantage of the technology, the concern has been dispelled. Certainly, there is an upfront learning curve for both surgeons and operating room staff; however, the literature suggests that as the utilization of CAN has increased at certain centers and institutions, their operative time has concurrently either remained unchanged or decreased. As an example, a study by Lang et al. using intraoperative 3D fluoroscopy-based navigation for treating Hangman fractures through a C2–C3 pedicle screw fixation construct, showed that CAN did not lengthen the operative time (134.2 ± 8.0 min in MISS vs. 139.3 ± 25.8 in open, $P > .01$).[5] In an effort to help address some of these concerns regarding intraoperative times, groups like Navarro-Ramirez et al., who have switched to a total navigation system for MISS and completely eliminated fluoroscopy in most surgeries, have developed algorithms to help with workflow.[6] Their eight-step surgical workflow for total navigation is just one example of how a systems approach can help make certain CAN procedures faster than open techniques, even in spine trauma cases.

Beyond the benefits of reducing operative time, there is a significant reduction in radiation exposure to both the patient and staff when using CAN.[7,8] The increased awareness of the hazardous effects of radiation exposure is changing the way surgeons, OR staff, and hospital administrators overseeing operating rooms perform surgeries in order to make the environment safer to all involved. A spine surgeon often experiences as much as 50 times the lifetime radiation dose of a surgeon in other orthopedic subspecialties, such as a hip surgeon.[9] More complex spine procedures like MISS, tumor, and trauma that rely on fluoroscopy, given the complicated anatomy or lack of visible anatomical landmarks, subject all parties to higher doses of radiation. CAN is uniquely positioned to help in reducing this effect as it does not rely on the same radiation doses. It has the added benefit of enhanced 3D visual experience in real time.

SURGICAL TREATMENT FOR SPINAL PATHOLOGY

Clinical Case Study 1

History/Clinical Presentation

- The patient is an 80-year-old man with a history of hypertension and osteopenia who sustained a fall from standing a month prior to his current hospitalization. From his original fall, a CT revealed a mild compression fracture at T12 that was treated conservatively with bracing, given its imaging features as well as the minimal subjective back pain (Fig. 3.1A). However, over the course of a month, his back pain worsened significantly and he was readmitted. The neurologic examination revealed normal strength, reflexes, and sphincter tone. However, he had substantial back pain with midline tenderness to palpation.

Preoperative Imaging

- His original CT scan from his fall a month prior revealed only a mild superior endplate fracture at T12 with no other bony fractures or associated focal kyphosis (Fig. 3.1A). There was also no fracture to the posterior elements or splaying of the posterior elements. An MRI obtained upon readmission a month later revealed progression of his T12 fracture, now with significant height loss, and a burst component into the canal with focal kyphosis (see Fig. 3.1B). The posterior ligamentous complex was without injury on MRI. On the axial view of the MRI, the T12/L1 space was moderately stenotic from the burst fragment abutting the conus (see Fig. 3.1C).

Surgical Plan

- In order to decompress the burst fragment and restore height and alignment, a decision was made for a right lateral decubitus transthoracic MISS approach for corpectomy of T12 followed by posterior percutaneous stabilization. The posterior percutaneous stabilization was done with CT-guided intraoperative navigation (BrainLab). Iliac pins with an array were placed for intraoperative navigation (see Fig. 3.1D). An intraoperative CT scan was obtained following the placement of the array. Four small incisions were made for the posterior percutaneous surgery, two on each side below and above the cage reconstruction at T12. These incisions were mapped out using our navigation to ensure they would encompass our screw trajectories.

Intraoperative Imaging

- An intraoperative CT scan of the thoracolumbar spine was rendered, ensuring at least three levels above and below the corpectomy level (i.e., T12). The fascia was opened above the pedicles of interest (T10–T11 and L1–L2). Our navigation wand was placed over each pedicle of interest and a trajectory was saved at each pedicle from T10 to L2 that included the axial plane angle, sagittal plane angle, screw length, and screw width. Once all the trajectories were obtained, we calibrated a navigated drill guide, navigated tap, and navigated screwdriver. The pedicles were cannulated and tapped and screws were placed according to their pre-planned trajectories. Following the placement of all screws, a new CT image was obtained using the BrainLab AIRO (see Fig. 3.1E). This was used to confirm the adequate placement of our screws. Following this, rods of appropriate size were obtained, contoured, passed through the fascia, and finally tightened into position. A final lateral x-ray was obtained with intraoperative fluoroscopy to confirm the proper placement of the rod along the screws and to confirm that the rod could be seen above and below our construct (see Fig. 3.1F).

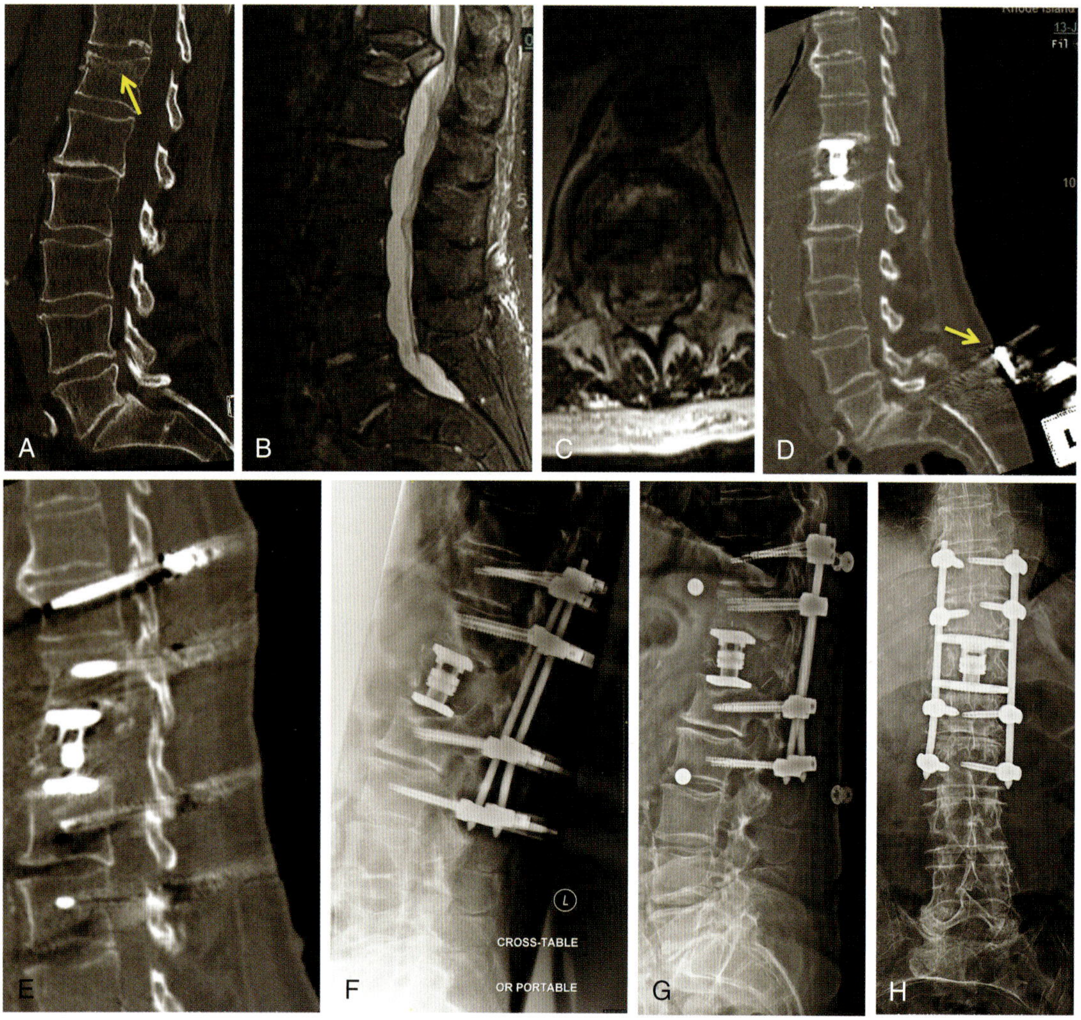

FIG. 3.1 An 80-year-old man who sustained a fall from standing at home. His initial CT scan on sagittal view shows a superior compression fracture of T12 (A, *yellow arrow* showing the fracture line). One month later, when he was readmitted with worsening back pain, his T12 fracture had progressed to a burst fracture with retropulsion and canal stenosis (B, C). Intraoperative CT (BrainLab AIRO) shows the cage reconstruction of T12 and iliac pins with the array (*yellow arrow*) for posterior percutaneous instrumentation (D). Intraoperative CT scan (BrainLab AIRO) post-placement of percutaneous screws (E). Intraoperative lateral x-rays showing the placement of percutaneous rods through the T10 to L2 construct (F). X-rays in the Antero-posterior (AP)/lateral dimensions at 6 months after surgery (G, H).

Postoperative Imaging

- The patient had Antero-posterior (AP) and lateral x-rays of the thoracolumbar spine at 6 months postoperatively that revealed stable cage reconstruction at T12 with stable posterior stabilization of percutaneous instrumentation from T10 to L2. His overall alignment appeared conserved with good height restoration (see Fig. 3.1G and H).

Postoperative Recovery and Follow-Up

- The patient has been followed up for 6 months postoperatively and resides in a nursing facility. He was supplied with a custom fit Thoraco Lumbar Sacral Orthosis (TLSO) brace for out-of-bed use for 3 months. He is ambulating without any issues and has good strength in both legs. His back pain has improved significantly.

Clinical Case Study 2

History/Clinical Presentation

- The patient is a 77-year-old woman with a history of hypertension and osteopenia who presented to the emergency department after slipping and falling on her bathroom floor at night. A CT scan revealed a T12 burst fracture with minimal retropulsion, minimal height loss, and no significant angulation (Fig. 3.2A). Her neurologic examination revealed full strength in her legs, no sensory deficits, and significant midline tenderness to her lumbar area.

Preoperative Imaging

- An MRI of her lumbar spine revealed a positive Short Tau Inversion Recovery (STIR) signal involving the T12 vertebral body but no evidence of posterior ligamentous complex injury. There was no stenosis at this level. Of note, she had a grade I spondylolisthesis at L4–L5 that was degenerative in nature, unrelated to her fall (see Fig. 3.2B).

Surgical Plan

- Given her imaging findings, the initial plan was made for conservative management involving a custom fitted brace. However, upright films in her custom brace revealed increased wedging of the anterior fracture at T12 with associated focal kyphosis (see Fig. 3.2C). Given these findings, there was concern that she would fail bracing and continue to develop further kyphosis. She also still had significant lower back pain despite medical management. Given these findings, a plan was made for surgical stabilization via a percutaneous method with cement augmentation given her osteopenia.
- Our planned incisions were identified using our navigation wand to ensure they would encompass our stabilization (T11–L1). The fascia was then opened above the pedicles of interest (T11–L1). Our navigation wand was placed over each pedicle and a trajectory was saved at each pedicle position from T11 to L1 that included the axial plane angle, sagittal plane angle, screw length, and screw width. Once all trajectories were obtained, we calibrated a navigated drill guide, navigated tap, and navigated screwdriver. The pedicles were cannulated and tapped and screws were placed according to their pre-planned trajectories. In addition, a navigated Jamshidi was cannulated into the T10 pedicles bilaterally above our construct for cement augmentation of the adjacent level to prevent further breakdown of the adjacent level given her osteoporosis. Following the placement of all the fenestrated screws, a new CT image was obtained using the BrainLab AIRO. This was used to confirm adequate placement of our screws as well as our Jamshidi cannulas (see Fig. 3.2E). Fluoroscopy was brought in for our cement augmentation of the pedicle screws and the Jamshidi (see Fig. 3.2F). Final AP/lateral films in the operating room were taken to ensure adequate placement and filling of our cement into the vertebral bodies from T10 to L1 (see Fig. 3.2G). Following this, rods of appropriate size were obtained, contoured, passed through the fascia, and finally tightened into position. A final lateral x-ray was obtained with intraoperative fluoroscopy to

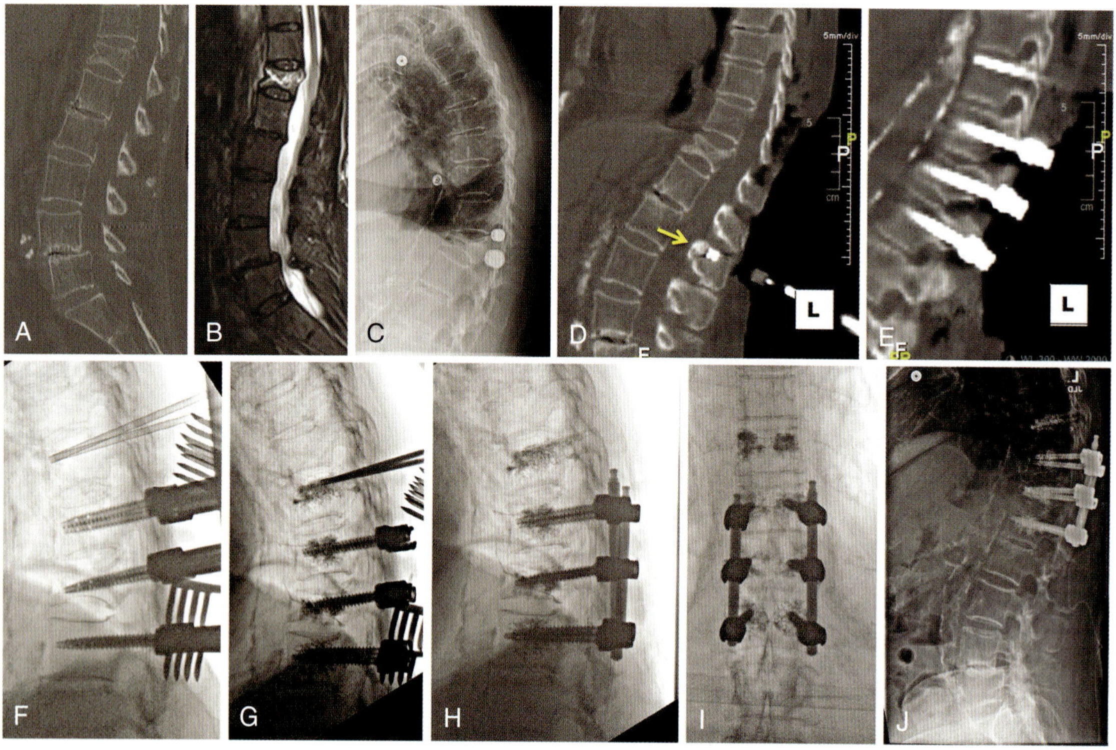

FIG. 3.2 A 77-year-old woman who fell from standing at home. The initial CT scan on sagittal view showed a T12 burst fracture with minimal height loss and no retropulsion (A). The MRI showed a STIR signal within the T12 body (B). Standing films in custom-fitted brace showed progressive angulation of her T12 fracture with associated kyphosis (C). Intraoperative CT (BrainLab AIRO) showing the placement of a spinous process clamp array at L2 (D, *arrow*). Intraoperative post-CT scan (BrainLab AIRO) showing the placement of fenestrated screws from T11 to L1, including in the fractured T12 body, as well as the placement of T10 Jamshidi cannulas bilaterally (E). Lateral fluoroscopy prior to cement augmentation of screws and Jamshidi cannulas. Final intraoperative fluoroscopy showing cement augmented fenestrated construct (G–I). Lateral x-ray at 6 months postoperatively (J).

confirm the proper placement of the rod and that enough rod could be found above and below our construct (see Fig. 3.2H and I).

Intraoperative Imaging

- The patient was positioned prone on the operating room table. The L2 spinous process was identified using lateral fluoroscopy (see Fig. 3.2D). A small midline incision was made with a periosteal dissection in order to clamp our navigation array on the spinous process of L2. Once clamped, we obtained a CT using the BrainLab AIRO for registration and navigating our screws. We obtained another CT scan after placing our screws to ensure the proper placement/position.

Postoperative Imaging

- The AP and lateral postoperative x-rays at 6 months revealed a stable construct from T11 to L1 with cement augmentation and no worsening of her kyphosis (see Fig. 3.2J).

Postoperative Recovery and Follow-Up

- The patient remained in the hospital for a few days recovering from her surgery and was discharged in stable condition to a short-term rehabilitation facility. She was supplied with a soft brace for use when out of bed for additional support for 3 months. At 6 months, she was seen as an outpatient and was found to have minimal back pain and to be ambulating without issues.

Procedural Concerns in Detail

With MISS procedures and the utilization of navigation, proper patient positioning and setup is paramount. Furthermore, preoperative planning with respect to levels requiring navigation, which tools will need to be registered with navigation to accomplish the surgery, and where the array will be placed to capture accurate real-time navigation need to be established in the preoperative planning phase to ensure smooth workflow. The surgeon must also account for alternative options if the instruments for navigation fail or cannot undergo troubleshooting (i.e., from using a navigated drill to then trying to use a navigated Jamshidi, etc.). The navigation array and accuracy must also be checked at all the phases of surgery and between instrument uses. If there is any doubt or concern, the accuracy should be checked before proceeding with the following step and/or a new CT scan should be obtained to re-register the system and check any instrumentation that has been placed. There can be a steep learning curve with navigating for spine trauma, but we have learned that significant preoperative planning along with attention to detail regarging accuracy during the surgery allows for good patient results in achieving the desired stabilization. Furthermore, the surgeon must also find their preference in the navigated tools and steps in which tools are used to assist with workflow.

Treatment Side Effects

The use of navigation and its accuracy for the correction of spinal trauma has allowed for a significant reduction in the deleterious side effects of surgery including significant blood loss, malpositioned screws, and injury to the neural/vascular elements. Nevertheless, these are the main concerns and side effects that can result even with the use of navigation. Usually, in our experience, this has occurred due to the loss of accuracy during the navigation phase of cannulating pedicles and/or placing screws. It is imperative that the proper accuracy be checked throughout the navigation process during surgery and that the surgeon not proceed with further steps until the accuracy has been verified. The other treatment side effects from navigation in spinal trauma include a lack of fusion in percutaneous stabilization cases. This can be a problem for patients who are elderly, who smoke, are on chronic steroids, and/or have pre-existing osteopenia/osteoporosis. The surgeon should weigh the risk/benefit of not decorticating and laying bone graft when navigating a percutaneous stabilization for spine trauma. It is important that the proper patient be selected for a navigated percutaneous instrumentation procedure and that the effects of not fusing be mitigated with such methods as bracing, cement augmentation, etc.

Potential Pitfalls

As previously alluded to, there can often be a steep learning curve for the surgeon in the incorporation of CAN. There can also often be a significant deleterious effect on the workflow of all operative team members. As such, efficiency on all levels of operative staff becomes imperative, including the anesthesia team that is taxed with navigating their equipment through the gantry of the scanner. With increased reliance on technology comes an increased number of opportunities for technologic malfunction, whether it be the scanner or navigation system, errors in data transfers, software bugs, or need for specially trained staff, these challenges can have detrimental effects. They not only slow down the workflow and increase operative time, but may also necessitate more spins (increasing radiation exposure) or be disorienting and result in patient harm. For example, if the reference clamp is not properly placed or is manipulated inadvertently, the registration process can be altered and lead to errors in stereotaxis between the instruments and the scan. If unrecognized, this could lead to misplaced screws or, worse, patient injury. Alternatively, in cases where there is a mismatch due to manipulation of the array, radiation exposure is increased as the patient will need to be rescanned to provide a new spinal map for accurate navigation.[1]

Management of Complications

Naturally, increased utilization of CAN helps all operating room staff familiarize themselves with the workflow and helps the surgeon with their individual learning curve.[6] With exposure, most of the challenges presented by navigation can be avoided or rapidly addressed, thus allowing for the benefits of this technology to far exceed the disadvantages. The surgeon should be ready to re-scan a patient if the accuracy appears off and/or monitoring changes occur. Being prepared ahead of time with the instruments that will be navigated as well as having familiarity with other tools that can be used in navigating can help mitigate the problems and complications that arise during the troubleshoot.

SUMMARY

Spinal navigation has revolutionized the way spine surgeons are performing spine surgery.[10] It is a powerful adjunct to the treatment of trauma patients with cervical, thoracic, lumbar, and sacral injuries. CAN provides accurate screw placement, minimizes blood loss, decreases operative time, and provides staff with reduced exposure to harmful radiation.[11] Although implementing the use of navigation involves a steep learning curve, it is certainly one that appears worth undertaking given the anticipated role of this tool in making surgeries safer for all involved.[12]

Future Directions

The efficacy and safety of CAN technologies for spine surgery has been well established. The future of this technology is difficult to anticipate given the increasing speed at which these applications are being developed. Still, it is safe to say that CAN is the future of surgical spine trauma management. A next step for device companies is to collaborate with spine surgeons on the incorporation of navigation for the placement of our interbody implants and corpectomy cages. Currently, navigation can be utilized for screw placement, planning trajectories of certain bony work, checking the correction, and evaluating the anatomy in real time.[4] When it comes time to placing a cage, however, fluoroscopy must still be employed in confirming accurate placement and depth. Once we are able to achieve this last piece confidently with CAN, navigation would stand to be involved in every case from start to finish, potentially eliminating all radiation exposure to staff.

How CAN will interact with the new advances in robotic spine surgery similarly remains unknown but is likely in our near future.[7] As its imaging capabilities continue to improve and novel imaging modalities continue to enter our practice, CAN will only enhance our ability as spine surgeons to perform safer, more accurate, and less invasive surgeries. Operating suites will inevitably need to be redesigned to accommodate these emerging technologies and to allow surgeons and staff to utilize these devices to their fullest potential. Importantly, in order to justify the cost of these new technologies, there will need to be better studies aimed at long-term patient outcomes, as well as long-term healthcare cost data.

REFERENCES

1. Gelalis ID, Paschos NK, Pakos EE, et al. Accuracy of pedicle screw placement: a systematic review of prospective in vivo studies comparing free hand, fluoroscopy guidance and navigation techniques. *Eur Spine J*. 2012;21(2):247–255. https://doi.org/10.1007/s00586-011-2011-3.
2. Kakarla UK, Little AS, Chang SW, Sonntag VK, Theodore N. Placement of percutaneous thoracic pedicle screws using neuronavigation. *World Neurosurg*. 2010;74(6):606–610. https://doi.org/10.1016/j.wneu.2010.03.028.
3. Wood KB, Li W, Lebl DR, Ploumis A. Management of thoracolumbar spine fractures. *Spine J*. 2014;14(1):145–164. https://doi.org/10.1016/j.spinee.2012.10.041.
4. Oh T, Scheer JK, Fakurnejad S, Dahdaleh NS, Smith ZA. Minimally invasive spinal surgery for the treatment of traumatic thoracolumbar burst fractures. *J Clin Neurosci*. 2015;22(1):42–47. https://doi.org/10.1016/j.jocn.2014.05.030.
5. Lang Z, Tian W, Liu Y, Liu B, Yuan Q, Sun Y. Minimally invasive pedicle screw fixation using intraoperative 3-dimensional fluoroscopy-based navigation (CAMISS Technique) for hangman fracture. *Spine (Phila Pa 1976)*. 2016;41(1): 39–45. https://doi.org/10.1097/BRS.0000000000001111.
6. Navarro-Ramirez R, Lang G, Lian X, et al. Total navigation in spine surgery; A concise guide to eliminate fluoroscopy using a portable intraoperative Computed Tomography 3-Dimensional Navigation System. *World Neurosurg*. 2017;100:325–335. https://doi.org/10.1016/j.wneu.2017.01.025.
7. Overley SC, Cho SK, Mehta AI, Arnold PM. Navigation and robotics in spinal surgery: where are we now? *Neurosurgery*. 2017;80(3S):S86–S99. https://doi.org/10.1093/neuros/nyw077.
8. Tinelli M, Matschke S, Adams M, Grützner PA, Münzberg M, Suda AJ. Correct positioning of pedicle screws with a percutaneous minimal invasive system in spine trauma. *Orthop Traumatol Surg Res*. 2014;100(4):389–393. https://doi.org/10.1016/j.otsr.2014.03.015.
9. Theocharopoulos N, Perisinakis K, Damilakis J, Papadokostakis G, Hadjipavlou A, Gourtsoyiannis N. Occupational exposure from common fluoroscopic projections used in orthopaedic surgery. *J Bone Jt Surg Am*. 2003;85(9):1698–1703. https://doi.org/10.2106/00004623-200309000-00007.
10. Fehlings MG, Ahuja CS, Mroz T, Hsu W, Harrop J. Future advances in spine surgery: the AOSpine North America perspective. *Neurosurgery*. 2017;80(3S):S1–S8. https://doi.org/10.1093/neuros/nyw112.
11. Harrop JS, Rymarczuk GN, Vaccaro AR, Steinmetz MP, Tetreault LA, Fehlings MG. Controversies in spinal trauma and evolution of care. *Neurosurgery*. 2017;80(3S):S23–S32. https://doi.org/10.1093/neuros/nyw076.
12. Moses ZB, Mayer RR, Strickland BA, et al. Neuronavigation in minimally invasive spine surgery. *Neurosurg Focus*. 2013; 35(2):E12. https://doi.org/10.3171/2013.5.FOCUS13150.

4

Navigated Spinal Deformity Correction

Brian Dial, MD, Richard Danilkowicz, MAT, MD, Melissa Erickson, MD, and Isaac Karikari, MD

INTRODUCTION OF TECHNOLOGY: ADULT SPINAL DEFORMITY

Background of Adult Spinal Deformity

Adult spinal deformity (ASD) is defined as an abnormal curvature or abnormal alignment of the vertebral column.[1] ASD has been demonstrated to limit a patient's quality of life significantly, and patients with both cervical and thoracolumbar deformity have predictable declines in health-related quality of life (HRQOL).[2,3] In the most severe cases, patients with lumbar scoliosis and sagittal malalignment have quality of life measures equal to patients who have lost the ability to use their upper or lower extremities.[4] The definition of scoliosis is a Cobb measurement greater than 10 degrees; however, in de novo adult degenerative scoliosis, coronal deformity is considered when Cobb measurements exceed 20 to 30 degrees. The Scoliosis Research Society (SRS) Schwab classification for spinal deformity classifies major coronal deformity as thoracic, thoracolumbar, or lumbar scoliosis greater than 30 degrees.[5]

A globally aligned spine allows for the least amount of energy expenditure necessary to maintain upright posture, bipedal gait, and horizontal gaze. In the globally aligned spine, a C7 plumb line should fall between the posterior superior corner of the sacrum and the center of femoral heads, and the central sacral vertical line (CSVL) should transect the C7 spinous process. While coronal imbalance greater than 4 cm has been associated with increased pain and decreased function, sagittal imbalance correlates more closely with HRQOL and is the primary focus of adult deformity correction.[6]

The importance of sagittal alignment was introduced with the conception of pelvic parameters and became the cornerstone for spinal deformity correction, as it was shown to correlate with the HRQOL measures.[7–9] The body attempts to compensate for sagittal imbalance through a series of mechanisms including reduction of thoracic kyphosis, retrolisthesis of lumbar vertebra, pelvic retroversion, and knee flexion.[10] It is important to identify these clinical and radiographic compensatory mechanisms as they can mask underlying spinal deformity. The most common spinopelvic parameters used to describe global sagittal alignment are pelvic incidence (PI), sacral slope (SS), pelvic tilt (PT), lumbar lordosis (LL), and sagittal vertical axis (SVA).[1,2] Similarly, the C2–C7 SVA and the chin-brow vertical angle (CBVA) are used to assess the degree of cervical spinal deformity.[3] In order to attain the greatest improvement in HRQOL, the following postoperative parameters should be achieved: PT < 25 degrees, PI-LL mismatch + 11 degrees, and SVA < 5 cm.[9] Historically, the treatment of spinal deformity had been supportive and aimed at delaying the progressive decline in a patient's overall health. However, currently, the treatment is corrective and aimed at improving the patient's quality of life. Significant evidence has been published demonstrating a clinically significant improvement in the HRQOL measure following the surgical correction of ASD.[11–14]

The potential to improve the quality of life of patients with spinal deformity significantly through surgery are well appreciated. However, it is biased to discuss the potential benefits of surgical intervention without discussing the high complication rate associated with performing these surgeries. In a two-year prospective multicenter study, the complication rate following ASD correction was approximately 70% and the revision surgery rate was approximately 28%.[15] The most frequent complications following ASD surgery include rod breakage, proximal junctional kyphosis (PJK), postoperative anemia, surgical site infection, and neurologic injury. Currently, predictive analytic models are being developed to identify patients with spinal deformity that would benefit from surgical correction and are at low risk for complication.[16] The use of modern technology with machine-based learning to predict success rates following ASD surgery is a perfect example of how modern technology is improving the field of spine surgery.

Spinal Navigation and Robotics in Spinal Deformity

Since 1911, when the first spinal fusion was performed, technology has been the fuel propelling advances in spine surgery. Engineers and like-minded inventors are perpetually advancing the field, and with developments in imaging modalities, interbody instrumentation, minimally invasive surgical (MIS) techniques, biologics, navigation software, and robotics, the face of spine surgery is constantly in flux. Despite the many avenues of technologic growth in spine, technologic advances in the last 30 years have been dominated by improving imaging modalities, redefining stereotactic image guidance, and introducing robotic assisted surgery.[17] The Oxford dictionary defines "navigation" as the process or activity of ascertaining one's position and planning or following a defined route. The concept of navigation is as much at the foundation of spine surgery as it is the basis for nautical or aerospace travel. At its core, spine surgery relies on visible anatomic landmarks and the mind's eye to recreate a three-dimensional (3D) mental representation of the spine to navigate surgery safely. Intraoperative imaging technologies have expanded the ability of the spinal surgeon to visualize the 3D anatomy of the spine, relying less on presumptions based on visible landmarks. Spinal navigation expands on intraoperative imaging, utilizing stereotactic technology to allow the surgeon to visualize their instrumentation in 3D radiographic images of the patient's spine.[18] Robotic shared control devices represent the current pinnacle in navigation technology. With robotic technology, the surgeon plans the pedicle screw trajectories on pre- or intraoperative imaging; these are subsequently produced by an automated robotic arm.

The ultimate goal of using computer assisted spinal navigation and robotics in ASD is to improve the precision and accuracy of the spine surgeon, which will lead to fewer complications and improved surgical outcomes. The theoretical advantages of navigation and robotics are (1) improved accuracy of pedicle screw placement, (2) improved ability to perform minimally invasive spine surgery, (3) decreased radiation exposure to the spine surgeon, and (4) avoiding surgeon fatigue and human error. The remainder of this chapter will focus on the application of navigation and robotics for use in ASD.

Accuracy of Pedicle Screw Placement

The accuracy of pedicle screw placement has been the most investigated topic for both spinal navigation and robotic assisted surgery. In deformity surgery, the placement of accurate pedicle screws becomes increasingly more difficult because of the loss of anatomic landmarks in revision settings, rotatory scoliosis requiring unique pedicle screw trajectories, and the presence of dysplastic pedicles (Fig. 4.1). Spinal navigation and robotics are tools that can facilitate accurate screw insertion in the aforementioned difficult clinical scenarios, and the use of CT spinal navigation has been shown to have equivalent pedicle screw insertion accuracy in primary and revision clinical cases.[19]

A number of studies have been performed comparing the accuracy of pedicle screw placement between free-hand techniques, fluoroscopic techniques, navigated techniques, and robotic techniques. A large meta-analysis compared pedicle screws placed using either conventional fluoroscopy, 2D fluoroscopic navigation, or 3D fluoroscopic navigation, and found accuracy rates of 68.1%, 84.3%, and 95.5%, respectively.[20] In a randomized controlled trial (RCT) that compared 100 consecutive patients with pedicle screws placed using either conventional techniques or navigation, the pedicle breach rate was 13.4% in the conventional group and 4.6% in the navigated group.[21] A prospective RCT of 1116 thoracolumbar pedicle screws demonstrated that robotic assisted pedicle screw placement was associated with better accuracy, a lower rate of violating the proximal facet capsule, and a lower rate of medial pedicle breach compared to the free-hand technique.[22] Similar results of improved accuracy with spinal navigation have been reported

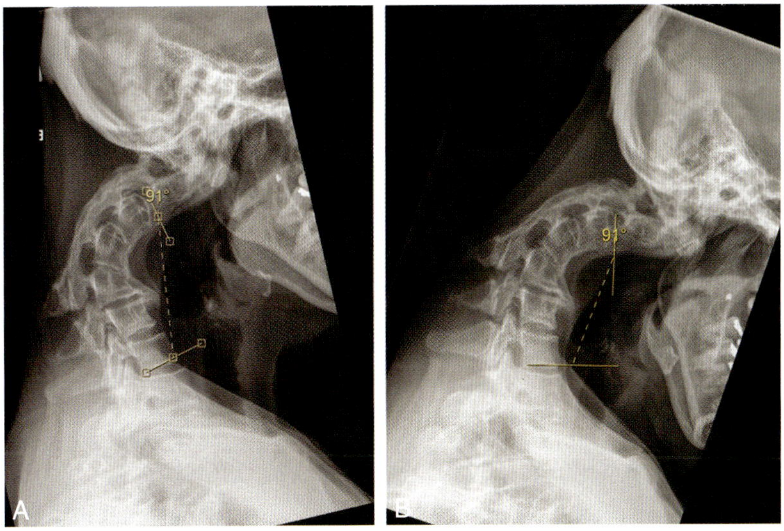

FIG. 4.1 Cervical spine flexion (A) and extension (B) radiographic images demonstrating the fixed cervical deformity.The post-laminectomy kyphosis does not correct with neck extension.

in the deformity setting. An RCT comparing navigated and nonnavigated pedicle screw accuracy in patients with spinal deformity demonstrated a pedicle breach rate of 2% with navigation and 23% without navigation.[23] In a review of patients with neuromuscular scoliosis and dysplastic apical pedicles, the accurate placement of apical pedicle screws was achieved in 79% of pedicles utilizing navigation and 67% of pedicles without navigation.[24] A systematic review compared navigated and non-navigated pedicle screw insertion in scoliosis patients and found a higher pedicle screw perforation rate without the use of navigation. However, no difference in revision treatment rates for screw malposition was seen between the groups.[25]

In addition to thoracolumbar pedicle screws, navigation has been shown to be effective for the instrumentation of cervical pedicle screws and lumbopelvic fixation. A number of technical guides and case series have demonstrated the usefulness of CT-guided navigation for the placement of S2-alar-iliac screws.[26–28] Cervical pedicle screws are technically demanding with a lateral breach threatening the vertebral artery and a medial breach placing the spinal cord at risk. The free-hand technique for subaxial cervical pedicle screws hm 14.3% to 29.1%.[29] Cervical pedicle screw placement using 3D navigation has an accuracy of 89.7%.[30] In the upper cervical spine, CT navigation has been shown to be an effective tool for the placement of C1 and C2 instrumentation.[31] However, the single head-to-head study comparing free-hand to navigated techniques for C2 pars screw placement found higher accuracy with the free-hand technique.[32]

Navigated MIS Applications in Deformity

In ASD there is a growing trend toward utilization of MIS techniques for deformity correction. MIS techniques decrease the intraoperative blood loss, overall complication rate, and length of hospitalization. However, it is important to select suitable patients, as under-restoration of deformity parameters compared to conventional open surgery is frequently reported.[33,34] A classification system has been developed to aid in the selection of appropriate patients whose spinal deformity can be corrected successfully with MIS techniques.[34] In general, fixed sagittal plane deformities should be considered cautiously for purely MIS techniques, and these deformities are best addressed with open or hybrid techniques. The most common MIS technique for deformity correction involves a two-position surgery with a lateral lumbar interbody fusion (LLIF) and percutaneous pedicle screws. A hybrid technique has been described with an LLIF followed by an open posterior fusion incorporating Smith Peterson osteotomies, allowing for greater sagittal correction. A relatively recent MIS technique, anterior column realignment (ACR), allows for greater restoration of LL by releasing the anterior longitudinal ligament (ALL).[35] A promising adoption of navigation and robotic assisted surgery allows for single-position surgery placing both the LLIF cage and percutaneous pedicle screw from the lateral decubitus position. Single-position surgery eliminates the need to stage the surgery, change the patient's position intraoperatively, or potentially require two intraoperative CT scans if navigating both the interbody cage and percutaneous pedicle screws.[36,37]

Visualization for the accurate placement of lateral interbody cages and percutaneous pedicle screws has traditionally, and successfully, been accomplished with conventional fluoroscopy. However, it has been demonstrated clearly that fluoroscopy in MIS surgery exposes the surgeon to high levels of ionizing radiation, and that 3D navigation greatly reduces the radiation exposure to the surgeon.[38] Initial studies investigating CT navigated LLIF demonstrated that navigation allows for successful and reproducible placement of the interbody cage.[39,40] With the use of CT navigation, the instruments required to prepare the disk space, trial different size cages, and place the actual cage can all be navigated in real time.[38]

Percutaneous pedicle screws can be inserted using conventional fluoroscopic imaging, 2D or 3D navigation, or robotic assisted navigation. The largest study to date reported an accuracy rate of 97% with robotic assisted placement of percutaneous pedicle screws.[41] One study compared conventional percutaneous screw placement, 2D navigated percutaneous screw placement, and 3D navigated percutaneous screw placement and reported screw malposition rates of 5.16%, 7.29%, and 1.23%, respectively.[42] In addition to the reduced radiation exposure with navigated percutaneous pedicle screw insertion, navigated and robotic assisted placement of screws minimize the risk of violating the proximal facet joint capsule. Damaging the proximal facet capsule can lead to increased rates of adjacent segment deterioration and PJK. A cadaver study demonstrated violation of the proximal facet joint capsule in 58% of those percutaneous screws placed with conventional fluoroscopy.[43] LLIF and percutaneous pedicle screw insertion can be performed safely and effectively with conventional fluoroscopic imaging or 3D navigated technologies. However, the utilization of navigation significantly lowers the radiation doses to both the operating surgeon and the patient, and preservation of the proximal facet joint capsule is more likely to occur when using robotics and navigation.

Unique Applications of Spinal Navigation and Robotics in Deformity

At present, robots are assistive tools for the accurate placement of percutaneous and open pedicle screws. Robotic technology can aid the deformity surgeon by allowing the accurate placement of pedicle screws in the challenging setting of rotated and dysplastic pedicles. While the current depth of utilization with robotics is pedicle screw insertion, the applications of spinal navigation for deformity surgery are much broader. In addition to pedicle screw insertion, spinal navigation has been used for the planning of cervicothoracic pedicle subtraction osteotomies (PSOs), for determining the resection planes for lumbar PSO, and for 3D visualization of the patient's head alignment in space. Case reports in the literature have described how spinal navigation can be used to plan resection planes and navigate osteotomes for the accurate execution of lumbar PSOs.[44,45] In the revision setting, previous fusion masses mask the lumbar anatomy, exponentially increasing the difficulty of performing three-column osteotomies. Navigation can assist in safely performing three-column osteotomies through previous fusion beds.[46] In addition to lumbar osteotomies, a case report demonstrated the utility of spinal navigation for cervical spine PSOs.[45] Multiple studies have reported the utility of spinal navigation with tumor resection; similarly, within the deformity literature, spinal navigation has been shown to assist with vertebrectomies of hemivertebra, resulting in congenital scoliosis.[47,48] As demonstrated in our case report, intraoperative CT can be utilized to create 3D representations of the patient's head in space. This application is useful when correcting cervical deformity or performing occipitocervical fusions. In our case, we were able to measure the CBVA successfully intraoperatively to ensure adequate restoration of horizontal gaze following deformity correction. It is of the utmost importance when fusing the patient's head in a fixed position or correcting cervical deformity to position the head such that the patient can visualize the world with the greatest ease. It has been reported that the CBVA following deformity correction should be between 10 and 20 degrees to provide the greatest functional outcome.[49] The ability to effectively measure the CBVA intraoperatively on a 3D image of the patient's head-neck relationship ensures the appropriate head position prior to spinal fusion.

Limitations of Spinal Navigation

Despite stereotactic navigation being invented in 1908 and spinal navigation coming onto the market in the 1990s, spinal navigation for spinal deformity remains in its infancy. Many surgeons are resistant to using the technology, and not without right cause. The navigation is based on referencing, and movement of the patient or referencing frame following registration will result in inaccuracy of the location of the navigated instrument in relation to the patient's anatomy. This limitation of the technology needs to be understood by the operating surgeon, and it remains imperative to assess the accuracy of the navigation frequently throughout a surgical case. The use of intraoperative navigation or robotic assisted surgery requires additional equipment and complexity for room setup and workflow. In order to not significantly delay operative times, the OR staff must become proficient in the workflow of using these technologies. In the current era of rapidly evolving technology, it is exciting to see where navigation and robotics will lead in the field of spinal deformity. With advances in technology, the goal remains to minimize complications and maximize patient outcomes following deformity correction.

CASE REPORT

History/Clinical Presentation

A 66-year-old female presented with the complaint of significant deformity of her neck and progressive symptoms of worsening balance and poor hand dexterity. Her previous surgical history was significant for a posterior cervical laminectomy for intramedullary spinal cord ependymoma in 1970. On examination she demonstrated intact motor and sensory function but exaggerated deep tendon reflexes and gait instability. She was unable to look upright.

Preoperative Imaging

Preoperative cervical radiographs demonstrated fixed kyphosis measuring 91.5 degrees (Fig. 4.2). A subsequent CT scan of the cervical spine confirmed fused facet joints from C1 to C5. A radiographic diagnosis of post-laminectomy kyphosis was confirmed. The patient's SVA was 1.7 cm, the C2–C7 SVA equaled 3.5 cm, and the CBVA was 22 degrees (Fig. 4.3).

Surgical Plan

The surgical objective was to address the cervical deformity to re-establish horizontal gaze and prevent the progression of her myelopathic symptoms. The patient was taken to the OR and placed prone on the OR table with a Mayfield (Integra LifeSciences©, Plainsboro, NJ) head positioner. Bolsters were placed at the nipple line and anterior superior iliac spines to decrease the abdominal pressure. The Airo Mobile Intraoperative CT-based Spinal Navigation (Brainlab©, Feldkirchen, Germany) was utilized. The intraoperative CT scanner was placed above the patient's head, between anesthesia and the operative field (Fig. 4.4). A collision check was performed to ensure that the patient could be moved through the CT scanner without coming into contact with it. The navigation array was secured to the Mayfield head positioner. The patient was prepared and draped in the standard fashion. A hole was cut in the drapes to allow the attachment of the sterile array to the array positioner shown in Fig. 4.4. The drapes were secured over the CT to scanner to create a sterile field. The spine was exposed from C2 to T1. Next, a sterile drape, "shower curtain,"

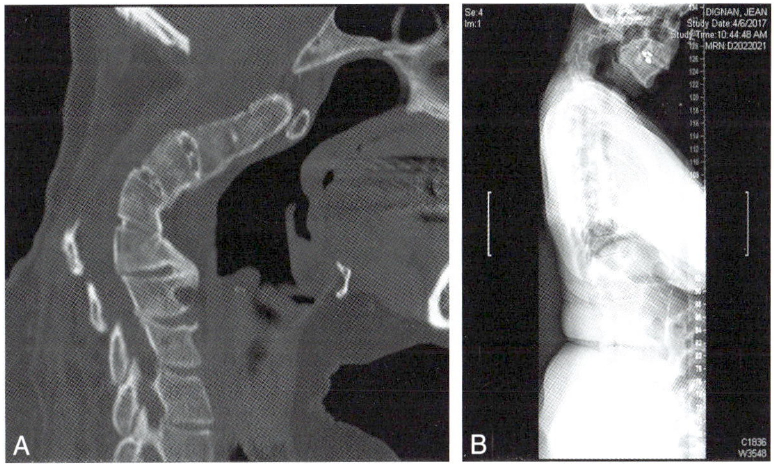

FIG. 4.2 (A) CT scan of the cervical spine demonstrating cervical kyphosis and a large syndesmophyte at C5/C6. B) Full-length standing radiographs with maintained global sagittal spinal alignment. The deformity was isolated to the cervical spine.

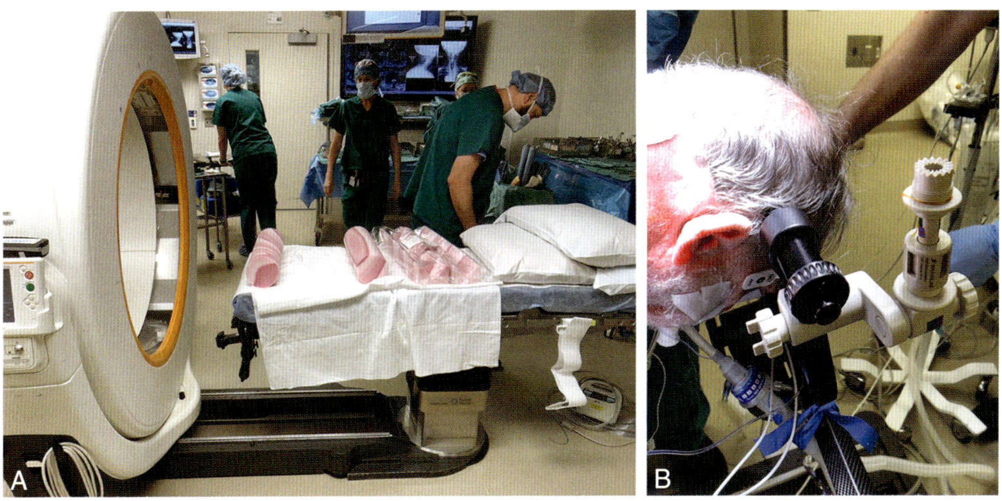

FIG. 4.3 (A) Typical room setup when utilizing intraoperative CT navigation for cervical deformity. (B) Clinical photograph demonstrating the position of the navigated array attached to the Mayfield head positioner.

was placed over the patient, and a CT scan was obtained. Accuracy of the CT scan was checked with a navigated pointer. Navigation was utilized for screw placement at C2, C7, and T1. Lateral mass screws from C3 to C6 were placed based on the anatomic landmarks. A Smith Peterson osteotomy was performed at C5/6 to restore cervical lordosis and horizontal gaze. Deformity correction was achieved through positioning of the Mayfield head positioner. Once the surgical team determined that the patient's head was in a good position, the Mayfield was locked in the extended position. Intraoperative neurologic monitoring was utilized to ensure no loss of motor-evoked potentials or somatosensory-evoked potentials following deformity correction. At this time, a second intraoperative CT scan

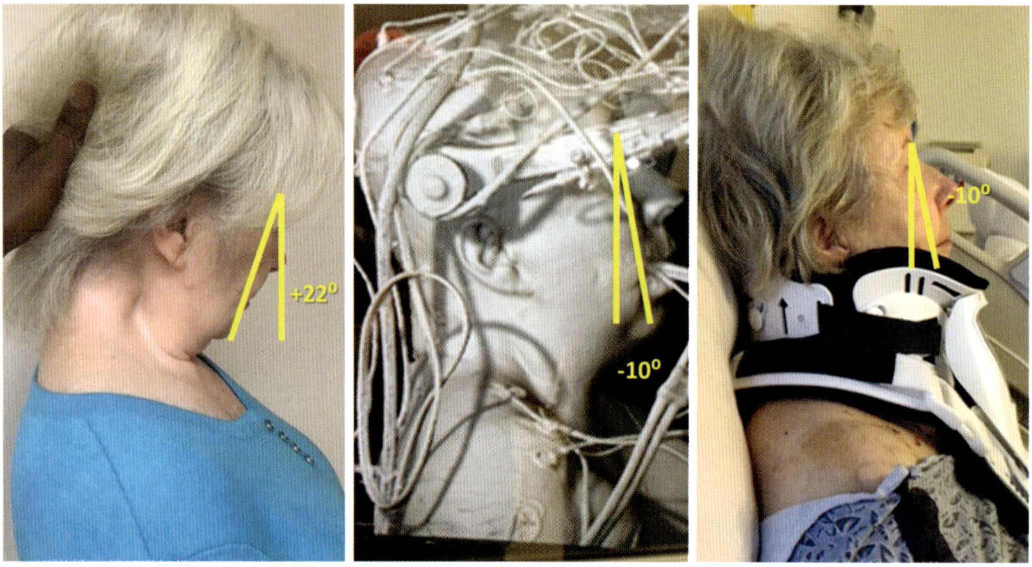

FIG. 4.4 (A) Clinical photograph demonstrating the CBVA of 22 degrees preoperatively. (B) Intraoperative 3D image of the position of the head. The CBVA can be measured from this 3D CT image to ensure adequate deformity correction prior to fusion. In this case the CBVA was corrected to −10 degrees following posterior Smith Peterson osteotomy at C5/6 and neck manipulation with the Mayfield held positioner. (C) Clinical photograph taken on post-operative day 2 demonstrating restoration of the patient's horizontal gaze.

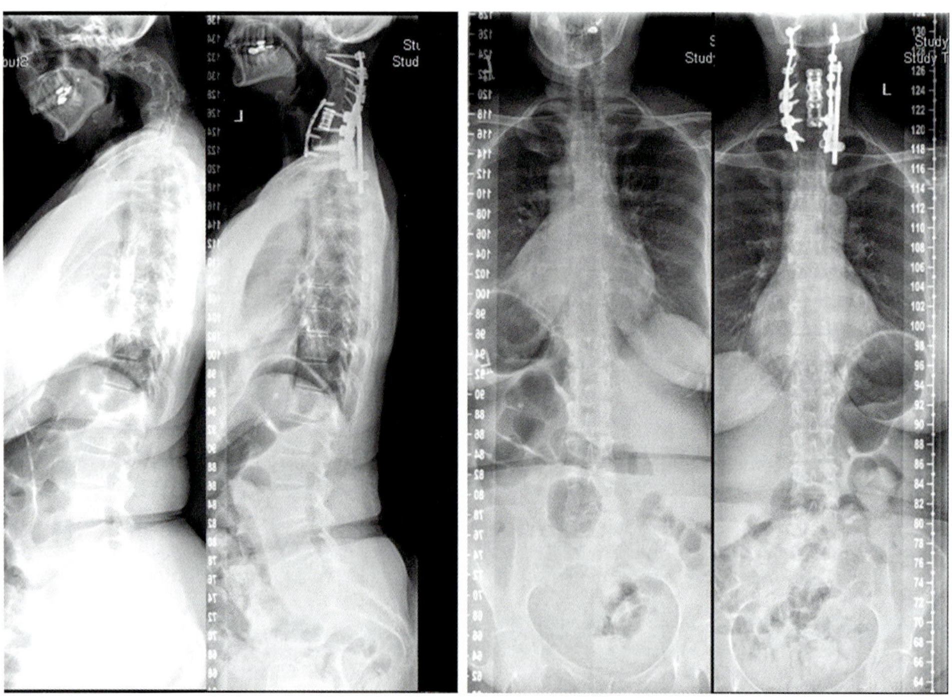

FIG. 4.5 Standing full-length spine radiographs demonstrating preoperative and 6-month postoperative cervical spine alignment. The C2 to C7 kyphosis was improved from 91 to 57 degrees. The CBVA was improved from 22 to −10 degrees.

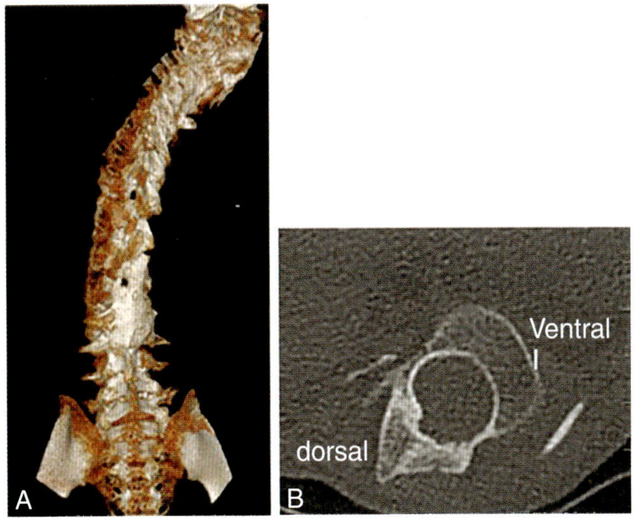

FIG. 4.6 An 8-yr old female with neuromuscular scolisis (A) 3D CT scan demonstrating the severe axial deformity of the patient's spine. (B) Axial CT image of the T12 vertebra demonstrating rotational deformity and dysplastic pedicles. Navigation allows for improved accuracy of pedicle screw placement in this clinical setting where free-hand placement would be extremely difficult.

was obtained. The CT scan was used first to check adequate screw position and second to create a 3D image of the position of the patient's head in space (Fig. 4.5). The patient's corrected CBVA was measured from the 3D image to ensure adequate deformity correction. Transition rods were then placed posteriorly. A single accessory rod was utilized to provide additional stability across the osteotomy site. Following completion of the posterior portion of the case, the patient was positioned supine and an anterior fusion from C5 to T1 with a C6 corpectomy was performed.

Postoperative Recovery and Follow-Up

The patient tolerated the surgery well without acute or delayed complications. Six-month postoperative radiographs demonstrate maintained deformity correction (Fig. 4.6).

REFERENCES

1. Ailon T, Smith JS, Shaffrey CI, et al. Degenerative spinal deformity. *Neurosurgery*. 2015;77(suppl 4):S75–S91. https://doi.org/10.1227/NEU.0000000000000938.
2. Ames CP, Scheer JK, Lafage V, et al. Adult spinal deformity: epidemiology, health impact, evaluation, and management. *Spine Deform*. 2016;4(4):310–322. https://doi.org/10.1016/j.jspd.2015.12.009.
3. Oe S, Togawa D, Nakai K, et al. The influence of age and sex on cervical spinal alignment among volunteers aged over 50. *Spine (Phila Pa 1976)*. 2015;40(19):1487–1494. https://doi.org/10.1097/BRS.0000000000001071.
4. Bess S, Line B, Fu KM, et al. The health impact of symptomatic adult spinal deformity: comparison of deformity types to United States population norms and chronic diseases. *Spine (Phila Pa 1976)*. 2016;41(3):224–233. https://doi.org/10.1097/BRS.0000000000001202.
5. Terran J, Schwab F, Shaffrey CI, et al. The SRS-Schwab adult spinal deformity classification: assessment and clinical correlations based on a prospective operative and nonoperative cohort. *Neurosurgery*. 2013;73(4):559–568. https://doi.org/10.1227/NEU.0000000000000012.
6. Glassman SD, Berven S, Bridwell K, Horton W, Dimar JR. Correlation of radiographic parameters and clinical symptoms in adult scoliosis. *Spine (Phila Pa 1976)*. 2005;30(6):682–688. https://doi.org/10.1097/01.brs.0000155425.04536.f7.

7. Legaye J, Duval-Beaupère G, Hecquet J, Marty C. Pelvic incidence: a fundamental pelvic parameter for three-dimensional regulation of spinal sagittal curves. *Eur Spine J.* 1998;7(2):99–103. https://doi.org/10.1007/s005860050038.
8. Glassman SD, Bridwell K, Dimar JR, Horton W, Berven S, Schwab F. The impact of positive sagittal balance in adult spinal deformity. *Spine (Phila Pa 1976).* 2005;30(18):2024–2029. https://doi.org/10.1097/01.brs.0000179086.30449.96.
9. Schwab FJ, Blondel B, Bess S, et al. Radiographical spinopelvic parameters and disability in the setting of adult spinal deformity: a prospective multicenter analysis. *Spine (Phila Pa 1976).* 2013;38(13):E803–E812. https://doi.org/10.1097/BRS.0b013e318292b7b9.
10. Barrey C, Roussouly P, Le Huec JC, D'Acunzi G, Perrin G. Compensatory mechanisms contributing to keep the sagittal balance of the spine. *Eur Spine J.* 2013;22(suppl 6):S834–S841. https://doi.org/10.1007/s00586-013-3030-z.
11. Bridwell KH, Baldus C, Berven S, et al. Changes in radiographic and clinical outcomes with primary treatment adult spinal deformity surgeries from two years to three- to five-years follow-up. *Spine (Phila Pa 1976).* 2010;35(20):1849–1854. https://doi.org/10.1097/BRS.0b013e3181efa06a.
12. Kelly MP, Lurie JD, Yanik EL, et al. Operative versus non-operative treatment for adult symptomatic lumbar scoliosis. *J Bone Joint Surg Am.* 2019;101(4):338–352. https://doi.org/10.2106/JBJS.18.00483.
13. Smith JS, Lafage V, Shaffrey CI, et al. Outcomes of operative and nonoperative treatment for adult spinal deformity: a prospective, multicenter, propensity-matched cohort assessment with minimum 2-year follow-up. *Neurosurgery.* 2016;78(6):851–861. https://doi.org/10.1227/NEU.0000000000001116.
14. Smith JS, Shaffrey CI, Glassman SD, et al. Risk-benefit assessment of surgery for adult scoliosis: an analysis based on patient age. *Spine (Phila Pa 1976).* 2011;36(10):817–824. https://doi.org/10.1097/BRS.0b013e3181e21783.
15. Smith JS, Klineberg E, Lafage V, et al. Prospective multicenter assessment of perioperative and minimum 2-year postoperative complication rates associated with adult spinal deformity surgery. *J Neurosurg Spine.* 2016;25(1):1–14. https://doi.org/10.3171/2015.11.SPINE151036.
16. Ames CP, Smith JS, Pellisé F, et al. Artificial intelligence based hierarchical clustering of patient types and intervention categories in adult spinal deformity surgery: towards a new classification scheme that predicts quality and value. *Spine (Phila Pa 1976).* 2019;44(13):915–926. https://doi.org/10.1097/BRS.0000000000002974.
17. Marcus HJ, Hughes-Hallett A, Kwasnicki RM, Darzi A, Yang GZ, Nandi D. Technological innovation in neurosurgery: a quantitative study. *J Neurosurg.* 2015;123(1):174–181. https://doi.org/10.3171/2014.12.JNS141422.
18. Kochanski RB, Lombardi JM, Laratta JL, Lehman RA, O'Toole JE. Image-guided navigation and robotics in spine surgery. *Neurosurgery.* 2019;84(6):1179–1189. https://doi.org/10.1093/neuros/nyy630.
19. Hsieh JC, Drazin D, Firempong AO, Pashman R, Johnson JP, Kim TT. Accuracy of intraoperative computed tomography image-guided surgery in placing pedicle and pelvic screws for primary versus revision spine surgery. *Neurosurg Focus.* 2014;36(3):E2. https://doi.org/10.3171/2014.1.FOCUS13525.
20. Mason A, Paulsen R, Babuska JM, et al. The accuracy of pedicle screw placement using intraoperative image guidance systems. *J Neurosurg Spine.* 2014;20(2):196–203. https://doi.org/10.3171/2013.11.SPINE13413.
21. Laine T, Lund T, Ylikoski M, Lohikoski J, Schlenzka D. Accuracy of pedicle screw insertion with and without computer assistance: a randomised controlled clinical study in 100 consecutive patients. *Eur Spine J.* 2000;9(3):235–240. https://doi.org/10.1007/s005860000146.
22. Han X, Tian W, Liu Y, et al. Safety and accuracy of robot-assisted versus fluoroscopy-assisted pedicle screw insertion in thoracolumbar spinal surgery: a prospective randomized controlled trial. *J Neurosurg Spine.* 2019;30(5):615–622. https://doi.org/10.3171/2018.10.SPINE18487.
23. Rajasekaran S, Vidyadhara S, Ramesh P, Shetty AP. Randomized clinical study to compare the accuracy of navigated and non-navigated thoracic pedicle screws in deformity correction surgeries. *Spine (Phila Pa 1976).* 2007;32(2):E56–E64. https://doi.org/10.1097/01.brs.0000252094.64857.ab.
24. Jin M, Liu Z, Liu X, et al. Does intraoperative navigation improve the accuracy of pedicle screw placement in the apical region of dystrophic scoliosis secondary to neurofibromatosis type I: comparison between O-arm navigation and free-hand technique. *Eur Spine J.* 2016;25(6):1729–1737. https://doi.org/10.1007/s00586-015-4012-0.
25. Tian W, Zeng C, An Y, Wang C, Liu Y, Li J. Accuracy and postoperative assessment of pedicle screw placement during scoliosis surgery with computer-assisted navigation: a meta-analysis. *Int J Med Robot.* 2017;13(1). https://doi.org/10.1002/rcs.1732.
26. Pham MH, Jakoi AM, Hsieh PC. S-1 and S-2-alar-iliac screw fixation via intraoperative navigation. *Neurosurg Focus.* 2016;41(Video suppl 1):1. https://doi.org/10.3171/2016.2.FocusVid.1693.
27. Ray WZ, Ravindra VM, Schmidt MH, Dailey AT. Stereotactic navigation with the O-arm for placement of S-2 alar iliac screws in pelvic lumbar fixation. *J Neurosurg Spine.* 2013;18(5):490–495. https://doi.org/10.3171/2013.2.SPINE12813.
28. Shin JH, Hoh DJ, Kalfas IH. Iliac screw fixation using computer-assisted computer tomographic image guidance: technical note. *Neurosurgery.* 2012;70(1)(suppl Operative):16–20, discussion 20. https://doi.org/10.1227/NEU.0b013e318230517a.
29. Yukawa Y, Kato F, Ito K, et al. Placement and complications of cervical pedicle screws in 144 cervical trauma patients using pedicle axis view techniques by fluoroscope. *Eur Spine J.* 2009;18(9):1293–1299. https://doi.org/10.1007/s00586-009-1032-7.
30. Rajasekaran S, Kanna PR, Shetty TA. Intra-operative computer navigation guided cervical pedicle screw insertion in thirty-three complex cervical spine deformities. *J Craniovertebr Junction Spine.* 2010;1(1):38–43. https://doi.org/10.4103/0974-8237.65480.

31. Czabanka M, Haemmerli J, Hecht N, et al. Spinal navigation for posterior instrumentation of C1-2 instability using a mobile intraoperative CT scanner. *J Neurosurg Spine*. 2017;27(3): 268–275. https://doi.org/10.3171/2017.1.SPINE16859.
32. Hlubek RJ, Bohl MA, Cole TS, et al. Safety and accuracy of freehand versus navigated C2 pars or pedicle screw placement. *Spine J*. 2018;18(8):1374–1381. https://doi.org/10.1016/j.spinee.2017.12.003.
33. Wang MY, Mummaneni PV. Minimally invasive surgery for thoracolumbar spinal deformity: initial clinical experience with clinical and radiographic outcomes. *Neurosurg Focus*. 2010;28(3):E9. https://doi.org/10.3171/2010.1.FOCUS09286.
34. Mummaneni PV, Shaffrey CI, Lenke LG, et al. The minimally invasive spinal deformity surgery algorithm: a reproducible rational framework for decision making in minimally invasive spinal deformity surgery. *Neurosurg Focus*. 2014;36(5):E6. https://doi.org/10.3171/2014.3.FOCUS1413.
35. Mundis GM Jr, Turner JD, Kabirian N, et al. Anterior column realignment has similar results to pedicle subtraction osteotomy in treating adults with sagittal plane deformity. *World Neurosurg*. 2017;105:249–256. https://doi.org/10.1016/j.wneu.2017.05.122.
36. Blizzard DJ, Thomas JA. MIS single-position lateral and oblique lateral lumbar interbody fusion and bilateral pedicle screw fixation: feasibility and perioperative results. *Spine (Phila Pa 1976)*. 2018;43(6):440–446. https://doi.org/10.1097/BRS.0000000000002330.
37. Quiceno E, Hartman C, Godzik J, Pacult MA, Hemphill C, Uribe JS. Single position spinal surgery for the treatment of grade II spondylolisthesis: a technical note. *J Clin Neurosci*. 2019;65:145–147. https://doi.org/10.1016/j.jocn.2019.03.016.
38. Oh T, Park P, Miller CA, Chan AK, Mummaneni PV. Navigation-assisted minimally invasive surgery deformity correction. *Neurosurg Clin N Am*. 2018;29(3):439–451. https://doi.org/10.1016/j.nec.2018.03.002.
39. Joseph JR, Smith BW, Patel RD, Park P. Use of 3D CT-based navigation in minimally invasive lateral lumbar interbody fusion. *J Neurosurg Spine*. 2016;25(3):339–344. https://doi.org/10.3171/2016.2.SPINE151295.
40. DiGiorgio AM, Edwards CS, Virk MS, Mummaneni PV, Chou D. Stereotactic navigation for the prepsoas oblique lateral lumbar interbody fusion: technical note and case series. *Neurosurg Focus*. 2017;43(2):E14. https://doi.org/10.3171/2017.5.FOCUS17168.
41. Kam JKT, Gan C, Dimou S, et al. Learning curve for robot-assisted percutaneous pedicle screw placement in thoracolumbar surgery. *Asian Spine J*. 2019:920–927. https://doi.org/10.31616/asj.2019.0033.
42. Tajsic T, Patel K, Farmer R, Mannion RJ, Trivedi RA. Spinal navigation for minimally invasive thoracic and lumbosacral spine fixation: implications for radiation exposure, operative time, and accuracy of pedicle screw placement. *Eur Spine J*. 2018;27(8):1918–1924. https://doi.org/10.1007/s00586-018-5587-z.
43. Patel RD, Graziano GP, Vanderhave KL, Patel AA, Gerling MC. Facet violation with the placement of percutaneous pedicle screws. *Spine (Phila Pa 1976)*. 2011;36(26):E1749–E1752. https://doi.org/10.1097/BRS.0b013e318221a800.
44. Fujibayashi S, Neo M, Takemoto M, et al. Computer-assisted spinal osteotomy: a technical note and report of four cases. *Spine (Phila Pa 1976)*. 2010;35(18):E895–E903. https://doi.org/10.1097/brs.0b013e3181dc5ed1.
45. Shin JH, Yanamadala V, Cha TD. Computer-assisted navigation for real time planning of pedicle subtraction osteotomy in cervico-thoracic deformity correction. *Oper Neurosurg (Hagerstown)*. 2019;16(4):445–450. https://doi.org/10.1093/ons/opy162.
46. Vital JM, Boissière L, Bourghli A, Castelain JE, Challier V, Obeid I. Osteotomies through a fusion mass in the lumbar spine. *Eur Spine J*. 2015;24(suppl 1):S107–S111. https://doi.org/10.1007/s00586-014-3657-4.
47. Kosterhon M, Gutenberg A, Kantelhardt SR, Archavlis E, Giese A. Navigation and image injection for control of bone removal and osteotomy planes in spine surgery. *Oper Neurosurg (Hagerstown)*. 2017;13(2):297–304. https://doi.org/10.1093/ons/opw017.
48. Takahashi J, Ebara S, Hashidate H, et al. Computer-assisted hemivertebral resection for congenital spinal deformity. *J Orthop Sci*. 2011;16(5):503–509. https://doi.org/10.1007/s00776-011-0134-3.
49. Song K, Su X, Zhang Y, et al. Optimal chin-brow vertical angle for sagittal visual fields in ankylosing spondylitis kyphosis. *Eur Spine J*. 2016;25(8):2596–2604. https://doi.org/10.1007/s00586-016-4588-z.

5

Navigation of Tumor and Metastatic Lesions in the Thoracolumbar Spine

Zach Pennington, MD, A. Karim Ahmed, MD, Jeff Ehresman, MD, Sheng-Fu Larry Lo, MD, MHS, and Daniel M. Sciubba, MD

INTRODUCTION OF TECHNOLOGY

Spine oncology is a broad field encompassing a wide array of pathologies. The vast majority are spinal metastases arising from the vertebral body,[1-3] most commonly in the thoracic (70%) or lumbar spine (30%),[4] secondary to breast, prostate, lung, and renal cell cancers.[5] The patients with these pathologies are often extremely frail[6] and benefit from more minimally invasive approaches.[7] Over the past 5 years, advances in spinal navigation in robotics have helped facilitate the development of these approaches. Additionally, they are increasingly being applied for the resection of primary vertebral column malignancies. Here, we review the application of both technologies in the field of spinal oncology.

Present Practice

For both primary vertebral column malignancies and spinal metastases with spinal cord compression, surgical intervention is considered the standard of care.[8-12] In isolated primary malignancies, the indication for surgery is curative resection, which has been shown to improve local control and disease-specific survival.[8-11] For spinal metastases, the indications for surgery are (1) neural element decompression and (2) fixation of an unstable tumor-affected segment.

Spinal metastases make up the core of the practices of most spinal oncologists and decision-making can be guided by either the **N**eurologic, **O**ncologic, **M**echanical, and **S**ystemic (NOMS)[13] or **L**ocation, **M**echanical instability, **N**eurology, **O**ncology, and **P**atient fitness, prognosis and response to prior therapy (LMNOP) frameworks.[14] In both systems, the epidural disease burden can be graded using the Epidural Spinal Cord Compression System (Table 5.1)[15] and mechanical instability can be graded using the Spinal Instability Neoplastic Score (SINS; Table 5.2).[16]

For these patients, advances in radiation treatment modalities have made it such that extensive tumor resection is not necessary to achieve durable long-term local control.[17] As a result, with the exception of patients with de novo deformity requiring anterior column

TABLE 5.1 Epidural spinal cord compression system for the classification of spinal cord impingement in patients with metastatic vertebral column disease.[15]

No Cord Compression		Cord Compression	
Grade	*Definition*	*Grade*	*Definition*
0	Bone-only disease	2	Epidural disease with cord compression, but only partial effacement of CSF space
1a	Epidural disease without deformation of thecal sac	3	Epidural disease with cord compression and complete effacement of CSF space
1b	Epidural disease with thecal sac deformation but no cord abutment		
1c	Epidural disease with thecal sac deformation and cord abutment without compression		

CSF, Cerebrospinal fluid.

reconstruction,[18] minimally invasive approaches such as separation surgery via a mini-open approach[19] are generally preferred due to their lower associated morbidity.[7] Such approaches employ either transcutaneous[19] or transfascial placement of instrumentation.[20] In both cases, the lack of direct visualization means that navigation of some sort must be used for instrumentation placement. Conventionally this has been done under the guidance of two-dimensional fluoroscopy; however, many surgeons are increasingly using stereotactic navigation systems (e.g., BrainLab, StealthStation) and robotic assisted instrumentation. Both strategies have the potential to reduce the overall radiation exposure to the surgeon and surgical staff.[21] Additionally, nearly a dozen published series have suggested that operative and clinical outcomes are superior for patients with spinal metastases treated using minimally invasive, navigation-assisted versus open techniques.[20,22-31] As indicated in two recent systematic reviews,[7,32] minimally invasive techniques appear to reduce intraoperative blood loss, hospital length of stay, and complication rates relative to open surgery. Equally as important, the pain-related and neurological outcomes appear to be equivalent.

Advances in intraoperative navigation have also allowed the application of nonsurgical interventions to the spinal metastasis population, such as radiofrequency ablation,[33,34] and have enhanced the ability to plan and execute osteotomies for primary malignancies.[35,36] In both primary and metastatic lesions of the vertebral column, intraoperative navigation systems may be useful for assessing the degree of tumor extraction,[35,37] an especially important benefit for primary lesions given the association of greater tumor excision with superior local control.[8,38]

Guidelines for Spinal Navigation

The common platforms used for cranial and spinal navigation mean that many of the techniques developed by trainees during cranial cases can be applied when learning how to apply navigation to spine oncology cases. Recently, the *International Society for Computer Assisted Orthopaedic Surgery* published a set of guidelines for how navigation can best be applied for spine surgery.[39] The core principles highlighted in the guidelines include (1) the importance of verifying navigation registration pre-instrumentation using known anatomic landmarks (Fig. 5.1A–D), (2) maintaining a clear line of sight between the infrared camera of the navigation system and the patient-fixed reference frame, (3) continuous verification of registration accuracy by comparing the image location with the known landmarks,

TABLE 5.2 The Spinal Instability Neoplastic Score (SINS) for classifying vertebral column instability in the context of metastatic spine disease.[16]

Component	Score
Alignment	
Subluxation/translation	4
Kyphosis/scoliosis only	2
Normal	0
Bone quality	
Lytic	2
Mixed lytic/blastic	1
Blastic	0
Location	
Junctional: O–C2, C7–T2, T11–L1, L5–S1	3
Mobile: C3–C6, L2–L4	2
Semirigid: T3–T10	1
Rigid: S2–S5	0
Pain	
Yes, mechanical	3
Yes, oncologic only	2
No	1
Posterolateral involvement	
Bilateral	3
Unilateral	1
No involvement	0
Vertebral body involvement	
>50% height loss	3
0%–50% height loss	2
No collapse, but >50% body involvement	1
None of the above	0
Categorization	**Score**
Unstable	13–18
Potentially unstable	7–12
Stable	1–6

and (4) minimizing changes in the locoregional alignment prior to the completion of navigation-assisted maneuvers, as alignment changes can result in significant registration inaccuracies. Along these lines, the group similarly indicated that the contraindications to navigation-assisted surgery include excessive spinal mobility, the inability to place a stable and rigid tracker, and poor preoperative image quality, the latter of which limits the accuracy of the navigation system. Within the realm of tumors, significant disruption of

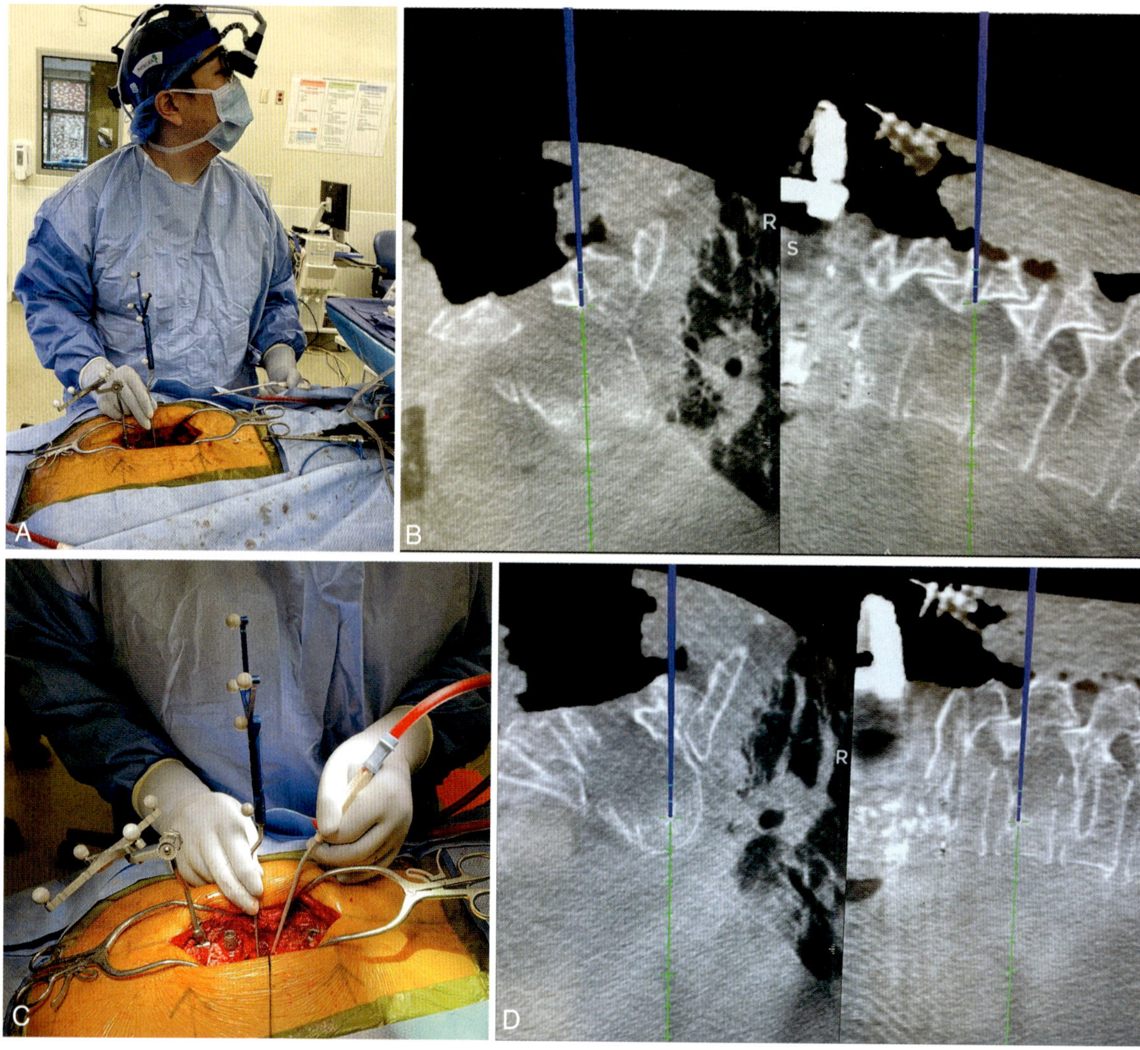

FIG. 5.1 **Illustration of the use of intraoperative navigation to verify positioning during en bloc spondylectomy.** (A) The navigated wand is placed in the field over the planned instrumentation or osteotomy site, and (B) the wand position is correlated with the projected position on the intraoperative navigation. Shown here is the wand being used to verify the position of the tumor in a patient undergoing a single-level piecemeal spondylectomy. The projected image is from an intraoperative cone-beam CT scan acquired following the posterior exposure. (C and D) Illustrate the use of the wand to monitor the extent of vertebral column resection.

the locoregional landmarks by oncologic disease may preclude the ability to employ spinal navigation effectively.

The group similarly acknowledged the existence of a learning curve, a finding corroborated by others.[40] As it pertains to the adoption of this program for spine oncology, our opinion is that navigation should be integrated into the surgical workflow in a staged approach. It should begin with application to more straightforward procedures, such as the placement of pedicle screws in normal, non-dysplastic vertebrae, and gradually move toward more complex maneuvers, culminating in its application to the guidance of osteotomy cuts. In all cases, it is our opinion that the surgeon should be acquainted with the execution of the procedure without navigation prior to attempting it under navigation guidance.

Applications of Spinal Navigation to Tumors and Present Outcomes

In spine tumor surgery, the main applications of navigation technology are instrumentation placement and tumor resection. The evidence for the former is relatively limited in the spine tumor population,[41,42] as the fundamentals of pedicle screw instrumentation are highly similar for patients with oncologic and degenerative disease. Within the degenerative literature, however, several series suggest that navigation-assisted instrumentation provides superior instrumentation accuracy. The recent series include those of Jing et al.,[43] Budu et al.,[44] and Yang et al.[45] In their series of 60 patients undergoing thoracolumbar instrumentation using either O-arm (n = 191) or fluoroscopy-assisted placement (n = 150), Jing et al.[43] found that screws placed under navigation were significantly more likely to have clinically acceptable placement. Budu et al.[44] similarly showed in their series of 831 screws (296 navigated using BrainLab and Orbic 3D, Siemens) that screws placed under navigation were half as likely to be misplaced. Additionally, they found that the use of navigation reduced the variability in misplacement rates across surgeons. Navigation was associated with improved accuracy in those who had greater inaccuracy using fluoroscopic assistance, suggesting that it may elevate the performance of surgeons who have subpar results using fluoroscopic assistance. These results reflect the findings of an earlier systematic review by Gelalis et al.[46] In a review of 26 prospective trials of 6617 screws, the authors found that navigation assistance was associated with superior instrumentation accuracy. They also found that, whereas free-hand placed screws tended to deviate medially (into the canal), those placed under CT-guided navigation more commonly perforated the lateral pedicle wall. Consequently, ceteris paribus, navigation-assisted placement may decrease the neurological risk profile associated with thoracic screw placement by biasing the screws laterally, away from the spinal canal and cord.

This improved accuracy offered by navigation may be even greater in deformity operations, where patients may have hypoplastic or obliquely oriented pedicles that are difficult to cannulate without navigation assistance.[47–49] As deformity is not uncommon in tumor patients, similar benefits may be observed within the oncology population. Additionally, as metastatic lesions frequently disrupt the local bony anatomy, intraoperative navigation may enable surgeons to identify more easily compromised bone and select more optimal screw trajectories. De la Garza Ramos et al.[42] recently provided evidence to support the superiority of navigation-assisted pedicle screw instrumentation in patients with spinal metastases. In a series of 62 patients instrumented with 547 total screws (249 navigated), they found that the utilization of navigation led to a significantly lower rate of pedicle breach compared to free-hand instrumentation.

By comparison, the support for navigation in facilitating tumor resection is unique to the oncology population. For the resection of primary tumors, several groups have described good results.[36,50–54] Most of the early descriptions were for benign pathologies. One of the first descriptions was reported by Moore and McLain,[55] who described their experience using the Viewpoint Stereotactic Navigation System (Z-kat) for the resection of an osteoid osteoma and osteoblastoma of the cervicothoracic junction. Rajasekaran et al.[56] also used navigation to treat benign lesions. They described the application of Iso-C 3D (Seimens) fluoroscopy-guided resection to four osteoid osteomas of the mobile spine.

All the lesions arose from the posterior elements and were successfully treated with piecemeal resection, leading to durable recurrence-free survival in all patients at an average of 2 years. Nagashima et al.[57] subsequently described the application of navigation to an osteoid osteoma of the C2 pedicle. Using the StealthStation (Medtronic) navigation system and a preoperative CT, they achieved piecemeal resection with minimal morbidity; the postoperative outcomes were not reported.

A contemporaneous description of the application of intraoperative navigation to primary vertebral column malignancies was reported by Dasenbrock et al.[36] The authors employed intraoperative navigation for partial sacrectomy and en bloc resection of three sacral chordomas. The group utilized a preoperative CT scan and the BrainLab (BrainLab) system to guide the osteotomy cuts for the partial sacrectomy. The imaging reference frame was affixed to the L5 spinous process and the superior articulating processes of S1 were used as locoregional landmarks during point-to-point mapping for registration of the system. To guide the cuts and monitor the trajectory of the high-speed drill, a tracking probe was attached to the drill. This facilitated tracking in the sagittal and axial planes in real time. The authors reported en bloc excision with negative margins and the patient remained disease free at the 44-month follow-up. The same group also applied intraoperative, image-guided navigation to resect a recurrent cervical chordoma via an endoscopic, transcervical approach with good results.[58]

Yang et al. subsequently employed a similar technique in their series of 26 patients undergoing computer navigation-aided resection of sacral chordoma. They reported achieving marginal (R1) or negative (R0) margins in 22 cases (85%); the overall recurrence rate was only 8% at a mean of 39 months.[50] Jeys et al. also reported good results in 23 patients treated for primary tumors of the pelvis or sacrum. Ninety-one percent of patients had clean bone and soft tissue margins and local recurrence was seen in only 13% of cases.[59] Perhaps more importantly, the authors found the navigation system to reflect the real-time position of their surgical instruments with respect to the patient's anatomy. The average registration error was less than 1 mm; although no comparisons were made to surgeons navigating by anatomy alone, it is likely that the navigation significantly improved surgeon accuracy. Examinations by the same group have found navigated procedures to be associated with reduced operative time, intraoperative blood loss, and iatrogenic neurological injury, suggesting that the use of navigation may also reduce the morbidity of surgical intervention.[60]

Subsequently, Nasser et al.[61] described their use of O-arm (Medtronic) assisted navigation for the biopsy or resection of 41 spinal column tumors of the mobile spine and sacrum. Seven patients with metastatic lesions and 13 with primary tumors underwent extensive bony resection with the assistance of navigation. Although no non-navigated group was included for comparison, the authors concluded that navigation assistance was highly useful and could improve the precision of resection margins and instrumentation placement.

More recently, Bosma et al. published results suggesting that intraoperative navigation may improve a surgeon's ability to achieve negative margins during the resection of primary tumors of the sacrum and pelvis.[62] Patients who underwent navigation-assisted surgery were four times more likely to have negative margins than were historic controls who underwent resection without navigation assistance. Similar comparisons have not been conducted for lesions of the mobile spine; however, Ando et al.[63] reported their experience of 18 patients with primary spine tumors (two sarcomas) and saw no incidence of recurrence at a median of 24.5 months. Additional experience comprised solely of patients with malignant neoplasms is required though.

SURGICAL TREATMENT FOR SPINAL PATHOLOGY

Owing to the overall rarity of primary vertebral column tumors, the practicing surgeon is more likely to employ navigation-based techniques in a patient with metastatic disease. Nevertheless, we illustrate here the integration of intraoperative navigation into the treatment of a primary lesion.

Clinical Case 1

History/Clinical Presentation

A 65-year-old male was referred to the clinic of the senior author from an outside hospital for the management of biopsy-proven sacral chordoma. The patient had begun to notice right-sided buttock pain roughly 5 months prior to presentation that was progressive and proved refractory to medical management. The patient also endorsed progressive bowel and bladder symptoms characterized by constipation and mild urinary retention. He also endorsed perianal numbness but denied radicular pain or weakness. On examination he was found to be neurologically non-focal with 5/5 strength in all major muscle groups of the bilateral upper and lower extremities; his sensation was intact to light touch and pinprick throughout all extremities and his reflexes were normoactive at the knee and ankle. Romberg and gait testing revealed no abnormalities.

Preoperative Imaging

Imaging conducted at an outside hospital revealed a large sacral mass that was hypointense on T1- and hyperintense on T2-weighted MRI sequences (Fig. 5.2A–F). The lesion had a large 5 × 6 × 7 cm presacral component encasing the bilateral S1–S3 roots. Repeat imaging with contrast-enhanced sequences revealed enhancing lesions of the bilateral posterior superior iliac spine consistent with skip metastases.

Surgical Plan

Consistent with the current literature, it was felt that the patient would benefit from multimodal management combining stereotactic radiation and en bloc surgical resection. The decision was made to employ neoadjuvant radiation, which comprised five fractions of 800 cGy delivered to the sacrum and bilateral medial pelvis.

Planning was then performed for en bloc resection of the lesion. Given the presence of the bilateral foci involving the PSIS = posterior superior iliac spine, the planned margins necessarily included the bilateral medial hemipelvis. The superior osteotomy was planned through the L5/S1 disk space and the lateral osteotomies were planned to include the medial 7 cm of the bilateral hemipelvis. As this would require complete disruption of the pelvic ring, the decision was made to include instrumentation, extending from L3 down to the pelvis. To improve the torsional strength of the planned construct, the decision was made to include a femoral strut allograft compressed between the two hemipelves. Fibular strut allograft was also planned for the construct to help facilitate fusion across the large defect that would result from the en bloc sacrohemipelvectomy.

Intraoperative Imaging

The surgery was performed in two stages, given the extent of the dissection planned. The first stage involved an anterior transperitoneal approach. A midline laparotomy incision was performed and the bowel contents were swept laterally to expose the posterior peritoneum,

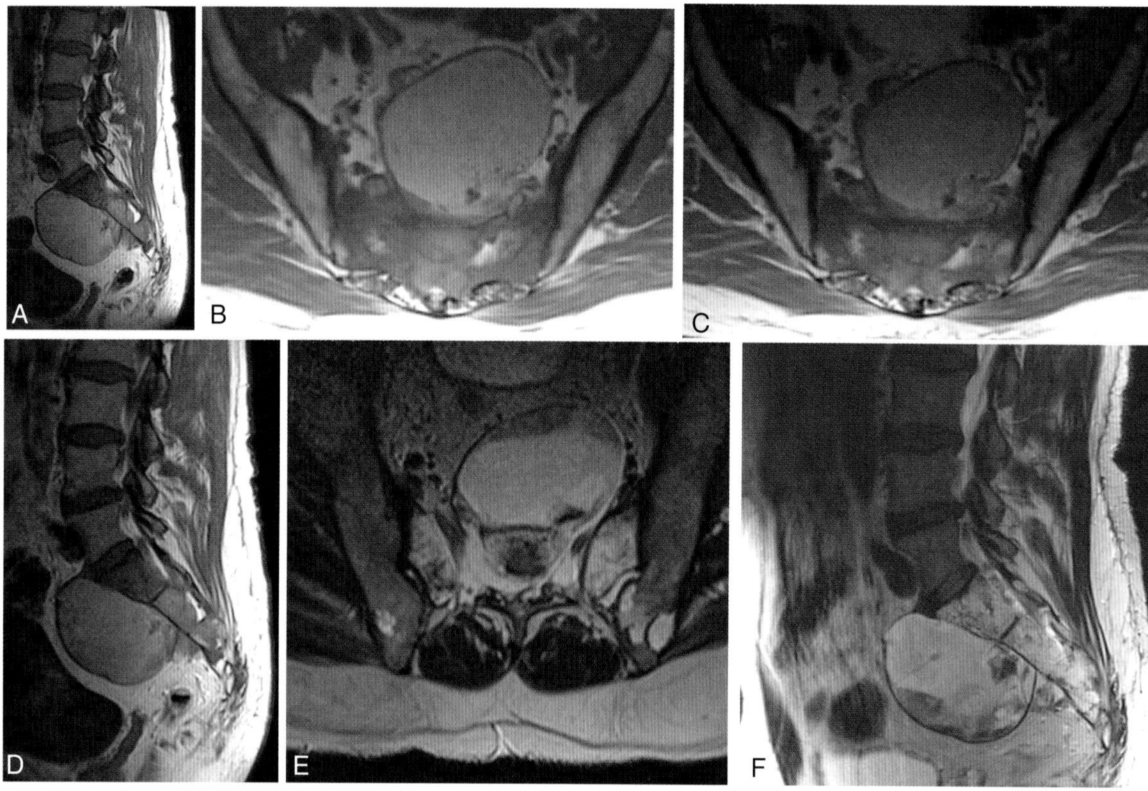

FIG. 5.2 Preoperative imaging demonstrating a large (8.2 × 10.4 × 7 cm) T1-hypointense, T2-hyperintense sacral mass invading the bilateral S1–S4 foramina. A biopsy of the lesion revealed chords of physaliphorous cells with a myxoid matrix, consistent with classical chordoma. The cells stained positively for Brachyury, S100, and pankeratin, and stained negative for TTF-1, Pax8, CK7, and RCC. (A and B) Precontrast T1 imaging shows a hypointense sacral mass with a large presacral component. (C and D) Postcontrast T1-imaging shows minimal enhancement. (E and F) T2-weighted imaging shows a large presacral mass isointense to surrounding adipose tissue and hyperintense to nonaffected bone.

which was divided to expose the presacral component of the lesion. Using a combination of sharp and electrocautery dissection, the iliac vessels were mobilized bilaterally, exposing the L5/S1 disk space. A L5/S1 anterior hemidiskectomy was performed, forming the superior border of the surgical specimen. A rectus flap was formed with the assistance of plastic surgery to assist with closure following the posterior portion. A silastic sheath was then placed (Fig. 5.3A) and the incision closed; the patient was neurologically intact upon awakening.

The second stage of the operation employed a posterior midline approach from L2 to the tip of the coccyx, with dissection extending over the bilateral hemipelvis to expose the PSIS and medial iliac crest. After the spinous processes were exposed, a reference frame was affixed to the L2 spinous process by way of a spinous process clamp. Registration of the patient anatomy to a preoperatively acquired CT image was then performed using the StealthStation (Medtronic) system. The acquired sequences in the preoperative CT included 0.75-mm and 3-mm slices; the 0.75-mm sequences with bone-windowing was employed for intraoperative navigation due to the higher special resolution. The L4 spinous process

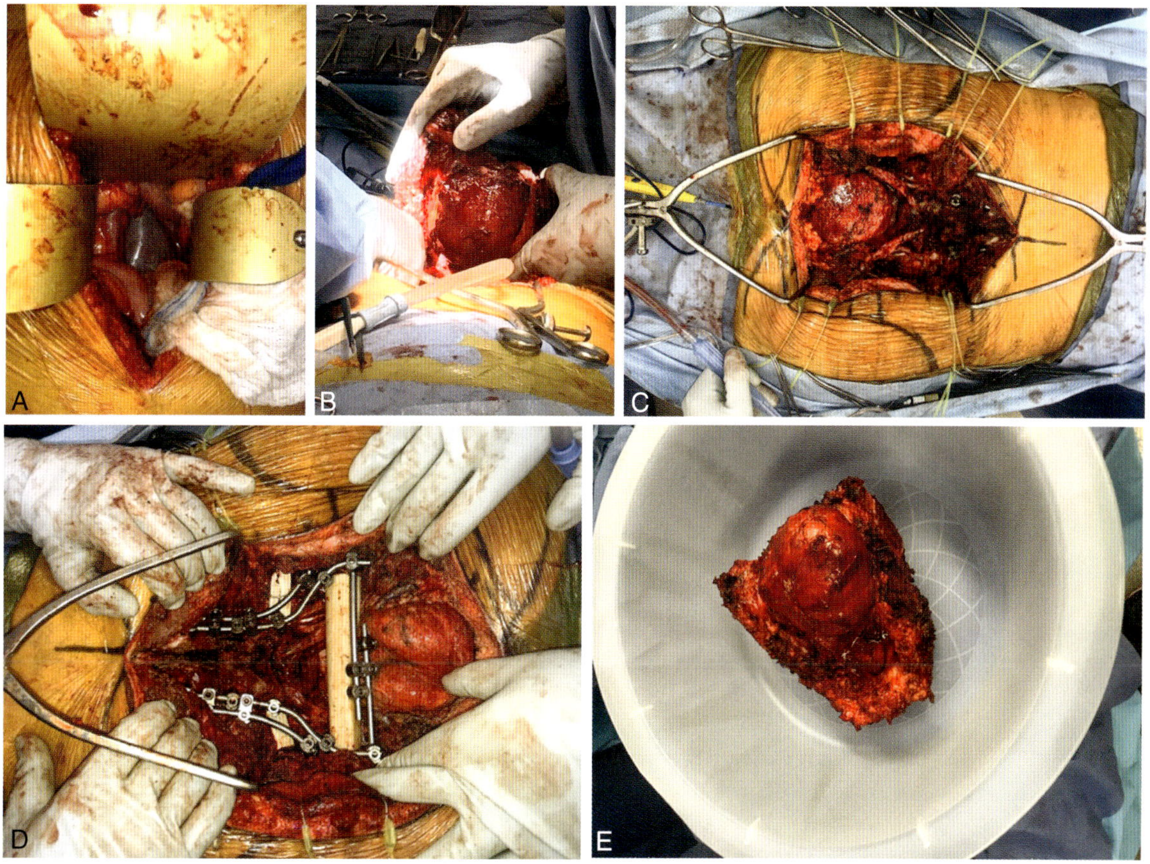

FIG. 5.3 Intraoperative imaging showing (A) the anterior approach following placement of the silastic sheath. (B) Delivery of the tumor specimen left (C) a large sacral defect. (D) Due to the post-resection instability, a quadruple rod construct with fibular and femoral strut allograft was employed. (E) Examination of the resected specimen shows the clean edges facilitated by intraoperative navigation.

and bilateral L4/5 facet joints were used as image registration points. After registering the reference frame to the preoperative image, registration accuracy was confirmed by touching the L5 spinous process and the S1 bilateral laminae and superior articulating processes.

Fenestrated screws were then placed bilaterally in the L3–L5 pedicles, the positions of which were confirmed using an intraoperative CT system (O-Arm, Medtronic, Minneapolis, MN). The gluteal muscles were detached from the medial iliac crest bilaterally, preserving a cuff of healthy muscle over the PSIS to allow for negative margins. With the sacrum and hemipelves exposed, an L5 laminectomy was then performed using an ultrasonic cutting device affixed with a clamp registered to the StealthStation system. After removing the laminae, the L5 roots and thecal sac were identified and the thecal sac was doubly ligated just below the level of the L5 roots. The decision was then made to perform a three-column osteotomy through the posterior half of the L5 vertebral body to avoid compromise of the S1 tumor capsule. The osteotomy was made using the same registered ultrasonic cutting device and was connected to the L5/S1 anterior hemidiskectomy from the first stage, completing the dissociation of the sacrum from the mobile spine. The ultrasonic cutting device was again employed to form osteotomies bilaterally through the medial hemipelves, extending from the iliac crest to the sciatic notch, roughly 7 cm lateral to the sacroiliac joints. When executing the osteotomies, care was taken to start at least 5 mm outside of the proposed tumor margin, so as to avoid an intracapsular dissection. In our experience, this is essential for chordoma, which has been demonstrated to have micro-skip metastases at a mean distance of 3 mm from the tumor in up to 43% of patients.[64] The L4 and L5 roots, and the rectum were then meticulously dissected off of the anterior face of the specimen. The specimen was delivered (see Fig. 5.3B), leaving a large defect for reconstruction (see Fig. 5.3C).

Given the potential shift in the locoregional anatomy, the image registration was confirmed using the bilateral iliac crests. After ensuring accurate registration, pelvic screws were placed with the assistance of the intraoperative navigation system. Vertebroplasty was performed through the L3–L5 screws bilaterally to reinforce them, and rods were contoured to the placed screws. To reinforce the sacral defect, a 20-cm femoral strut graft was placed and attached to the quadruple rod construct via crosslink; the hemipelves were collapsed onto the femoral strut graft to maximize the torsional strength of the patient's pelvic ring. A fibular strut allograft was placed to define the final construct (see Fig. 5.3D) and the rectus flap formed during stage 1 was completed to help eliminate dead space in the sacrectomy defect. Examination of the delivered specimen showed well-defined osteotomies (see Fig. 5.3E), which were confirmed on postoperative histology to have produced negative margins.

Postoperative Imaging

Postoperative imaging at the 6-month visit demonstrated a residual seroma from the surgical procedure. However, no evidence of tumor recurrence was noted on MRI (Fig. 5.4A–D), nor were signs of instrumentation failure noted on the postoperative CT image.

Postoperative Recovery and Follow-Up

The patient tolerated the initial procedure well with only mild neurological deficit, as was expected based upon the decision to sacrifice the sacral roots. His main deficits were 0/5 strength in dorsiflexion and plantarflexion with accompanying sensory loss in the S1–C0 dermatomes. He also required periodic self-catheterization for a neurogenic bladder secondary to sacrifice of the sacral roots.

Unfortunately, the patient did experience a postoperative ileus as well as a deep wound infection with mixed anaerobes and gram-negative species requiring washouts and surgical revision. Despite this, the patient continues to make a good recovery and shows no evidence of recurrence as of his 24-month follow-up.

Clinical Case 2

History/Clinical Presentation

A 64-year-old male with a known history of widely disseminated renal cell carcinoma presented to the clinic of the senior author for the evaluation of severe mechanical back pain and progressive deficits of the bilateral lower extremity. The patient had previously undergone conventional external beam radiation of his spine lesions and had been evaluated for percutaneous cementoplasty. Given his past history of unsuccessful vertebroplasty and his progressive neurological decline secondary to epidural disease, it was felt that he might benefit from surgical evaluation.

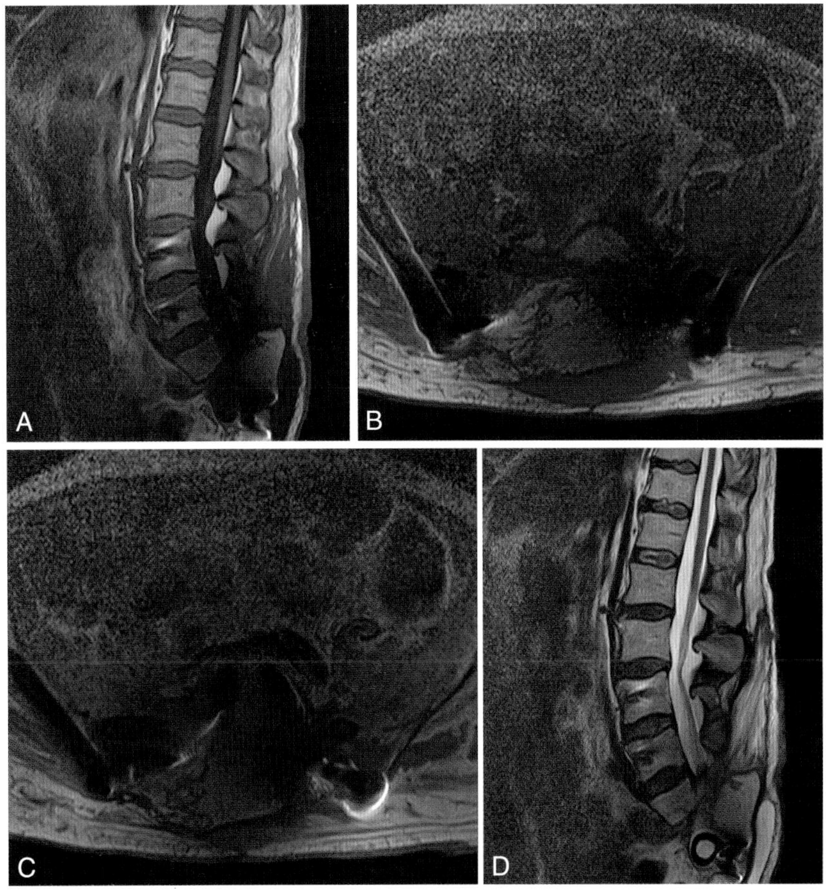

FIG. 5.4 Postoperative imaging demonstrating no evidence of recurrence. (A) Sagittal and (B) axial precontrast T1 images and (C) noncontrast T2-weighted images show no evidence of lesion recurrence. (D) Postcontrast T1-weighted imaging shows no evidence of an enhancing lesion. Significant metal artifact is noted.

On examination, the patient was grossly 4+/5 in his bilateral lower extremities, but endorsed subjective weakness throughout. He similarly endorsed paresthesias throughout his bilateral lower extremity, although no focal sensory deficits were noted in the light touch or pinprick modalities. His gait was mildly myelopathic, although he was able to tandem walk with assistance. He endorsed mild pain with palpation of the lumbar spine and moderate to severe pain with axial loading.

Preoperative Imaging

CT imaging demonstrated a previously cemented T12 lytic lesion with anterior column height loss and de novo deformity at the thoracolumbar junction (Fig. 5.5A and B). Multifocal thoracolumbar disease was noted, recommending against aggressive surgical realignment. MRI demonstrated a T1-hypointense, mildly T2-hypointense mass of the T12 (Fig. 5.5C and D) with mild abutment of the left-sided anterolateral cord.

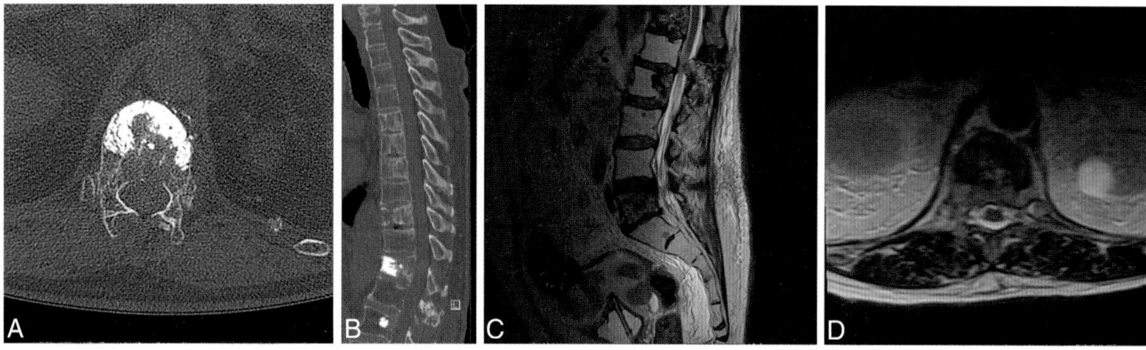

FIG. 5.5 Preoperative CT imaging of the patient in case 2 demonstrated a previously cemented lytic T12 mass with significant anterior column height loss and **de novo** deformity (A and B). T2-weighted MR imaging (C and D) of the mass demonstrated a small amount of epidural disease without obvious cord compression.

Surgical Plan

In light of the patient's widespread disease, it was felt that his prognosis was too poor for conventional open surgery. Additionally, as it was felt that his epidural disease would be amenable to stereotactic radiosurgery, the decision was made to offer a minimally invasive procedure involving percutaneous instrumentation and a mini-open approach for focal decompression of the L1 and L2 segments. The goal was to alleviate the patient's mechanical pain by stabilizing the L1 and L2 segments and to provide a margin between the tumor and spinal cord for the delivery of stereotactic radiation.

Procedure

The patient was placed prone and, after scrubbing and draping, a registration array was percutaneously affixed to the patient's posterior superior iliac spine. As described by others,[65] we target a penetration depth of approximately 2.5 cm to ensure that the reference marker is firmly seated in the iliac bone. Poor seating of the reference frame will lead to intraoperative reference frame drift and accordant inaccuracy of the navigation system. A navigated probe was then used to register the reference frame to the preoperative CT in the StealthStation system; as with the previous case, we employed the volume with bone-windowing and 0.75 mm slice thickness. A preliminary registration confirmation was then performed by palpating the spinous processes and contralateral PSIS to confirm system accuracy.

The surgical tools were then registered by affixing them with clamps registered to the StealthStation system. These included a tap, standard drill, and screwdriver. Under navigation, stab incisions were planned and formed over the bilateral pedicles at the T10–L3 levels. The incisions were planned using the tip of the navigated probe, which was extended on the stealth system by approximately 4 cm to reflect the definitive pedicle screw. While plotting incision points, the probe was angled to reflect the trajectory of the planned screw. This resulted in stab incisions being formed 3 to 4 cm lateral to the midline. When forming the incisions, we attempted to make them colinear to help facilitate rod passing at the end of the procedure.

Starting at the T10 level, a Jamshidi needle was then inserted through the paraspinal muscles and docked on the interarticular process of the target vertebrae. A mallet was then used to advance the Jamshidi needle through the pedicle into the posterior vertebral body (roughly 2–3 cm). The advancement of the needle can be monitored under fluoroscopic visualization, although we elected not to do so in this case. The inner stylet of the Jamshidi was then removed and Kirschner wires (K-wires) were placed and advanced through the Jamshidi trochar until they contacted the anterior cortex. The Jamshidi trochar was then exchanged for a series of dilators, which retracted the paraspinal musculature. An undersized pedicle tap was then passed over the K-wire and used to cannulate the pedicle. For each screw, the tap was slightly undersized relative to the planned screw to optimize screw-bone interface in the final construct. After cannulating the pedicle, the awl was removed and the fenestrated pedicle screw passed over the K-wire and inserted into the pedicle.

After instrumenting all the pedicles, an intraoperative CT using the second-generation O-arm (Medtronic) was performed to confirm the screw positioning. For intraoperative O-arm capture, we employ a standard dosing protocol (120 kVp, 80 mA, 391 projections, 0.415-mm pixel size, 0.83-mm slice thickness).[66] Once the screw positions were confirmed, vertebroplasty was performed through the fenestrated screw. A small 3- to 4-cm incision was then formed over the L1–L2 lamina and a subperiosteal dissection was performed, extending laterally out to the medial facets. Laminectomy was performed at L1 and L2 and the epidural tumor was removed with a combination of pituitary rongeur, suction, and curettes. A probe registered to the navigation system was used to help confirm adequate decompression, after which the midline incision was closed in the typical fashion. The rods were then passed subfascially through the distal stab incision bilaterally and set screws were placed to secure the rod. After confirming the position on a cross-table radiograph, the stab incisions were closed with figure-of-eight sutures.

Postoperative Imaging

The postoperative standing films demonstrated good positioning of all screws, which was confirmed on CT. The repeat CT at 3 months showed no evidence of hardware loosening (Fig. 5.6A and B).

Postoperative Recovery and Follow-Up

The patient experienced good recovery following the surgery. He had near-immediate improvement in his mechanical back pain and remained neurologically intact relative to his preoperative condition. The patient unfortunately experienced progressive decline over the subsequent six months, resulting in death from his systemic disease burden.

Procedural Concerns

As with all new technologies, one of the major concerns with navigated tumor surgery is learning to integrate the technology into one's workflow. Prior studies have suggested that for experienced bone oncology surgeons with minimal experience with navigation-assisted surgery, at least 20 cases are required before navigation can be integrated into the workflow smoothly.[52] Similar investigations examining the learning curve for navigation-assisted surgery in the degenerative population have estimated it to be between 6 months[67] and 40 cases.[68] Notably, these investigations were for pedicle screw placement and did not involve extensive bone work, which may add to the learning curve.

Ensuring accurate system registration is also key to a successful surgery, especially for primary tumors undergoing en bloc resection, where small discrepancies in registration may mean the difference between negative and positive margins. The factors to consider during registration are the strategy of registration employed and movement between the patient and table that may occur during registration. Of the two main registration

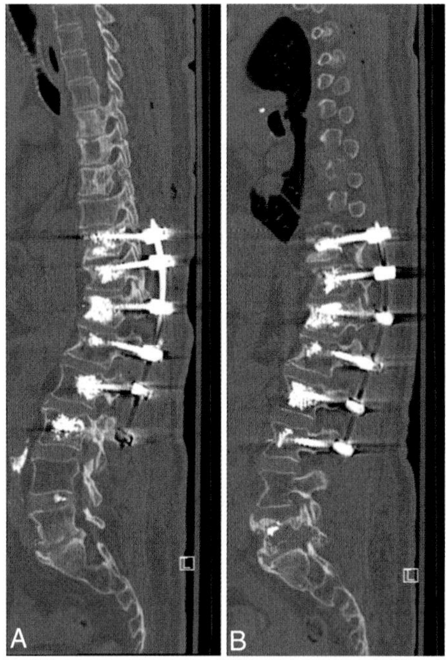

FIG. 5.6 Postoperative CT imaging (A and B) demonstrating the percutaneously placed T10–L3 construct.

techniques—paired-point registration and surface mapping[69]—we prefer paired-point mapping. Use of this technique allows for faster registration[70] and data from the skull base literature suggests there to be no statistically or clinically significant difference in the mean registration error.[71] By comparison, a study by Holly et al. suggested that the addition of surface mapping to paired-point matching significantly increases registration accuracy.[72] However, the actual navigation accuracy was not statistically or clinically different between the two techniques. Accordingly, for both technologies it is recommended that the treating surgeon confirm mapping accuracy following registration by comparing the navigation system images to the known patient anatomy at several identifiable landmarks.

Regarding table-patient movement during registration, there are three main concerns: (1) surgical staff leaning on the table, (2) table position change during registration, and (3) patient respiration, which necessarily shifts all patient-fixed fiducials. The former two errors are easily addressed by fixing the operating table throughout the procedure and ensuring that no surgical team members are contacting the table during the registration process. The third source of error—patient respiration-induced movement—ultimately produces roughly 2 mm of error in navigation registration, with the error increasing with increasing distance from the fiducial.[73] This error is positively correlated with the tidal volume, positive end expiratory pressure, and mean arterial pressure. Consequently, working with anesthesia during navigation to optimize these parameters may help to produce more accurate patient-image mapping.

Surgical manipulation additionally imparts error to the image-patient mapping, albeit to a lesser extent.[74] If extensive bony work or manipulation is done, however, the acquisition of an intraoperative CT volume of the working area and re-registration may improve overall navigation accuracy. It also allows for the incorporation of placed hardware into the navigation system. Re-registration may also compensate for movement in the fiducial marker, which can occur due to slippage of the spinous process clamp or accidental contact by a member of the surgical team.

Another key consideration when using navigation is the operating room setup. This includes both equipment selection and position. Of chief concern in equipment selection is the use of a radiolucent frame, such as the Jackson or Wilson frame. We regularly employ the Jackson frame due to institutional availability, although, to our knowledge, there is no strong evidence supporting the use of one over the other. Second, the placement of the guidance system is crucial to its ability to function throughout the case; namely, the system's infrared sensor must be able to visualize the patient-fixed reference frame and registered instruments throughout the case. We generally prefer placement of the sensor at the head of the bed. Along these same lines, when using tracked instruments, surgeons must take care to ensure that the instrument-mounted reflectors are in view of the infrared sensor. Loss of the line of sight between the sensor and instrument means that the position of the instrument is no longer being tracked and can lead to erroneous manipulations.

Treatment Side Effects

One of the most widely discussed side effects of navigated surgery is radiation exposure. Without question, the addition of intraoperative image acquisition to preoperative image acquisition increases patient radiation exposure. However, intraoperative navigation based upon preoperative acquired images likely decreases the radiation exposure relative to conventional fluoroscopy-guided procedures. This is supported by the findings of a recent systematic review that observed radiation exposure to the surgeon and surgical staff to be reduced in cases using intraoperative navigation based upon preoperatively acquired images.[21] However, depending upon how the imaging for intraoperative navigation is acquired, the overall radiation exposure to the patient may be increased, as the addition of an intraoperative CT volume (O-arm, Medtronic, Minneapolis, MN) increases radiation exposure relative to fluoroscopy alone. If these images are used in place of preoperatively acquired CT, radiation exposure across the treatment course may actually be decreased, even relative to free-hand surgery. Of note, although the included studies from the review all focused on thoracolumbar instrumentation for degenerative procedures, the results are likely directly translatable.[21] The techniques employed for pedicle screw placement are highly similar in tumor and non-tumor cases, so we believe that these results can be generalized to the tumor population, at least for instrumentation in en bloc procedures and for the percutaneous instrumentation of patients with symptomatic metastases.

Another side effect of navigation is that it can add time to the surgical case. This is most notable for surgeons inexperienced with intraoperative navigation. Evidence suggests that for surgeons who are experienced with intraoperative navigation, the surgical times may actually be shorter.[67,74] To this end, the use of navigation may also help to reduce the total care costs, as operating room time and facility costs comprise more than one-third of the total costs in spine surgery admissions.[75]

Potential Pitfalls

The pitfalls of a navigated spine tumor case include both the errors innate to the use of the imaging system and those errors associated with operating on a patient with cancer. As discussed above, the successful use of navigation begins by ensuring accurate registration.

Errors in navigation system registration at the start of the case will be carried throughout the procedure and inevitably lead to poorer outcomes. Even if registration is meticulously performed, there is inevitable error in anatomy-image mapping, which only increases with surgical manipulation.[73] Consequently, it is incumbent upon the surgeon to remain cognizant of the local anatomy and to be willing to re-register the system or revert to free-hand, anatomically-guided surgery when the navigation system mapping becomes inaccurate. For this reason, intraoperative navigation should be thought of more as a strategy for confirming the patient's appreciation of the local anatomy. Additionally, by using navigation in this role, never events for example, wrong-level surgery, can be avoided.

The second group of complications comprise those associated with the patient's disease and prior therapeutic regimen, which occur at a rate of 19% to 28%.[76] The intraoperative complications include hemorrhage secondary to neoplasm-induced coagulopathies, cerebral spinal fluid leak, neurological injury, injury to the adjacent viscera, myocardial infarction, venous thromboembolic events, and death. Excessive bleeding is especially common among those with liver primary lesions or metastatic disease involving the long bones.[77] The postoperative complications include wound infection, hardware failure, and, in the case of operations seeking oncologic cure, local recurrence. Of these, wound infection is the most common, occurring in up to one in every five patients operated for metastatic disease.[76] It is especially common among those undergoing revision operations, those who have been previously irradiated at the surgery site, those who are obese, and those with diabetes mellitus.[76]

Complication Management

While the preventative strategies are numerous, none can ensure complication avoidance. With regard to the image navigation, the primary strategies are (1) to be meticulous during system registration, (2) to avoid contact with the reference frame intraoperatively, and (3) to appraise the mapping suggested by the system regularly to ensure it agrees with the surgeon's impression of their current location. As registration imparts the majority of uncorrectable errors, meticulous registration minimizes inaccuracies occurring secondary to mapping issues. Where the reference frame is contacted intraoperatively, or where the registration is felt to have lost accuracy, registration should be repeated before continuing under image guidance.

The strategies for the avoidance of cancer-related complications are outlined in Table 5.3. In short, complications can be minimized by employing a multidisciplinary approach that focuses on controlling medical comorbidities and tailors the surgical strategy to both the patient's robustness and the oncologic surgical goals.

Future Advancements

Although the application of navigation to spinal oncology is still relatively new, further advancements are already on the horizon in the form of spine robots and augmented reality. Spine robots, of which there are currently three systems on the market—Mazor Stealth X (Medtronic), ExcelsiusGPS (Globus), and ROSA ONE Spine (Zimmer Biomet)—are similar to conventional navigation in that they use reference frames to correlate the intraoperative anatomy with either preoperative or intraoperative CT volumes. Additionally, they help to potentially improve accuracy by stabilizing the proposed screw trajectory and eliminating surgeon tremor. A meta-analysis by Zhou et al.,[78] comparing patients instrumented using either computer assisted navigation or robotic guidance with the Mazor system,

TABLE 5.3 Complications associated with spine tumor surgery and strategies for avoidance.

Complication Class and Types		Avoidance
Preoperative	Neurological • Spinal cord or nerve root compression	• Avoid nerve root and cord compression during positioning • Consider preoperative steroid administration
Intraoperative	Neurological • Nerve root or cord injury	• Careful manipulation of cord, roots, and adjoining tissues • Ensure sufficient surgical window • Intraoperative monitoring • Maintain mean arterial pressure ≥ 85 mm Hg
	Hemorrhage • Excessive intraoperative bleeding	• Obtain preoperative coagulation studies (PT, INR, fibrinogen), CBC (esp., platelet count) • Cross and type preoperatively; have blood products available • Preoperative embolization of tumor • Employ vascular surgeon/access surgeon for anterior approaches
	CSF Leak • Incidental dural rent	• Avoid preoperative radiation • Careful manipulation of cord and roots • Primary repair of detected rent
	Visceral Organ Injury	• Protect organs during dissection • Include general surgery for repair of injury
Postoperative	Neurological • New onset postoperative neurological deficit	• Consider postoperative steroids • Maintain mean arterial pressure ≥ 85 mm Hg
	Thromboembolic • New deep venous thrombosis or pulmonary embolism	• Postoperative VTE prophylaxis (e.g., LMWH, DOAC)
	Hemorrhage • Continued postoperative hemorrhage	• Image patients with continued postoperative Hgb drop
	Wound • Infection • Dehiscence	• Postoperative blood sugar control • Avoid operation in irradiated tissue • Consider plastic surgery closure • Encourage smoking cessation • Use of minimally invasive approach
	Hardware Failure • Rod fracture • Screw pullout	• Carefully consider need for wound site irradiation • PMMA screw augmentation intraoperatively • Consider addition of outrigger rods/second rod sets • Consider structural allograft (e.g., fibular, femur) • Regular radiographic follow-up • Use of large endplate cage to ensure adequate load sharing • Encourage smoking cessation

CBC, Complete blood count; *CSF*, cerebrospinal fluid; *DOAC*, direct oral anticoagulant (e.g., apixaban, rivaroxaban); *Hgb*, hemoglobin; *INR*, international normalized ratio; *LMWH*, low molecular weight heparin (e.g., enoxaparin, dalteparin); *PMMA*, poly(methyl methacrylate); *PT*, prothrombin time; *VTE*, venous thromboembolism.

found that robotic-guided screws had great odds of achieving optimal or clinically acceptable placement. The screws placed with robotic assistance were also associated with lower intraoperative blood loss without any appreciable differences in complications, intraoperative placement time, or rates of surgical revision. Similar comparisons specific to the spine oncology population are pending.

Augmented reality is considered by some to represent the pinnacle of computer assisted navigation.[79] Although only one system—the Augmedics xvision (Augmedics)[80–83]—has currently attained FDA approval, several systems have been described over the past half-decade.[80–86] These augmented reality devices work by projecting preoperatively acquired images onto partially reflective lenses worn by the surgeon. As with conventional navigation, the image is registered to a reference frame affixed to the spinous process of a vertebra adjacent to the working field. The surgeon can then simultaneously view the patient imaging and surgical anatomy, avoiding the disruptions caused by having to look up to verify positioning on the navigation screen. While the augmented reality systems lack the ability to stabilize surgeon tremor that is possessed by the robotic systems, they are far cheaper and require minimal modifications to the pre-existing workflows used for computer assisted navigation. They are also compatible with all available instrumentation sets,[84] whereas many robotic systems require that the disposables be purchased from the same manufacturer.

SUMMARY

Image guidance represents an exciting development in the field of spine tumor surgery. Such systems carry with them the potential to increase instrumentation accuracy and dissection accuracy, which for primary tumors may mean higher odds of oncologic resection. Additionally, by allowing for more efficient dissections, they can be used to facilitate minimally invasive approaches for spine tumor resection, which have been associated with shorter hospitalizations, lower blood loss, and fewer complications. The description of these techniques is still relatively sparse in the spine tumor literature, but will doubtless increase in the next decade as the field moves more toward minimally invasive separation surgery for spinal metastases.

REFERENCES

1. Sohn S, Kim J, Chung CK, et al. A nationwide epidemiological study of newly diagnosed spine metastasis in the adult Korean population. *Spine J.* 2016;16(8):937–945. https://doi.org/10.1016/j.spinee.2016.03.006.
2. Sohn S, Kim J, Chung CK, Lee NR, Sohn MJ, Kim SH. A nation-wide epidemiological study of newly diagnosed primary spine tumor in the adult Korean population, 2009-2011. *J Korean Neurosurg Soc.* 2017;60(2):195–204. https://doi.org/10.3340/jkns.2016.0505.011.
3. Sohn S, Kim J, Chung CK, et al. Nationwide epidemiology and healthcare utilization of spine tumor patients in the adult Korean population, 2009-2012. *Neurooncol Pract.* 2015;2(2):93–100. https://doi.org/10.1093/nop/npv006.
4. Klimo P, Schmidt MH. Surgical management of spinal metastases. *Oncologist.* 2004;9(2):188–196. https://doi.org/10.1634/theoncologist.9-2-188.
5. Wright E, Ricciardi F, Arts M, et al. Metastatic spine tumor epidemiology: comparison of trends in surgery across two decades and three continents. *World Neurosurg.* 2018;114:e809–e817. https://doi.org/10.1016/j.wneu.2018.03.091.
6. Ehresman J, Pennington Z, Feghali J, et al. Predicting nonroutine discharge in patients undergoing surgery for vertebral column tumors. *J Neurosurg Spine.* 2020;1–10. https://doi.org/10.3171/2020.6.SPINE201024.
7. Pennington Z, Ahmed AK, Molina CA, Ehresman J, Laufer I, Sciubba DM. Minimally invasive versus conventional spine surgery for vertebral metastases: a systematic review of the evidence. *Ann Transl Med.* 2018;6(6):103. https://doi.org/10.21037/atm.2018.01.28.
8. Gokaslan ZL, Zadnik PL, Sciubba DM, et al. Mobile spine chordoma: results of 166 patients from the AOSpine Knowledge Forum Tumor database. *J Neurosurg Spine.* 2016;24(4):644–651. https://doi.org/10.3171/2015.7.SPINE15201.
9. Charest-Morin R, Dirks MS, Patel S, et al. Ewing sarcoma of the spine: prognostic variables for survival and local control in surgically treated patients. *Spine (Phila Pa 1976).* 2018;43(9):622–629. https://doi.org/10.1097/BRS.0000000000002386.
10. Dekutoski MB, Clarke MJ, Rose P, et al. Osteosarcoma of the spine: prognostic variables for local recurrence and overall survival, a multicenter ambispective study. *J Neurosurg*

Spine. 2016;25(1):59–68. https://doi.org/10.3171/2015.11.SPINE15870.

11. Fisher CG, Versteeg AL, Dea N, et al. Surgical management of spinal chondrosarcomas. *Spine (Phila Pa 1976)*. 2016;41(8):678–685. https://doi.org/10.1097/BRS.0000000000001485.
12. Patchell RA, Tibbs PA, Regine WF, et al. Direct decompressive surgical resection in the treatment of spinal cord compression caused by metastatic cancer: a randomised trial. *Lancet*. 2005;366(9486):643–648. https://doi.org/10.1016/S0140-6736(05)66954-1.
13. Laufer I, Rubin DG, Lis E, et al. The NOMS framework: approach to the treatment of spinal metastatic tumors. *Oncologist*. 2013;18(6):744–751. https://doi.org/10.1634/theoncologist.2012-0293.
14. Paton GR, Frangou E, Fourney DR. Contemporary treatment strategy for spinal metastasis: the "LMNOP" system. *Can J Neurol Sci*. 2011;38(3):396–403. https://doi.org/10.1017/S031716710001177X.
15. Bilsky MH, Laufer I, Fourney DR, et al. Reliability analysis of the epidural spinal cord compression scale. *J Neurosurg Spine*. 2010;13(3):324–328. https://doi.org/10.3171/2010.3.SPINE09459.
16. Fisher CG, DiPaola CP, Ryken TC, et al. A novel classification system for spinal instability in neoplastic disease: an evidence-based approach and expert consensus from the Spine Oncology Study Group. *Spine (Phila Pa 1976)*. 2010;35(22):E1221–E1229. https://doi.org/10.1097/BRS.0b013e3181e16ae2.
17. Laufer I, Bilsky MH. Advances in the treatment of metastatic spine tumors: the future is not what it used to be. *J Neurosurg Spine*. 2019;30(3):299–307. https://doi.org/10.3171/2018.11.SPINE18709.
18. Pennington Z, Sciubba DM. Commentary: minimally invasive tubular separation surgery for metastatic spinal cord compression. *Oper Neurosurg (Hagerstown)*. 2021;20(5):E357–E358. https://doi.org/10.1093/ons/opaa438.
19. Barzilai O, Laufer I, Robin A, Xu R, Yamada Y, Bilsky MH. Hybrid therapy for metastatic epidural spinal cord compression: technique for separation surgery and spine radiosurgery. *Oper Neurosurg (Hagerstown)*. 2019;16(3):310–318. https://doi.org/10.1093/ons/opy137.
20. Lau D, Chou D. Posterior thoracic corpectomy with cage reconstruction for metastatic spinal tumors: comparing the mini-open approach to the open approach. *J Neurosurg Spine*. 2015;23(2):217–227. https://doi.org/10.3171/2014.12.SPINE14543.
21. Pennington Z, Cottrill E, Westbroek EM, et al. Evaluation of surgeon and patient radiation exposure by imaging technology in patients undergoing thoracolumbar fusion: systematic review of the literature. *Spine J*. 2019;19(8):1397–1411. https://doi.org/10.1016/j.spinee.2019.04.003.
22. Lu DC, Chou D, Mummaneni PV. A comparison of mini-open and open approaches for resection of thoracolumbar intradural spinal tumors. *J Neurosurg Spine*. 2011;14(6):758–764. https://doi.org/10.3171/2011.1.SPINE09860.
23. Jung JM, Chung CK, Kim CH, Yang SH. Minimally invasive surgery without decompression for hepatocellular carcinoma spinal metastasis with epidural spinal cord compression Grade 2. *J Korean Neurosurg Soc*. 2019;62(4):467–475. https://doi.org/10.3340/jkns.2018.0199.
24. Chou D, Lu DC. Mini-open transpedicular corpectomies with expandable cage reconstruction. Technical note. *J Neurosurg Spine*. 2011;14(1):71–77. https://doi.org/10.3171/2010.10.SPINE091009.
25. Fang T, Dong J, Zhou X, McGuire Jr RA, Li X. Comparison of mini-open anterior corpectomy and posterior total en bloc spondylectomy for solitary metastases of the thoracolumbar spine. *J Neurosurg Spine*. 2012;17(4):271–279. https://doi.org/10.3171/2012.7.SPINE111086. http://thejns.org/doi/abs/10.3171/2012.7.SPINE111086?url_ver=Z39.88-2003&rfr_id=ori:rid:crossref.org&rfr_dat=cr_pub%3Dpubmed.
26. Hansen-Algenstaedt N, Kwan MK, Algenstaedt P, et al. Comparison between minimally invasive surgery and conventional open surgery for patients with spinal metastasis: a prospective propensity score-matched study. *Spine (Phila Pa 1976)*. 2017;42(10):789–797. https://doi.org/10.1097/BRS.0000000000001893.
27. Hikata T, Isogai N, Shiono Y, et al. A retrospective cohort study comparing the safety and efficacy of minimally invasive versus open surgical techniques in the treatment of spinal metastases. *Clin Spine Surg*. 2017;30(8):E1082–E1087. https://doi.org/10.1097/BSD.0000000000000460.
28. Huang TJ, Hsu RW-W, Li YY, Cheng CC. Minimal access spinal surgery (MASS) in treating thoracic spine metastasis. *Spine (Phila Pa 1976)*. 2006;31(16):1860–1863. https://doi.org/10.1097/01.brs.0000225995.56028.46.
29. Kumar N, Malhotra R, Maharajan K, et al. Metastatic spine tumor surgery: a comparative study of minimally invasive approach using percutaneous pedicle screws fixation versus open approach. *Clin Spine Surg*. 2017;30(8):E1015–E1021. https://doi.org/10.1097/BSD.0000000000000400.
30. Miscusi M, Polli FM, Forcato S, et al. Comparison of minimally invasive surgery with standard open surgery for vertebral thoracic metastases causing acute myelopathy in patients with short- or mid-term life expectancy: surgical technique and early clinical results. *J Neurosurg Spine*. 2015;22(5):518–525. https://doi.org/10.3171/2014.10.SPINE131201. http://thejns.org/doi/full/10.3171/2014.10.SPINE131201.
31. Saadeh YS, Elswick CM, Fateh JA, et al. Analysis of outcomes between traditional *open versus mini-open* approach in surgical treatment of spinal metastasis. *World Neurosurg*. 2019;130:e467–e474. https://doi.org/10.1016/j.wneu.2019.06.121.
32. Lu VM, Alvi MA, Goyal A, Kerezoudis P, Bydon M. The potential of minimally invasive surgery to treat metastatic spinal disease versus open surgery: a systematic review and meta-analysis. *World Neurosurg*. 2018;112:e859–e868. https://doi.org/10.1016/j.wneu.2018.01.176.
33. Tatsui CE, Stafford RJ, Li J, et al. Utilization of laser interstitial thermotherapy guided by real-time thermal MRI as

an alternative to separation surgery in the management of spinal metastasis. *J Neurosurg Spine*. 2015;23(4):400–411. https://doi.org/10.3171/2015.2.SPINE141185.

34. Tatsui CE, Lee SH, Amini B, et al. Spinal laser interstitial thermal therapy: a novel alternative to surgery for metastatic epidural spinal cord compression. *Neurosurgery*. 2016;79(suppl 1):S73–S82. https://doi.org/10.1227/NEU.0000000000001444.
35. Pennington Z, Ahmed AK, Cottrill E, Westbroek EM, Goodwin ML, Sciubba DM. Systematic review on the utility of magnetic resonance imaging for operative management and follow-up for primary sarcoma—Lessons from extremity sarcomas. *Ann Transl Med*. 2019;7(10). https://doi.org/10.21037/atm.2019.01.59. 225-225.
36. Dasenbrock HH, Clarke MJ, Bydon A, et al. En bloc resection of sacral chordomas aided by frameless stereotactic image guidance: a technical note. *Neurosurgery*. 2012;70(1). (suppl Operative):82–87; discussion 87–88. https://doi.org/10.1227/NEU.0b013e31822dd958.
37. Kelly PD, Zuckerman SL, Yamada Y, et al. Image guidance in spine tumor surgery. *Neurosurg Rev*. 2020;43(3):1007–1017. https://doi.org/10.1007/s10143-019-01123-2.
38. Pennington Z, Westbroek EM, Ahmed AK, et al. Surgical management of giant presacral schwannoma: systematic review of published cases and meta-analysis. *J Neurosurg Spine*. 2019;31(5):1–12. https://doi.org/10.3171/2019.4.SPINE19240.
39. Tian W, Liu B, He D, et al. Guidelines for navigation-assisted spine surgery. *Front Med*. 2020;14(4):518–527. https://doi.org/10.1007/s11684-020-0775-8.
40. Venier A, Croci D, Robert T, Distefano D, Presilla S, Scarone P. Use of intraoperative computed tomography improves outcome of minimally invasive transforaminal lumbar interbody fusion: a single-center retrospective cohort study. *World Neurosurg*. 2021;148:e572–e580. https://doi.org/10.1016/j.wneu.2021.01.041.
41. Arand M, Hartwig E, Kinzl L, Gebhard F. Spinal navigation in tumor surgery of the thoracic spine: first clinical results. *Clin Orthop Relat Res*. 2002;399(399):211–218. https://doi.org/10.1097/00003086-200206000-00026.
42. De la Garza Ramos RDLG, Echt M, Benton JA, et al. Accuracy of freehand versus navigated thoracolumbar pedicle screw placement in patients with metastatic tumors of the spine. *J Korean Neurosurg Soc*. 2020;63(6):777–783. https://doi.org/10.3340/jkns.2020.0001.
43. Jing L, Wang Z, Sun Z, Zhang H, Wang J, Wang G. Accuracy of pedicle screw placement in the thoracic and lumbosacral spines using O-arm-based navigation versus conventional freehand technique. *Chin Neurosurg J*. 2019;5(1):6. https://doi.org/10.1186/s41016-019-0154-y.
44. Budu A, Sims-Williams H, Radatz M, et al. Comparison of navigated versus fluoroscopic-guided pedicle screw placement accuracy and complication rate. *World Neurosurg*. 2020;144:e541–e545. https://doi.org/10.1016/j.wneu.2020.08.207.
45. Yang P, Chen K, Zhang K, Sun J, Yang H, Mao H. Percutaneous short-segment pedicle instrumentation assisted with O-arm navigation in the treatment of thoracolumbar burst fractures. *J Orthop Transl*. 2020;21:1–7. https://doi.org/10.1016/j.jot.2019.11.002.
46. Gelalis ID, Paschos NK, Pakos EE, et al. Accuracy of pedicle screw placement: a systematic review of prospective in vivo studies comparing free hand, fluoroscopy guidance and navigation techniques. *Eur Spine J*. 2012;21(2):247–255. https://doi.org/10.1007/s00586-011-2011-3.
47. Liu Z, Jin M, Qiu Y, Yan H, Han X, Zhu Z. The superiority of intraoperative O-arm navigation-assisted surgery in instrumenting extremely small thoracic pedicles of adolescent idiopathic scoliosis: a case-control study. *Med (Baltim)*. 2016;95(18):e3581. https://doi.org/10.1097/MD.0000000000003581.
48. Jin M, Liu Z, Liu X, et al. Does intraoperative navigation improve the accuracy of pedicle screw placement in the apical region of dystrophic scoliosis secondary to neurofibromatosis type I: comparison between O-arm navigation and free-hand technique. *Eur Spine J*. 2016;25(6):1729–1737. https://doi.org/10.1007/s00586-015-4012-0. http://doi.org/10.1007/s00586-015-4053-4.
49. Perdomo-Pantoja A, Ishida W, Zygourakis C, et al. Accuracy of current techniques for placement of pedicle screws in the spine: a comprehensive systematic review and meta-analysis of 51,161 screws. *World Neurosurg*. 2019;126:664–678. https://doi.org/10.1016/j.wneu.2019.02.217. e3.
50. Yang YK, Chan CM, Zhang Q, Xu HR, Niu XH. Computer navigation-aided resection of sacral chordomas. *Chin Med J (Engl)*. 2016;129(2):162–168. https://doi.org/10.4103/0366-6999.173465.
51. Jentzsch T, Vlachopoulos L, Fürnstahl P, Müller DA, Fuchs B. Tumor resection at the pelvis using three-dimensional planning and patient-specific instruments: a case series. *World J Surg Oncol*. 2016;14(1):249. https://doi.org/10.1186/s12957-016-1006-2.
52. Farfalli GL, Albergo JI, Ritacco LE, Ayerza MA, Milano FE, Aponte-Tinao LA. What is the expected learning curve in computer-assisted navigation for bone tumor resection? *Clin Orthop Relat Res*. 2017;475(3):668–675. https://doi.org/10.1007/s11999-016-4761-z.
53. Drazin D, Bhamb N, Al-Khouja LT, et al. Image-guided resection of aggressive sacral tumors. *Neurosurg Focus*. 2017;42(1):E15. https://doi.org/10.3171/2016.6.FOCUS16125.
54. Abraham JA, Kenneally B, Amer K, Geller DS. Can navigation-assisted surgery help achieve negative margins in resection of pelvic and sacral tumors? *Clin Orthop Relat Res*. 2018;476(3):499–508. https://doi.org/10.1007/s11999.0000000000000064.
55. Moore T, McLain RF. Image-guided surgery in resection of benign cervicothoracic spinal tumors: a report of two cases. *Spine J*. 2005;5(1):109–114. https://doi.org/10.1016/j.spinee.2004.06.020.
56. Rajasekaran S, Kamath V, Shetty AP. Intraoperative Iso-C three-dimensional navigation in excision of spinal osteoid osteomas. *Spine (Phila Pa 1976)*. 2008;33(1):E25–E29. https://doi.org/10.1097/BRS.0b013e31815e6308.

57. Nagashima H, Nishi T, Yamane K, Tanida A. Case report: osteoid osteoma of the c2 pedicle: surgical technique using a navigation system. *Clin Orthop Relat Res*. 2010;468(1):283–288. https://doi.org/10.1007/s11999-009-0958-8.
58. Hsu W, Kosztowski TA, Zaidi HA, Gokaslan ZL, Wolinsky JP. Image-guided, endoscopic, transcervical resection of cervical chordoma: technical note. *J Neurosurg Spine*. 2010;12(4):431–435. https://doi.org/10.3171/2009.10.SPINE09393.
59. Jeys L, Matharu GS, Nandra RS, Grimer RJ. Can computer navigation-assisted surgery reduce the risk of an intralesional margin and reduce the rate of local recurrence in patients with a tumour of the pelvis or sacrum? *Bone Jt J*. 2013;95-B(10):1417–1424. https://doi.org/10.1302/0301-620X.95B10.31734.
60. Laitinen MKK, Parry MCC, Albergo JI, Grimer RJ, Jeys LM. Is computer navigation when used in the surgery of iliosacral pelvic bone tumours safer for the patient? *Bone Jt J*. 2017;99-B(2):261–266. https://doi.org/10.1302/0301-620X.99B2.BJJ-2016-0149.R2.
61. Nasser R, Drazin D, Nakhla J, et al. Resection of spinal column tumors utilizing image-guided navigation: a multicenter analysis. *Neurosurg Focus*. 2016;41(2):E15. https://doi.org/10.3171/2016.5.FOCUS16136.
62. Bosma SE, Cleven AHG, Dijkstra PDS. Can navigation improve the ability to achieve tumor-free margins in pelvic and sacral primary bone sarcoma resections? A historically controlled study. *Clin Orthop Relat Res*. 2019;477(7):1548–1559. https://doi.org/10.1097/CORR.0000000000000766.
63. Ando K, Kobayashi K, Machino M, et al. Computed tomography-based navigation system-assisted surgery for primary spine tumor. *J Clin Neurosci*. 2019;63:22–26. Epub 2019 Feb 28. PMID: 30827883. https://doi.org/10.1016/j.jocn.2019.02.015.
64. Akiyama T, Ogura K, Gokita T, et al. Analysis of the infiltrative features of chordoma: the relationship between micro-skip metastasis and postoperative outcomes. *Ann Surg Oncol*. 2018;25(4):912–919. https://doi.org/10.1245/s10434-017-6268-6.
65. Baaj AA, Beckman J, Smith DA. O-arm-based image guidance in minimally invasive spine surgery: technical note. *Clin Neurol Neurosurg*. 2013;115(3):342–345. https://doi.org/10.1016/j.clineuro.2012.05.007.
66. Casiraghi M, Scarone P, Bellesi L, et al. Effective dose and image quality for intraoperative imaging with a cone-beam CT and a mobile multi-slice CT in spinal surgery: a phantom study. *Phys Med*. 2021;81:9–19. https://doi.org/10.1016/j.ejmp.2020.11.006.
67. Bai YS, Zhang Y, Chen ZQ, et al. Learning curve of computer-assisted navigation system in spine surgery. *Chin Med J (Engl)*. 2010;123(21):2989–2994. http://www.ncbi.nlm.nih.gov/pubmed/21162943.
68. Sasso RC, Garrido BJ. Computer-assisted spinal navigation versus serial radiography and operative time for posterior spinal fusion at L5-S1. *J Spinal Disord Tech*. 2007;20(2):118–122. https://doi.org/10.1097/01.bsd.0000211263.13250.b1.
69. Kalfas IH. Image-guided spinal navigation: application to spinal metastases. *Neurosurg Focus*. 2001;11(6):e5. https://doi.org/10.3171/foc.2001.11.6.6. http://thejns.org/doi/pdfplus/10.3171/foc.2001.11.6.6.
70. Nottmeier EW, Crosby TL. Timing of paired points and surface matching registration in three-dimensional (3D) image-guided spinal surgery. *J Spinal Disord Tech*. 2007;20(4):268–270. https://doi.org/10.1097/01.bsd.0000211282.06519.ab.
71. Mohebbi S, Sadrehosseini SM, Mohammadi S, Lenarz T, Mucha D, Majdani O. Accuracy assessment of different registration and imaging methods on image-guided surgery of lateral skull base. *Arch Neurosci*. 2018:e74051 https://doi.org/10.5812/ans.74051. In(Press).
72. Holly LT, Bloch O, Johnson JP. Evaluation of registration techniques for spinal image guidance. *J Neurosurg Spine*. 2006;4(4):323–328. https://doi.org/10.3171/spi.2006.4.4.323.
73. Guha D, Jakubovic R, Gupta S, et al. Intraoperative error propagation in 3-dimensional spinal navigation from nonsegmental registration: a prospective cadaveric and clinical study. *Global Spine J*. 2019;9(5):512–520. https://doi.org/10.1177/2192568218804556.
74. Rajasekaran S, Vidyadhara S, Ramesh P, Shetty AP. Randomized clinical study to compare the accuracy of navigated and non-navigated thoracic pedicle screws in deformity correction surgeries. *Spine (Phila Pa 1976)*. 2007;32(2):E56–E64. https://doi.org/10.1097/01.brs.0000252094.64857.ab.
75. Twitchell S, Karsy M, Reese J, et al. Assessment of cost drivers and cost variation for lumbar interbody fusion procedures using the value driven outcomes database. *Neurosurg Focus*. 2018;44(5):E10. https://doi.org/10.3171/2018.1.FOCUS17724.
76. Carl HM, Ahmed AK, Abu-Bonsrah N, et al. Risk factors for wound-related reoperations in patients with metastatic spine tumor. *J Neurosurg Spine*. 2018;28(6):663–668. https://doi.org/10.3171/2017.10.SPINE1765.
77. Clarke MJ, Vrionis FD. Spinal tumor surgery: management and the avoidance of complications. *Cancer Control*. 2014;21(2):124–132. https://doi.org/10.1177/107327481402100204.
78. Zhou LP, Zhang RJ, Sun YW, Zhang L, Shen CL. Accuracy of pedicle screw placement and four other clinical outcomes of robotic guidance technique versus computer-assisted navigation in thoracolumbar surgery: a meta-analysis. *World Neurosurg*. 2021;146:e139–e150. https://doi.org/10.1016/j.wneu.2020.10.055.
79. Burström G, Persson O, Edström E, Elmi-Terander A. Augmented reality navigation in spine surgery: a systematic review. *Acta Neurochir (Wien)*. 2021;163(3):843–852. https://doi.org/10.1007/s00701-021-04708-3.
80. Dibble CF, Molina CA. Device profile of the XVision-spine (XVS) augmented-reality surgical navigation system: overview of its safety and efficacy. *Expert Rev Med Devices*. 2021;18(1):1–8. https://doi.org/10.1080/17434440.2021.1865795. December 24, 2020.
81. Molina CA, Sciubba DM, Greenberg JK, Khan M, Witham T. Clinical accuracy, technical precision, and workflow

of the first in human use of an augmented-reality head-mounted display stereotactic navigation system for spine surgery. *Oper Neurosurg (Hagerstown)*. 2021;20(3):300–309. https://doi.org/10.1093/ons/opaa398.

82. Molina CA, Theodore N, Ahmed AK, et al. Augmented reality-assisted pedicle screw insertion: a cadaveric proof-of-concept study. *J Neurosurg Spine*. 2019:1–8. https://doi.org/10.3171/2018.12.SPINE181142.
83. Molina CA, Phillips FM, Colman MW, et al. A cadaveric precision and accuracy analysis of augmented reality-mediated percutaneous pedicle implant insertion. *J Neurosurg Spine*. 2020:1–9. https://doi.org/10.3171/2020.6.SPINE20370.
84. Urakov TM. Augmented reality-assisted pedicle instrumentation: versatility across major instrumentation sets. *Spine (Phila Pa 1976)*. 2020;45(23):E1622–E1626. https://doi.org/10.1097/BRS.0000000000003669.
85. Xu B, Yang Z, Jiang S, Zhou Z, Jiang B, Yin S. Design and validation of a spinal surgical navigation system based on spatial augmented reality. *Spine (Phila Pa 1976)*. 2020;45(23):E1627–E1633. https://doi.org/10.1097/BRS.0000000000003666.
86. Burström G, Nachabe R, Homan R, et al. Frameless patient tracking with adhesive optical skin markers for augmented reality surgical navigation in spine surgery. *Spine (Phila Pa 1976)*. 2020;45(22):1598–1604. https://doi.org/10.1097/BRS.0000000000003628.

6

Navigated Oblique Lumbar Interbody Fusion

Rory R. Mayer, MD, Praveen V. Mummaneni, MD, MBA, Jeremy Huang, BS, and Dean Chou, MD

BACKGROUND

Present Practice

There are several well-described approaches for interbody fusion, and these include posterior lumbar interbody fusion (PLIF), transforaminal lumbar interbody fusion (TLIF), lateral lumbar interbody fusion (LLIF), and anterior lumbar interbody fusion (ALIF). More recently, the oblique lumbar interbody fusion (OLIF) has been added to the surgeon's armamentarium (Fig. 6.1).[1,2] There are advantages of the OLIF over other interbody techniques, but there are also challenges. The use of navigation for OLIF creates further advantages for this technique. The OLIF approach allows for the placement of a large interbody graft that spans the apophyseal ring and minimizes tissue damage and potential lumbar plexus injury by accessing the disk space through a prepsoas approach instead of a direct lateral transpsoas approach. Some of the well-described complications of the lateral approach including lumbar plexus injury and genitofemoral, iliohypogastric, or ilioinguinal nerve injury are minimized, but not eliminated, via a pre-psoas approach.[3] In addition, the oblique lateral approach at the L4–L5 level can avoid the difficulty that may arise in accessing the disk space via a true lateral approach with a high-riding iliac crest. Furthermore, the L5–S1 OLIF can be performed in the lateral position, eliminating the need for repositioning that needs to be done for an ALIF or the need for TLIF, which may not be optimal in certain cases (previous scar tissue, extremely collapsed space, or loss of lordosis).

The OLIF is appropriate for any patient who meets the diagnostic and clinical criteria for interbody fusion, which includes the diagnoses of degenerative spondylolisthesis, degenerative disk disease with foraminal stenosis necessitating indirect decompression, extension of fusion in adjacent segment degeneration, or coronal plane deformity and scoliosis. The contraindications to the OLIF include the need for a right-sided approach due to the proximity to the inferior vena cava and high risk for vascular injury. The other contraindications include anatomic constraints such as a narrow or absent operative corridor between the aorta and the psoas due to vascular or visceral structures that prevent easy access to the disk space.[1,2]

Literature on Outcomes

There have been numerous studies in the literature comparing both the radiographic and clinical outcomes between interbody techniques; however, there is no level I evidence to

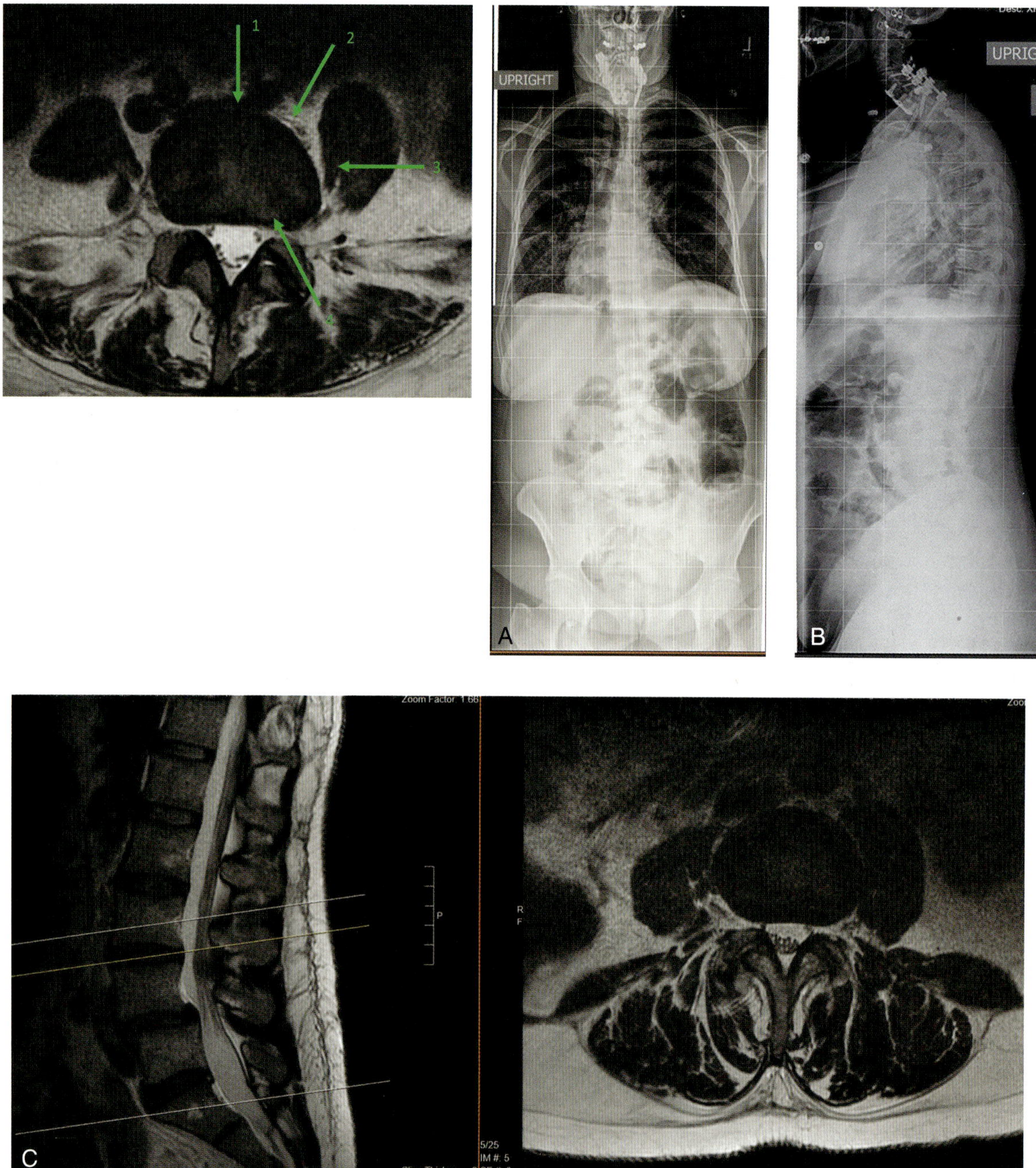

FIG. 6.1 Axial T2 MRI demonstrating the four interbody approach trajectories: 1, anterior interbody approach; 2, oblique lumbar interbody approach; 3, lateral lumbar interbody approach; 4, transforaminal lumbar interbody approach. (A, B) Standing radiographs demonstrated a pelvic incidence of 54 degrees, lumbar lordosis of 46 degrees, pelvic tilt of 16 degrees, sagittal vertical axis of 5.5 cm, coronal vertical axis of −2.6 cm, and a mobile L4–L5 grade I spondylolisthesis. (C) An MRI of the lumbar spine demonstrated severe L4–L5 foraminal stenosis.

support one approach over another.[4–10] Despite the limited rigorous comparative outcome studies, the OLIF technique demonstrates comparable radiographic outcomes[11–14] and evidence for biomechanical superiority relative to the TLIF due to the interbody cage spanning the entire apophyseal ring.[15] In our published experience, 94.86% of cages were accurately placed using navigation and only 1 of 214 patients required revision for a malpositioned cage.[16] Recent studies have demonstrated significant correction of the spinopelvic parameters during multilevel OLIF including L5–S1 in the correction of adult deformity.[13,14] The oblique approach also has distinct advantages over the transpsoas approach with regard to the neurologic complications, which have been reported to be as high as 20% with the transpsoas approaches.[17,18] Recent studies demonstrate an incidence of neurologic complications of approximately 1% to 4% with OLIF, and the vast majority of neurologic deficits tend to resolve within 8 weeks of surgery.[19] Finally, the use of navigation with an OLIF dramatically decreases the intraoperative radiation exposure to the operating room staff and is similar to a navigated TLIF approach with regard to the reduction in radiation exposure compared to conventional fluoroscopy.[20]

SURGICAL TREATMENT FOR SPINAL PATHOLOGY

Clinical Studies

Case 1

History and Clinical Presentation

This is a 54-year-old woman with adult scoliosis and debilitating back and leg pain refractory to conservative measures.

Preoperative Imaging

Prior to surgery, an MRI of the thoracic and lumbar spine was obtained to evaluate for neural compression, and 36-inch standing AP and lateral radiographs with flexion-extension films were also obtained to assess sagittal and coronal alignment, evaluate for instability, and assess spinopelvic parameters. Standing radiographs demonstrated a pelvic incidence of 54 degrees, lumbar lordosis of 46 degrees, pelvic tilt of 16 degrees, sagittal vertical axis of 5.5 cm, coronal vertical axis of −2.6 cm, and a mobile L4–L5 grade I spondylolisthesis (Fig. 6.1A and B). An MRI of the lumbar spine demonstrated severe L4–L5 foraminal stenosis (see Fig. 6.1C). MRI is useful to evaluate for disk degeneration and a central, lateral recess, or foraminal stenosis. In addition, the prepsoas retroperitoneal corridor for an oblique approach can be assessed on MRI with an appreciation for the relationship of the psoas to the great vessels.

Surgical Plan

The surgical plan was to proceed with L2–L3, L3–L4, and L4–L5 oblique lateral interbody fusion followed by a stage II posterior decompression with osteotomies and instrumentation at L2–L5.

Intraoperative Imaging

Intraoperative O-arm imaging demonstrates the placement of the navigation reference array in the iliac crest (Fig. 6.2A); the use of navigation to denote the true lateral projection for use in marking the incision approximately 5 cm anterior to this point (see Fig. 6.2B and C); blunt muscle dissection (see Fig. 6.2D) to identify retroperitoneal fat (see Fig. 6.2E);

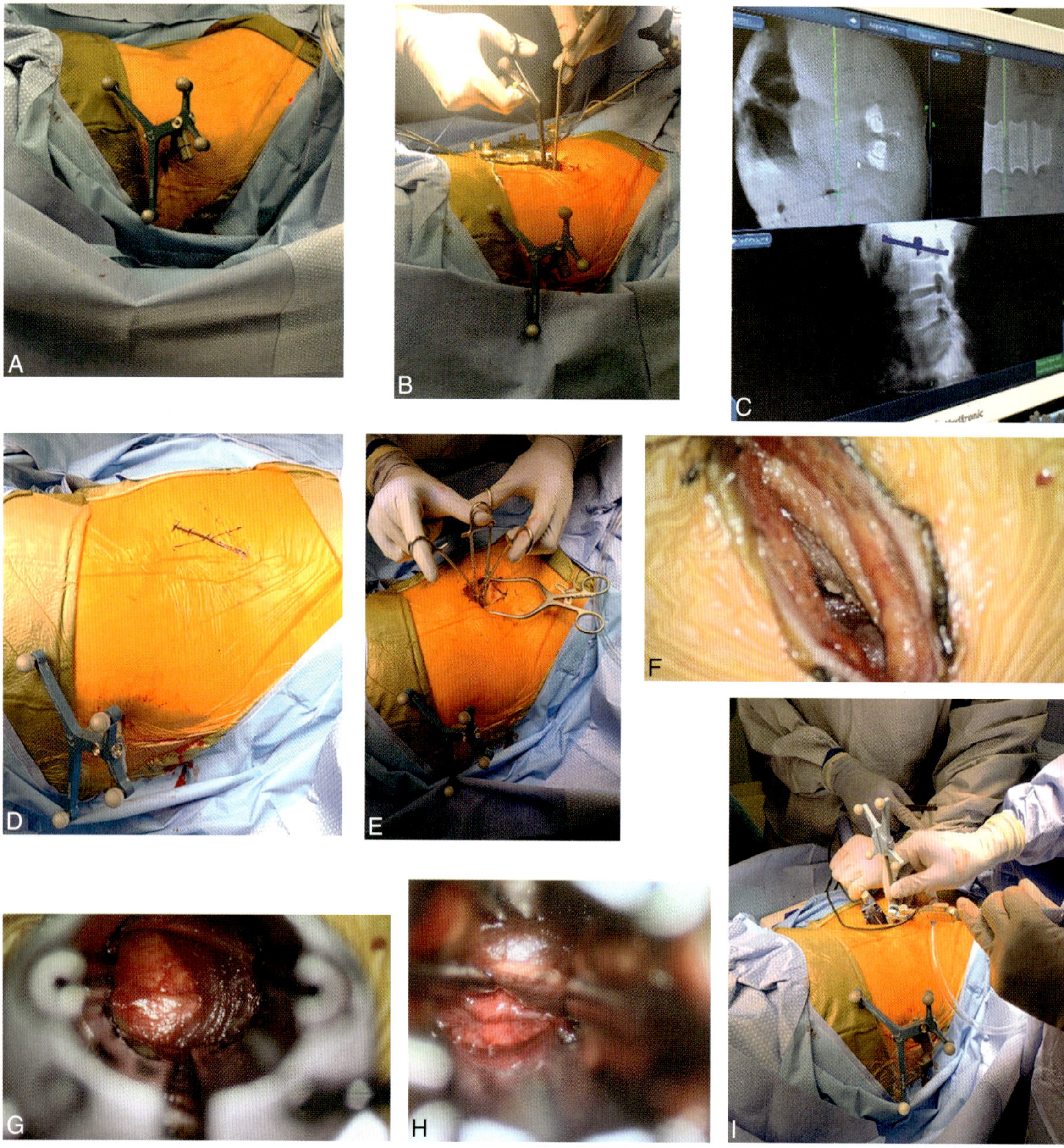

FIG. 6.2 (A) Intraoperative imaging demonstrates placement of the navigation reference array in the iliac crest. (B, C) Use of navigation to denote true lateral projection for use in marking incision approximately 5 cm anterior to this point. (D) Blunt muscle dissection with visualized external and internal oblique muscles. (E) Identification of retroperitoneal fat. (F) Identification of the psoas and disk space. (G) Use of navigation for confirmation of disk space level. (H) Use of sequential dilation and placement of table-mounted retractor blades. (I) Discectomy and endplate preparation.

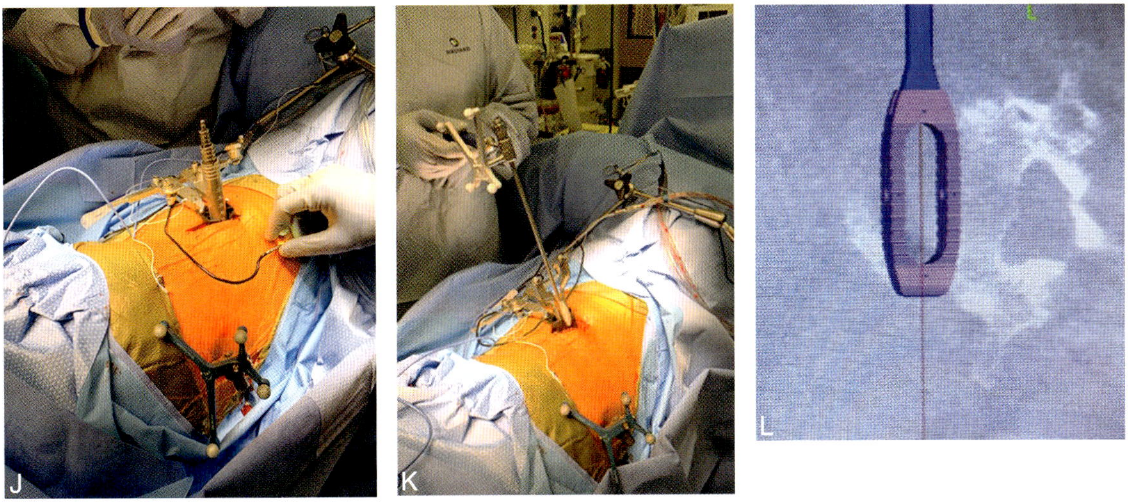

FIG. 6.2, cont'd. (J, K, L) Placement of the interbody device using navigation.

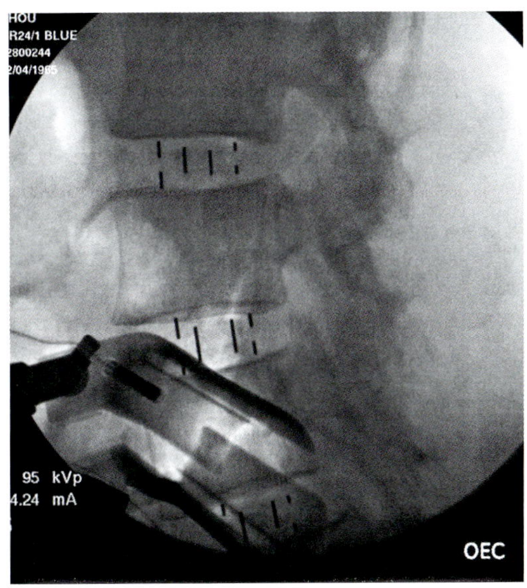

FIG. 6.3 Lateral x-ray demonstrating appropriate placement of interbody devices.

identification of the psoas and presumptive disk space (see Fig. 6.2F), which is then confirmed with navigation (see Fig. 6.2G); sequential dilation and placement of table-mounted retractor blades (see Fig. 6.2H); discectomy and endplate preparation (see Fig. 6.2I); and placement of the interbody device using navigation (see Fig. 6.2J and K). A lateral x-ray demonstrating appropriate placement of interbody devices is shown in Fig. 6.3.

Postoperative Imaging

Postoperative standing 36-inch radiographs were obtained with AP and lateral views (Fig. 6.4A and B) that demonstrate appropriate interbody device placement and posterior fixation.

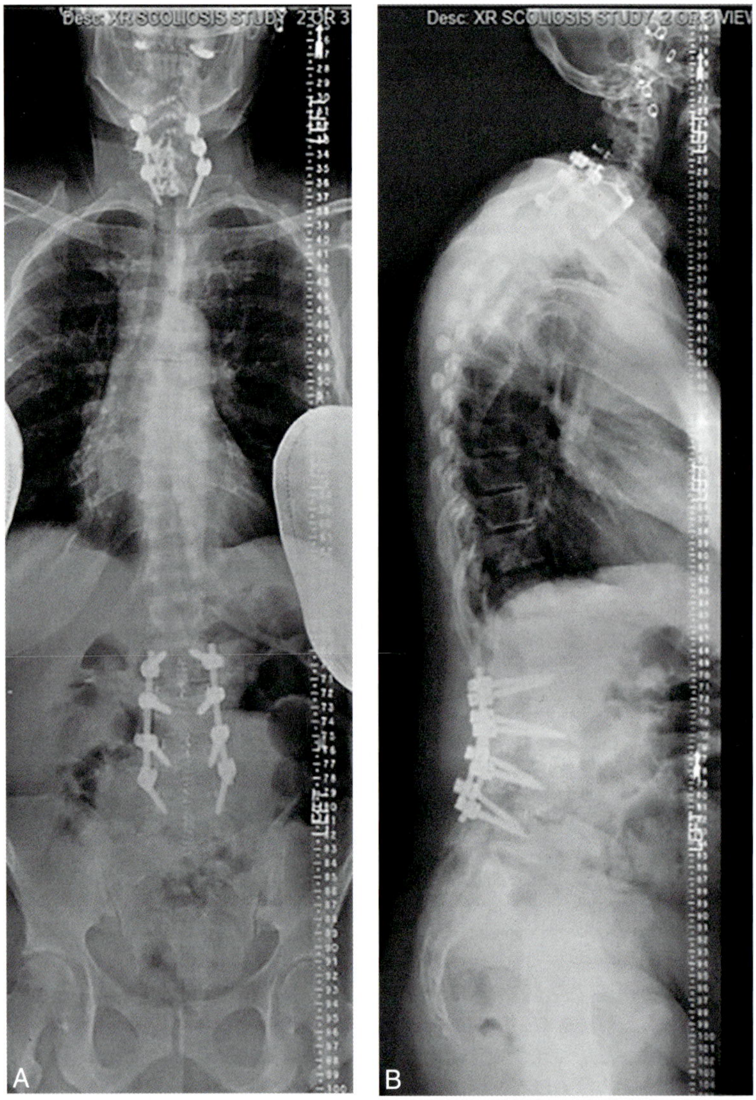

FIG. 6.4 (A, B) Postoperative standing 36-inch radiographs were obtained with AP and lateral views that demonstrate appropriate interbody device placement and posterior fixation.

Postoperative Recovery and Follow-Up

The patient was quickly mobilized and discharged home.

Case 2

History and Clinical Presentation

This is a 69-year-old man with a history of two prior lumbar decompressions who presented with a diagnosis of lumbar spondylolisthesis and symptoms of neurogenic claudication and foraminal stenosis refractory to conservative care.

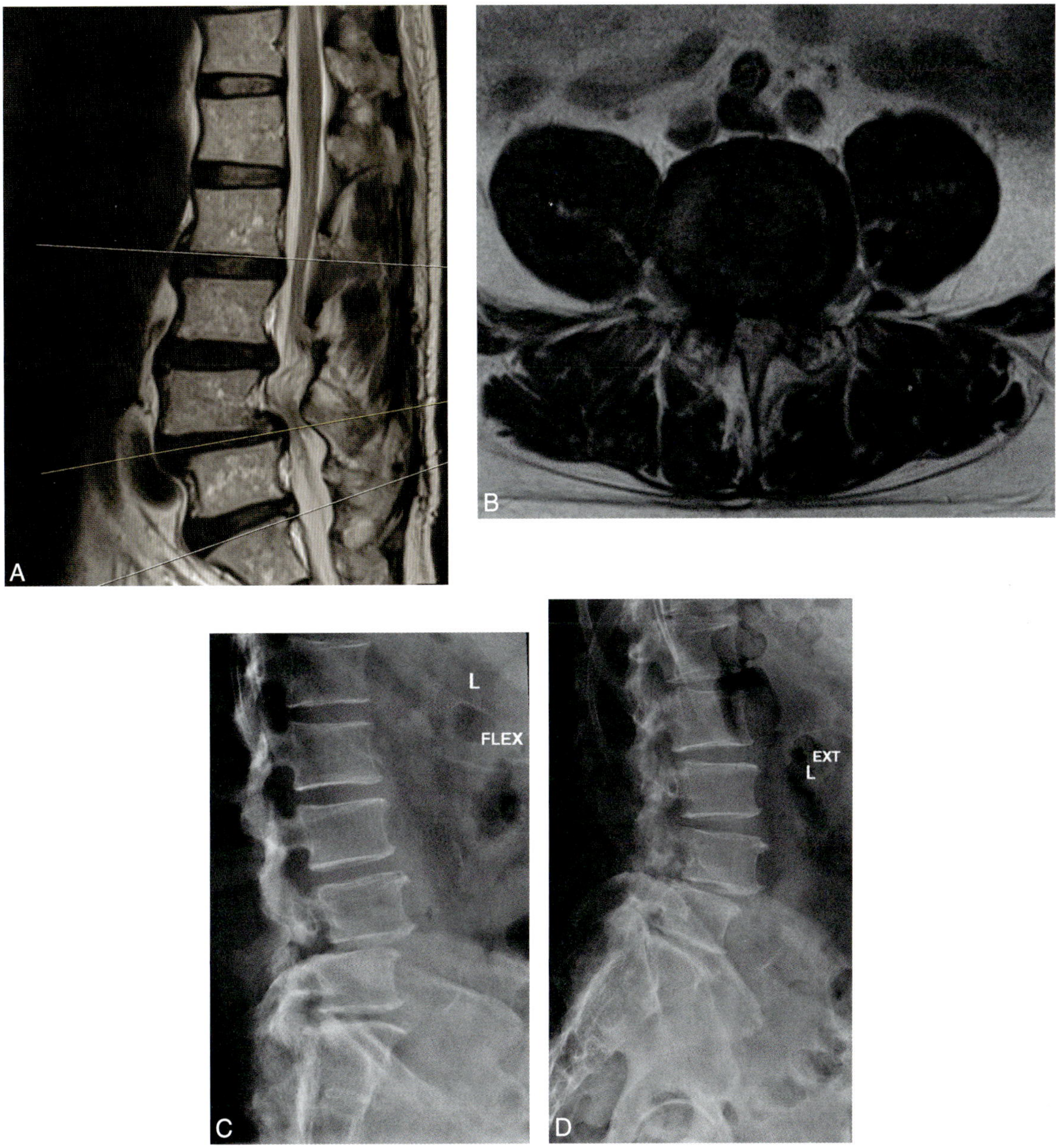

FIG. 6.5 (A–D) Preoperative magnetic resonance imaging of the lumbar spine demonstrates severe L4–L5 central and lateral recess stenosis secondary to worsening spondylolisthesis and up-down foraminal stenosis. Standing lumbar radiographs demonstrate a mobile L4–L5 spondylolisthesis.

Preoperative Imaging

Preoperative MRI of the lumbar spine demonstrates severe L4–L5 central and lateral recess stenosis secondary to worsening spondylolisthesis and up-down foraminal stenosis. Standing lumbar radiographs demonstrate a mobile L4–L5 spondylolisthesis (Fig. 6.5A–D).

Surgical Plan

The surgical plan was to proceed with L4–L5 oblique lateral interbody fusion followed by a stage II posterior percutaneous screw fixation at L4–L5.

Intraoperative Imaging

Fig. 6.6A demonstrates the oblique incision after dissection through the external oblique, internal oblique, and transversus abdominus. The incision was marked approximately 5 cm anterior to the midpoint of the L4–L5 disk space. Following the muscle dissection, identification of the retroperitoneal fat and disk space is performed with the navigation probe at the level of the disk space (see Fig. 6.6B). After sequential dilation, the retractor blades are placed for visualization over the disk space, and the level is confirmed with navigation. Subsequently, using navigated instruments, the disk is removed and the disk space prepared in the standard fashion. Similarly, after adequate preparation of the disk space and using trial sizers therein, an interbody cage packed with rib autograft is placed under navigation into the disk space (see Fig. 6.6C). The intraoperative x-rays confirm appropriate position of the interbody devices prior to closure (see Fig. 6.6D and E).

Postoperative Imaging

After the patient has been mobilized, standing AP and lateral 36-inch radiographs are obtained to evaluate the implants prior to discharge (Fig. 6.7A and B).

Postoperative Recovery and Follow-Up

Aggressive mobilization after OLIF is encouraged. For patients who are undergoing a two-stage procedure with posterior instrumentation, ambulation prior to the second stage is encouraged in order to evaluate for continued radicular symptoms that may warrant additional decompression during posterior fixation. The patients are typically advanced from a clear liquid diet to a regular diet if the return of bowel function is noted. Patients with extensive multilevel surgery, typically inclusive of L5–S1 interbody placement, have a clear liquid diet, but they are not given solid food until the return of bowel function to mitigate the effects of an ileus.

PROCEDURAL CONCERNS IN DETAIL

The development and adoption of the OLIF technique utilizing intraoperative navigation goes back to its original description by Mayer in 1997 as a prepsoas approach in combination with fluoroscopy.[21] The oblique trajectory and need to make an orthogonal move during disk space preparation and cage placement into a more lateral trajectory is not immediately intuitive; navigation improves comfort and sense of orientation relative to a pure fluoroscopic-based approach. These difficulties contrast with the ALIF (direct anterior) and extreme lateral interbody fusion (direct lateral) approaches that did not warrant such developments in navigation due to the relative straightforward anatomic trajectories of these techniques. In our institutional experience, we immediately adopted the navigated OLIF technique over a fluoroscopic-based approach due to prior studies demonstrating significant reduction in radiation exposure and what we felt would have been unnecessary radiation exposure to the surgical team.[20] Further, with increased experience, a navigated setup has allowed us to begin performing single-position L1–L5

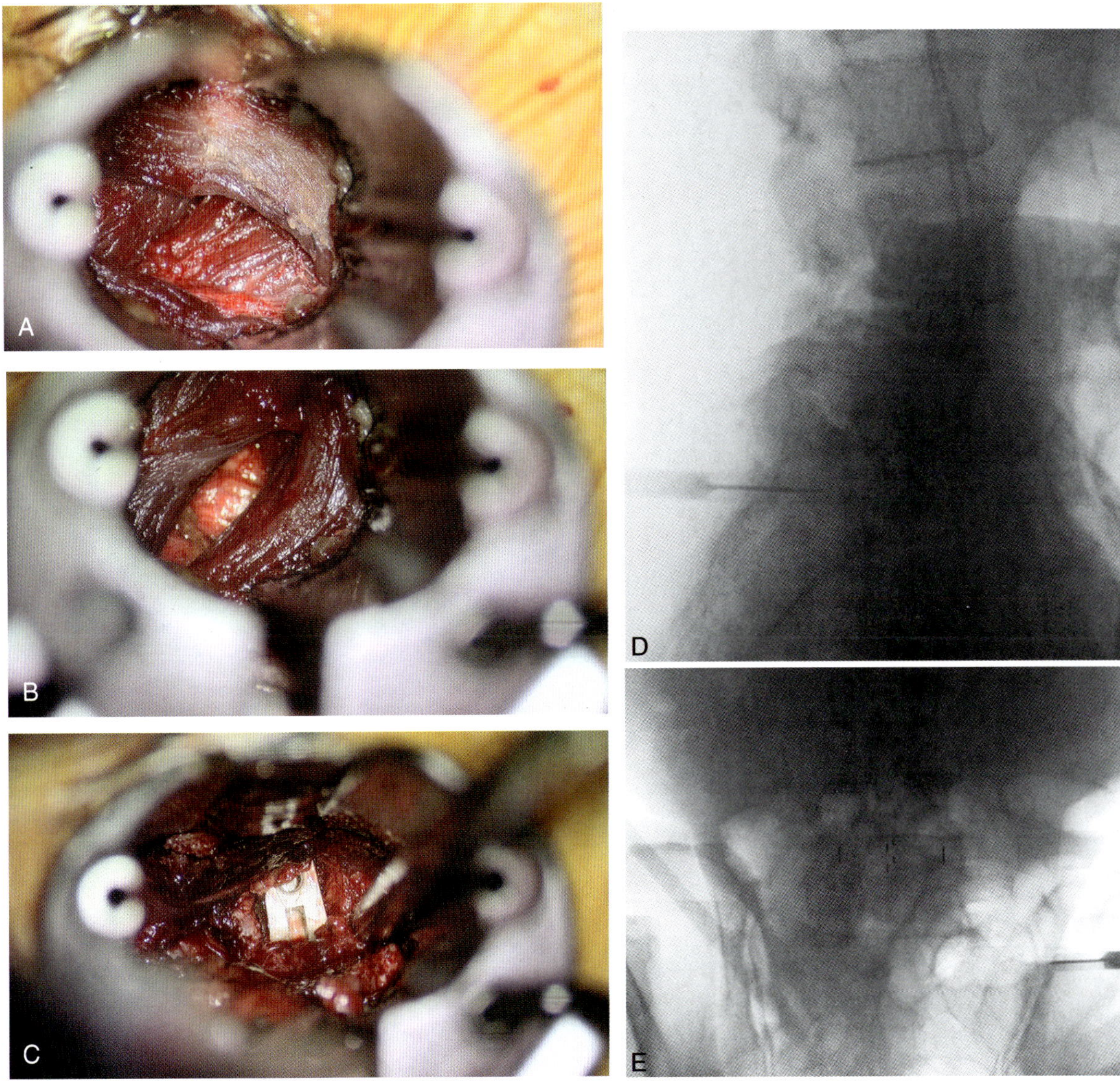

FIG. 6.6 (A) Visualization of the oblique incision after dissection through the external oblique, internal oblique and transversus abdominus. The incision was marked approximately 5 cm anterior to the midpoint of the L4–L5 disk space. (B) Following muscle dissection, identification of the retroperitoneal fat and disk space is performed with the navigation probe at the level of the disk space. (C) After adequate prepping of the disk space and using trial sizers in the disk space, an interbody cage packed with rib autograft is placed under navigation into the disk space. (D, E) Intraoperative x-rays confirm appropriate position of the interbody devices prior to closure.

OLIF and lateral position L5–S1 interbody fusion as well as single-position OLIF with percutaneous pedicle screw fixation.

Although a detailed description of our surgical technique has previously been published,[2] the important considerations are highlighted here. The patient is positioned with the left side up in a right lateral decubitus position on a flat top Jackson table with side-rail

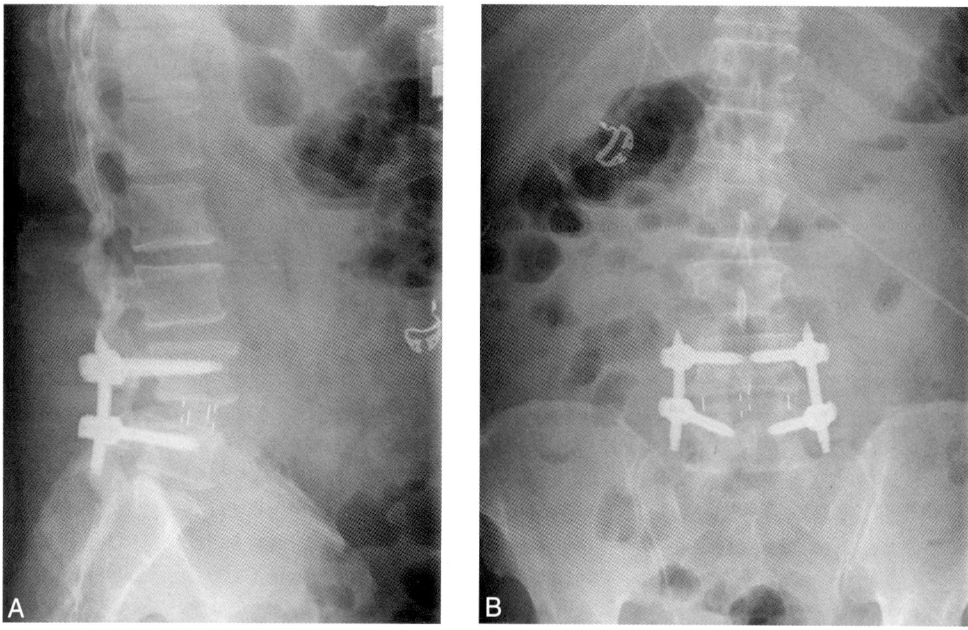

FIG. 6.7 (A, B) Postoperative standing AP and lateral 36-inch radiographs demonstrating appropriate placement of implants.

attachments and the reference array is malleted into the ilium approximately 2 to 3 cm superolateral to the posterior superior iliac spine (PSIS). A lateral entry point is important to prevent skiving of the reference arc off the bone medially into the soft tissues or dorsal sacral foramina. The O-arm CT navigation system (O-arm, Medtronic, Memphis, TN) is then brought into the room and the patient and array are registered to the navigation system after the imaging is complete. For every disk space of interest, using the axial and sagittal views on the navigation system, a true lateral projection as a virtual extension of the navigation probe is obtained to identify the midpoint of the disk space of interest (see Fig. 6.2B). We then measure 5 cm anterior to this location and mark an approximately 3 to 4 cm oblique incision. The incision is fashioned obliquely to parallel the path of the abdominal wall nerves to avoid nerve injury. Injury to these nerves may result in abdominal wall bulging or a pseudohernia. Throughout our dissection, we limit our use of electrocautery after completion of the initial dissection through the subcutaneous soft tissue and strictly adhere to blunt tissue dissection to mitigate this risk.

We utilize the navigation probe throughout the approach to confirm our position and trajectory toward the disk space. Using handheld retractors, we then identify and split the external and internal obliques, as well as the transversus abdominus muscle, using Mayo clamps. At the depth of the dissection, the transversalis fascia is encountered and opened to identify the retroperitoneal fat, after which we place a second finger into the opening and bluntly spread the opening to increase our working space. Then, utilizing finger dissection, the retroperitoneal fat and contents of the peritoneum are swept off the psoas muscle anteriorly. We then place the navigation probe into the cavity to confirm our trajectory and help identify the anterior border of the psoas. A 4 Penfield dissector is then used to sweep the psoas posteriorly. The disk space is further cleared using blunt instruments and direct visualization confirms no overlying neural structures, peritoneum, ureter, or blood vessels. Thereafter, sequential dilators are placed over the navigation probe, which we insert into the disk space to a depth of approximately 1 cm. Although the OLIF approach is a prepsoas technique without direct risk of injury to the lumbar plexus, our hospital and regional care patterns dictate the use of triggered electromyography (EMG), which we utilize in all cases. The disk space can be stimulated for EMG response prior to the sequential dilation process to ensure there are no overlying nerves. A table-mounted retractor is then placed over the dilators and secured in place. The dilators are removed and the annulotomy and discectomy performed. It is important to enter the disk space at an oblique angle and then rotate the instruments into a more posteriorly-based position to create a true lateral trajectory. A direct oblique approach may result in contralateral nerve root injury and thus, an orthogonal move with the surgeon's hand moved dorsally into a true lateral position is critical to avoid this complication.

After complete discectomy and endplate preparation, which may be done using navigated instruments, interbody template trials are placed with navigation. Once the correct trial size is determined, the interbody cage is filled with graft material and placed into the disk space via navigation. In our experience, the graft should be difficult to dislodge but not overly distracting of the disk space such that it requires significant force to impact into position. In our experience with the majority of degenerative cases, an 8-mm or 10-mm cage height is appropriate. For a disk space without significant collapse, a 10-mm or 12-mm interbody cage height is acceptable. The placement of a 14-mm cage height or higher is usually indicative of endplate violation during endplate preparation or interbody trialing. The interbody cage is placed in a navigated fashion into a precise location via an appropriate trajectory into the disk space to minimize endplate disruption and to impact to the appropriate depth, such that the cage spans the apophyseal ring. Following navigated cage placement, we use C-arm fluoroscopy to confirm acceptable implant position. Thereafter, our retractors are removed, hemostasis is obtained, and the wound is closed in a standard layered fashion.

Approach-Related Sequelae

There are expected postoperative sequelae associated with the oblique lumbar interbody fusion. Ileus is a common treatment-related sequelae that results from mobilization of the peritoneal contents, and ileus is frequently seen postoperatively not only from mobilization of the abdominal contents, but also from anesthesia and narcotic administration. In the event that intraoperative violation of the peritoneum occurs, this opening should be repaired primarily. Usually, a figure-of-eight 2–0 or 3–0 vicryl suffices, but any larger rents may require the consultation of general surgery. One consideration is to provide a bowel preparation preoperatively in order to empty the colon of all stool. Not only does this help with postoperative colonic distention by decreasing the bacterial count in the colon, it can help the patient with the nearly inevitable constipation that occurs postoperatively from anesthesia and narcotics. In addition, repleting electrolytes postoperatively promotes normal bowel function. Transient left-sided hip flexor weakness is a treatment-related sequela that may occur with the prepsoas approach, either due to muscle hematoma from the surgery or posterior retraction of the psoas muscle; this weakness typically improves rapidly and patients are counseled on this expectation prior to surgery.

Potential Downfalls

There are several potential challenges that the OLIF approach presents. When utilizing the navigation, there is a potential for inaccuracy to develop, and the likelihood of this becoming an issue is more common with multilevel surgeries. Because of the potential for inaccuracy with subsequent interbody graft placement, it is generally recommended that the most proximal (cephalad) level be treated first, prior to the more distal levels. This is because the reference array is placed distally in the pelvis, and, as interbody grafts are placed, the cephalad vertebral body is mobilized away from the reference arc. In addition, when performing more distal (caudal) levels, the surgical arc is closer to the reference arc, decreasing the inaccuracy factor by being in close proximity to the reference arc. Moreover, periodic confirmation of the accuracy of navigation with identifiable landmarks is important. Despite the advantages of navigation relative to fluoroscopy for OLIF, including decreased radiation exposure and improved workflow, it is important to remember that fluoroscopy provides real-time information at each surgical level and is a clear advantage if there are concerns regarding the accuracy of the navigation system at any point in the procedure.

There are a number of significant potential complications associated with this procedure that warrant an awareness of the potential pitfalls, both intraoperatively and in the early postoperative period. Delayed vascular injury can be identified on early postoperative examination, and a retroperitoneal hematoma may also be identified on serial trending of hemoglobin if there is concern by examination or vitals. A computed tomography (CT) scan can easily identify a psoas hematoma if present. Most psoas hematomas resolve over time, and as long as active bleeding is not present, expectant management with serial imaging is usually the treatment of choice. An important anatomic concept relates to accessing the upper lumbar spine. In the event that the lower thoracic ribs preclude easy access to the L1–L2 or L2–L3 disk spaces, partial rib resection is sometimes necessary to facilitate the approach. As long as the surgeon stays in the retropleural space, there is usually no need for a chest tube. However, if the pleural cavity is violated, a small drain can be placed up to the apex to evacuate any pneumothorax, and it is critical that the anesthesiologist not let the patient breathe separately from the machine until the wound is closed in order to avoid drawing in a pneumothorax. Finally, as a general principle of interbody work, subsidence of the interbody graft is an important structural concern when performing the disk preparation. Generally, this can be avoided by using extreme care when it comes to forces against the endplate while acknowledging tactile feedback; additionally, limiting direct sharp contact with forceful instruments during disk space preparation is critical. We also obtain a lateral fluoroscopic image after cage insertion to confirm appropriate cage placement and indirect decompression.

Management of Complications

Although there is a growing body of evidence to suggest low overall complication rates with the oblique interbody lateral fusion (OLIF) approach, with the complication profile at least equivalent to that of TLIF or XLIF, it is important to recognize that complications are inherent to lumbar fusion operations, even during minimally invasive OLIF.[3,22] Besides approach- or implant-related complications common to all interbody approaches, such as wound infection, cage migration or misplacement, pseudarthrosis, or implant subsidence, vascular injury is the most common category of intraoperative complications for OLIF procedures. Because OLIF involves a prepsoas procedure with an exclusively left-sided approach, the surgical entry corridor between the aorta and the psoas increases the risk of serious vascular injury.[3,23] Abe et al. reported a 2.6% incidence of segmental artery injury complications in a retrospective study of 155 OLIF surgeries.[24] However, direct visualization during the approach and real-time assessment of the surgical trajectory mitigates the risk of vascular injury.[1,2,25] The aorta and segmental vessels are not the only vascular structures that must be considered; injury to the iliac vein and vena cava must also be considered. In addition, there is a risk of arterial occlusion from retractors, and this warrants lower extremity pulse oximetry to monitor for such events, particularly when retracting the iliac vessels at L5–S1.

The other major category of complications associated with OLIF procedures is the specific approach-related complications. Injury to the genitofemoral nerve, iliohypogastric nerve, and ureter must be prevented, and this can be done with direct visualization during the approach and shallow docking. The use of bovie electrocautery should be avoided when exposing the disk space in order to decrease the risk of thermal injury to the surrounding structures and the inadvertent spread of the electrical current beyond the confines of the retractors. Genitofemoral nerve injury generally presents as numbness in the groin and anterior thigh[26]. It is critical not to damage any nerves that lay on the surface of the psoas muscle in order to avoid such an issue. In addition, loose taping of the legs to the bed is critical to minimize pressure on the right common peroneal nerve at the knee. Ultimately, a review of published literature on complication rates of interbody fusion procedures shows that the complication rate of OLIF compares favorably to those of similar procedures.[27]

SUMMARY

The oblique lumbar interbody fusion provides the spine surgeon with an additional technique to address lumbar spine pathology. The use of navigation has facilitated the ease of use of this technique while minimizing the radiation exposure to the operating surgeon. There are distinct advantages to this technique, including avoiding the lumbar plexus within the psoas muscle, the use of navigation to avoid radiation exposure to the operating room staff, and the ability to include L5–S1 interbody placement while in a lateral position. However, the OLIF has a unique complication profile that warrants thorough understanding of the anatomy and the approach when implementing this technique in practice.

Future Directions

Further refinements of the oblique lateral approach will expand the applications of this technique to treat even more thoracolumbar pathology, minimize morbidity, and push the boundaries of minimally invasive surgery using navigation and potentially robotic technology. Some authors are now advocating for simultaneous oblique lateral approach for interbody fusion with posterior fixation, potentially implementing both navigation and robotic surgery.[28]

REFERENCES

1. DiGiorgio AM, Edwards CS, Virk MS, Chou D. Lateral Prepsoas (oblique) approach nuances. *Neurosurg Clin N Am*. 2018;29(3):419–426. https://doi.org/10.1016/j.nec.2018.02.003.
2. DiGiorgio AM, Edwards CS, Virk MS, Mummaneni PV, Chou D. Stereotactic navigation for the prepsoas oblique lateral lumbar interbody fusion: technical note and case series. *Neurosurg Focus*. 2017;43(2):E14. https://doi.org/10.3171/2017.5.FOCUS17168.
3. Walker CT, Farber SH, Cole TS, et al. Complications for minimally invasive lateral interbody arthrodesis: a systematic review and meta-analysis comparing prepsoas and transpsoas approaches. *J Neurosurg Spine*. 2019:1–15. https://doi.org/10.3171/2018.9.SPINE18800.
4. Kim JS, Lee KY, Lee SH, Lee HY. Which lumbar interbody fusion technique is better in terms of level for the treatment of unstable isthmic spondylolisthesis? *J Neurosurg Spine*. 2010;12(2):171–177. https://doi.org/10.3171/2009.9.SPINE09272.
5. Madan SS, Boeree NR. Comparison of instrumented anterior interbody fusion with instrumented circumferential

lumbar fusion. *Eur Spine J*. 2003;12(6):567–575. https://doi.org/10.1007/s00586-002-0516-5.
6. Min JH, Jang JS, Lee SH. Comparison of anterior- and posterior-approach instrumented lumbar interbody fusion for spondylolisthesis. *J Neurosurg Spine*. 2007;7(1):21–26. https://doi.org/10.3171/SPI-07/07/021.
7. Pradhan BB, Nassar JA, Delamarter RB, Wang JC. Single-level lumbar spine fusion: a comparison of anterior and posterior approaches. *J Spinal Disord Tech*. 2002;15(5):355–361. https://doi.org/10.1097/00024720-200210000-00003.
8. Sears W. Posterior lumbar interbody fusion for degenerative spondylolisthesis: restoration of sagittal balance using insert-and-rotate interbody spacers. *Spine J*. 2005;5(2):170–179. https://doi.org/10.1016/j.spinee.2004.05.257.
9. Yan DL, Pei FX, Li J, Soo CL. Comparative study of PILF and TLIF treatment in adult degenerative spondylolisthesis. *Eur Spine J*. 2008;17(10):1311–1316. https://doi.org/10.1007/s00586-008-0739-1.
10. Faundez AA, Schwender JD, Safriel Y, et al. Clinical and radiological outcome of anterior–posterior fusion versus transforaminal lumbar interbody fusion for symptomatic disc degeneration: a retrospective comparative study of 133 patients. *Eur Spine J*. 2009;18(2):203–211. https://doi.org/10.1007/s00586-008-0845-0.
11. Li HM, Zhang RJ, Shen CL. Radiographic and clinical outcomes of oblique lateral interbody fusion versus minimally invasive transforaminal lumbar interbody fusion for degenerative lumbar disease. *World Neurosurg*. 2019;122:e627–e638. https://doi.org/10.1016/j.wneu.2018.10.115.
12. Mobbs RJ, Phan K, Malham G, Seex K, Rao PJ. Lumbar interbody fusion: techniques, indications and comparison of interbody fusion options including PLIF, TLIF, MI-TLIF, OLIF/ATP, LLIF and ALIF. *J Spine Surg*. 2015;1(1):2–18. https://doi.org/10.3978/j.issn.2414-469X.2015.10.05.
13. Patel RS, Suh SW, Kang SH, et al. The radiologic and clinical outcomes of oblique lateral interbody fusion for correction of adult degenerative lumbar deformity. *Indian J Orthop*. 2019;53(4):502–509. https://doi.org/10.4103/ortho.IJOrtho_655_17.
14. Anand N, Alayan A, Agrawal A, Kahwaty S, Nomoto E, Khandehroo B. Analysis of spino-pelvic parameters and segmental lordosis with L5-S1 oblique lateral interbody fusion at the bottom of a long construct in circumferential minimally invasive surgical correction of adult spinal deformity. *World Neurosurg*. 2019;130:e1077–e1083. https://doi.org/10.1016/j.wneu.2019.07.091.
15. Lu T, Lu Y. Comparison of biomechanical performance among posterolateral fusion and transforaminal, extreme, and oblique lumbar interbody fusion: a finite element analysis. *World Neurosurg*. 2019;129:e890–e899. https://doi.org/10.1016/j.wneu.2019.06.074.
16. Xi Z, Chou D, Mummaneni PV, Burch S. The navigated oblique lumbar interbody fusion: accuracy rate, effect on surgical time, and complications. *Neurospine*. 2020;17(1):260–267. https://doi.org/10.14245/ns.1938358.179.
17. Bergey DL, Villavicencio AT, Goldstein T, Regan JJ. Endoscopic lateral transpsoas approach to the lumbar spine. *Spine (Phila Pa 1976)*. 2004;29(15):1681–1688. https://doi.org/10.1097/01.brs.0000133643.75795.ef.
18. Cummock MD, Vanni S, Levi AD, Yu Y, Wang MY. An analysis of postoperative thigh symptoms after minimally invasive transpsoas lumbar interbody fusion. *J Neurosurg Spine*. 2011;15(1):11–18. https://doi.org/10.3171/2011.2.SPINE10374.
19. Liu C, Wang J, Zhou Y. Perioperative complications associated with minimally invasive surgery of oblique lumbar interbody fusions for degenerative lumbar diseases in 113 patients. *Clin Neurol Neurosurg*. 2019;184:105381. https://doi.org/10.1016/j.clineuro.2019.105381.
20. Zhang YH, White I, Potts E, Mobasser JP, Chou D. Comparison perioperative factors during minimally invasive pre-psoas lateral interbody fusion of the lumbar spine using either navigation or conventional fluoroscopy. *Glob Spine J*. 2017;7(7):657–663. https://doi.org/10.1177/2192568217716149.
21. Mayer HM. A new microsurgical technique for minimally invasive anterior lumbar interbody fusion. *Spine (Phila Pa 1976)*. 1997;22(6):691–699, discussion 700. https://doi.org/10.1097/00007632-199703150-00023.
22. Abbasi A, Khaghany K, Orandi V, Abbasi H. Clinical and radiological outcomes of oblique lateral lumbar interbody fusion. *Cureus*. 2019;11(2):e4029. https://doi.org/10.7759/cureus.4029.
23. Abbasi H, Abbasi A. Oblique lateral lumbar interbody fusion (OLLIF): technical notes and early results of a single surgeon comparative study. *Cureus*. 2015;7(10):e351. https://doi.org/10.7759/cureus.351.
24. Abe K, Orita S, Mannoji C, et al. Perioperative complications in 155 patients who underwent oblique lateral interbody fusion surgery: perspectives and indications from a retrospective, multicenter survey. *Spine (Phila Pa 1976)*. 2017;42(1):55–62. https://doi.org/10.1097/BRS.0000000000001650.
25. Quillo-Olvera J, Lin GX, Jo HJ, Kim JS. Complications on minimally invasive oblique lumbar interbody fusion at L2-L5 levels: a review of the literature and surgical strategies. *Ann Transl Med*. 2018;6(6):101. https://doi.org/10.21037/atm.2018.01.22.
26. Woods KR, Billys JB, Hynes RA. Technical description of oblique lateral interbody fusion at L1-L5 (OLIF25) and at L5-S1 (OLIF51) and evaluation of complication and fusion rates. *Spine J*. 2017;17(4):545–553.
27. Walker CT, Farber S, Cole TS, et al. Complications for minimally invasive lateral interbody arthrodesis: a systematic review and meta-analysis comparing prepsoas and transpsoas approaches. *J Neurosurg Spine*. 2019;30(4):446–460.
28. Sellin JN, Mayer RR, Hoffman M, Ropper AE. Simultaneous lateral interbody fusion and pedicle screws (SLIPS) with CT-guided navigation. *Clin Neurol Neurosurg*. 2018;175:91–97. https://doi.org/10.1016/j.clineuro.2018.10.013.

7

Navigation in Non-Instrumented Spine Surgery

Adriel Barrios-Anderson, BSc, and Adetokunbo 'Toki' Oyelese, MD, PhD

OVERVIEW

Since its emergence about 25 years ago, significant technological advancements have been made in spinal navigation and computer assisted spine surgery. Most of these advancements and the resulting wider spread adoption of the technology have occurred only more recently within the last decade.[1] Some of the reasons for the delayed adoption of the technology in the spine despite early progress with intracranial navigation may relate to the technical challenges with the implementation in a mobile, multisegmented anatomical structure, in contrast to intracranial navigation where the fixed bony anatomy serves as a reference. Additionally, while intracranial stereotaxy and navigation were initially designed for the targeting of deep brain structures,[2] the utilization of the technology very quickly evolved into a tool for the localization of surface and deep brain structures.[3] By contrast, navigation in the spine was designed for targeting, specifically, the delivery of pedicle screws through a precise desired anatomic trajectory of the pedicle into the vertebral body. The challenge for navigation technology companies was thus to effect a paradigm shift in the design and development of spinal instrumentation technology. Paradoxically, most interventions in the spine involve non-instrumented procedures. Recently, the technology has been more widely implemented in the course of non-instrumented spine surgery where the objective is precise localization rather than target delivery.

Spinal navigation in non-instrumented spine cases confers two distinct advantages to the surgeon. The first is the superior intraoperative anatomical localization of the critical structures of surgical interest either in the course of decompression (defining limits and extent) or in the resection of critical lesions and foci. The 3D radiographic and anatomical imaging upon which intraoperative CT (iCT) and 3D fluoroscopic spinal navigation are based is superior to the 2D imaging of fluoroscopy and x-ray guidance. Moreover, when this is coupled with techniques that allow for autofusion of iCT acquired imaging with preoperative MR or CT myelogram imaging, the surgeon has an impressive ability to localize and navigate through critical anatomical structures during decompressive and lesion resection procedures. This technique of fused CT-MRI based navigation has been particularly useful in the treatment of spinal vertebral column and intradural tumors.[4–6]

The second advantage conferred by spinal navigation is the superior radiographic localization that obviates the need for fluoroscopic guidance, thereby reducing harmful cumulative radiation exposure to the surgeon and operating room staff. The hazardous ionizing radiation to which spine surgeons are exposed is significantly greater than that for most other specialties and may be several times greater than that for non-spine orthopedic surgeons who also utilize significant fluoroscopic guidance in the operating room.[7–9] While CT- and 3D fluoroscopic-based spinal navigation results in increased one-time exposure to the patient, it decreases the exposure of the surgeon and operating room staff,[10] potentially reducing the cumulative lifetime radiation exposure and potential for risk of cataracts, skin erythema, and oncogenesis with malignancies such as thyroid cancer, leukemia, and lymphoma.

PRESENT PRACTICE: UTILIZATION OF SPINAL NAVIGATION IN NON-INSTRUMENTED SURGERY

Intraoperative spinal navigation technology has been utilized for a wide variety of surgical procedures including tubular minimally invasive disk surgery, endoscopic spine surgery, and spinal tumor resection surgery. Here, we discuss how navigation is presently utilized in several operative techniques and highlight the reported data on the feasibility and efficacy of integrating this technology in each surgical procedure.

Tubular Minimally Invasive Spine Microdiscectomy Surgery

Tubular minimally invasive spine (MIS) microdiscectomy surgical techniques are utilized for degenerative disk disease and herniation throughout the spinal cord for numerous approaches including cervical, lumbar, far lateral lumbar, transthoracic, and thoracolumbar discectomy. Notably, it has been demonstrated that tubular MIS microdiscectomy in the cervical and lumbar spine results in diminished blood loss, reduced postoperative pain, and shorter hospital stays compared with the traditional open techniques.[11] The procedure involves percutaneous localization of the anatomical segment and focus of interest, typically under fluoroscopic guidance, followed by serial dilation of the paraspinal musculature and soft tissues and insertion of a tubular port or retractor over the dilators and through which the surgical decompression is performed.[12] Radiographic localization is essential not only for identifying the appropriate level of the pathology but also for the anatomical localization of the bony elements to optimize the bony exposure, both for adequate decompressive access as well as to limit and avoid iatrogenic instability from overly aggressive bony resection. In this regard, the 3D anatomical representation afforded by iCT-based spinal navigation is far superior to 2D-fluoroscopic guidance.

Navigated Cervical and Lumbar MIS Surgery

The use of spinal navigation, such as with iCT, has been effective in both cervical and lumbar MIS discectomy and offers improved real-time visualization of the operative anatomy.[13] Disk herniation in the cervical and lumbar spine represents the vast majority of symptomatic disk herniation cases.[14,15]

In the cervical spine, spinal navigation technology has proven efficacious and highly valuable in performing posterior cervical foraminotomy (PCF), unilateral laminotomy for bilateral decompression (ULBD), and posterior facet joint fusion (PFJF).[16]

PCF, typically utilized for unilateral cervical radiculopathy, was initially developed as an open procedure; however, the tubular, minimally invasive approach often used today offers similar efficacy while reducing blood loss, postoperative analgesic use, and length of hospital stay.[17,18] This tubular MIS approach involves the placement of a small paramedian incision on the localized level and side of pathology, dilation, and ultimately placement of a tubular retractor through which the lateral aspect of the lamina and medial portion facet joint are removed to complete the foraminotomy.[16] In PCF, 3D intraoperative navigation is often used successfully to identify the precise location of the primary incision and docking site to perform the foraminotomy with the highest degree of safety.[16] Often, both the ipsi- and contralateral foramina can be accessed using this procedural approach, for patients with bilateral radiculopathy, and improved visualization of the contralateral side using intraoperative 3D navigation can prepare the surgeon for optimal positioning and docking for this procedure.[16,18]

ULBD, a unilateral approach for bilateral decompression of the spinal cord, was initially developed in lumbar spine procedures but has since been utilized effectively as an MIS procedure in all levels of the spine column.[16,19,20] Of note, it is a particularly useful procedure in patients with cervical spondylotic myelopathy.[16] In ULBD, intraoperative spinal navigation is used to determine the precise entry point for the placement of a 2 to 3-mm incision at the affected level.[16] After the incision and placement of a tubular retractor, the ipsilateral lamina is accessed and drilled away and the retractor is realigned, and, using an "over-the-top" approach, the spinal cord is safely bypassed to perform the contralateral laminotomy.[16,19] Navigation is used successfully to guide both the trajectory and extent of the laminotomy.[16] The MIS tubular ULBD is equally in efficacy to its open counterpart and reduces exposure, blood loss, muscle manipulation, and removal of bone, making it an often-preferred approach in some elderly or obese patients.[16,21,22]

The PFJF is a procedure aimed at treating cervical spondylotic radiculopathy and myelopathy by percutaneously placing bilateral cervical facet joint cages from a posterior approach, as opposed to the more traditional lateral mass fusion.[16,23–25] Spinal navigation is critical in this procedure, as it allows the surgeon to identify the medial and lateral aspects of the facet and safely enter the facet joint without injuring the nerve root.[16,25] Finally, a cage is placed in the facet joint and secured to the inferior articulating facet, thereby stabilizing the joint space and allowing for the introduction of graft material into the joint.[16] This approach may be similarly efficacious to lateral screw fixation as a successful indirect decompression and fusion method for single-level radiculopathy with high rates of radiographic fusion[25] and similar postoperative cervical segmental stability.[24]

Lumbar MIS Surgery

An estimated 95% of herniated disks occur in the lumbar spine at either L4–L5 or L5–S1; thus, non-instrumented spinal navigation may offer the most significant epidemiological benefit in the treatment of lumbar spine disease.[14,15]

Navigated Lumbar Far-Lateral MIS Discectomy

Extraforaminal or far-lateral lumbar disk herniations (FLDH), first described by Abdullah et al., in 1974,[26] represent 0.3% to 11% of lumbar disk herniations and pose a significant challenge to the spine surgeon.[27–30] The proportion of patients presenting preoperatively with symptoms of sensory dysesthesia has been observed to be greater with FLDH than with other types of disk herniations and the dysesthesia is often significantly more severe. This is thought to be related to the direct compression of the dorsal root ganglion (DRG) by the disk fragment.[31,32]

Foley et al. developed a tubular MIS approach based upon a modification of the earlier Wiltse paramedian approach to reduce approach-related muscle trauma with improved postoperative pain.[33] The technique involves the early identification of the exiting nerve inferior to the rostral pedicle, followed by visualization and resection of the disk herniation.[33] However, this technique involves dissection and manipulation of the exiting nerve root and DRG and may contribute to painful postoperative dysesthesia, potentially leading to poor postoperative outcomes, as has been suggested by cadaveric dissection studies.[34] An alternate technique in which the Kambin triangle (formed by the exiting nerve, the lateral border of the traversing nerve root, and the superior endplate of the caudal vertebral body)[35] is targeted for direct access to the disk has been proposed.[36] While this latter approach presumes a fixed relationship of the exiting nerve root to the disk space and traversing nerve root, it has been shown that this relationship may be quite variable with as many as 83% of patients having a reduced or non-identifiable Kambin triangle.[37] Thus, a challenge of the tubular MIS approach for FLDH surgery is the early identification of the exiting nerve root. A second major challenge is the proper anatomical localization of the bony elements and the disk space lateral to the spine given the paucity of familiar osseous landmarks such as the spinous process and lamina, through which a surgical corridor of safety may be negotiated. While fluoroscopy has been used in MIS surgery as the standard imaging modality for localization, it has the drawbacks of 2D anatomical representation, which is less accurate, and increased radiation exposure to the surgeon and operating room staff.[38,39] We recently demonstrated the utility of iCT navigational guidance for accurate bony anatomical localization in combination with Electromyography stimulation for early localization of the exiting nerve in the MIS tubular, microscopic paramedian approach for resection of far lateral disk herniations.[40]

Transthoracic MIS Discectomy

Thoracic central disk herniations may be calcified and present with myelopathy, often requiring an anterior transthoracic approach for surgical intervention. However, this approach is fraught with complexities including the precise localization of the level of the pathology of interest. Wrong-level thoracic spine surgery is not uncommon and may result in significant neurological morbidity and litigation.[41] Localization is challenging in part because of the similarity of thoracic vertebral segments and their remoteness from fixed identifiable landmarks such as the skull base or the sacrum.

The surgical technique for transthoracic approaches for central disk herniations may be divided into two parts: The approach technique involving the transthoracic/retropleural exposure and the decompressive technique involving the removal of the rib head and pedicle, creation of a trough in the adjacent vertebral bodies extending to the contralateral pedicle, and, finally, decompression of the central canal by removal of the centrally herniated disk material. The 3D anatomical representation of iCT spinal navigation offers superior localization and guidance in these two critical portions of this surgical approach compared with fluoroscopic guidance.

In our technique for the procedure, we percutaneously place a pedicle marker consisting of aneurysm endovascular coils at the level of interest, following which we obtain a CT or post-myelogram CT scan of the thoracic spine to confirm the relationship between the marker and the level of interest. The patient is then taken to the operating room, and, following induction with provision for potential lung isolation, positioned in the lateral decubitus position and secured in place rigidly with 3-inch tape to minimize motion. The posterior and lateral torso is prepared and draped widely in the standard surgical fashion. A DRA is mounted either into the iliac crest or sutured to the flat of the back and an iCT scan is obtained with auto-registration on the Brainlab Curve navigation system. The scan may be autofused with the post-myelogram CT scan or high-resolution MRI scan. The pedicle marker is localized and used to plan the skin incision. A mini-open incision (4–6 cm) is created and a thoracotomy is performed with rib resection if required, with a retropleural approach to obviate the need for a chest tube. An expandable MIS retractor (NuVasive or Globus) is inserted over dilators for visualization of the anatomy of interest. We use a navigable ultrasonic bone scalpel (Misonix) to remove the rib head and to create the trough in the vertebral bodies of the segments adjacent to the disk at the level of pathology. The neural foramen is used to identify the canal and, using a navigable high-speed drill with a coarse 5-mm diamond burr, the pedicle is drilled back to reveal the spinal canal. The remainder of the posterior wall of the vertebral body is then removed with the decompression extending from pedicle to pedicle and exposing the posterior longitudinal ligament (PLL) craniad and caudad to the disk space. The PLL is divided and the disk material removed by peeling it away from the spinal cord. iCT navigational guidance is a very useful adjunct in the confirmatory localization of the surgical level as well as anatomical localization of critical structures such as the rib head, pedicle, and spinal canal during the decompressive phase of the procedure. This is achieved while minimizing radiation exposure to the surgeon and OR staff from fluoroscopic guidance.

MIS Lateral Approach for Central Thoracolumbar Microdiscectomy

Like central thoracic disk herniations, large central disk herniations at the thoracolumbar junction (T11–T12, T12–L1) and in the upper lumbar spine (L1–L2, L2–L3) may represent a management dilemma for the spine surgeon.[42] Given the high density of neural elements located in this anatomical region (conus medullaris, upper cauda equina), the presenting symptoms in patients with upper lumbar disk herniations tend to be more varied than the clear-cut lumbosacral radiculopathy with which patients experiencing lower lumbar disk herniations present.[42–44] Additionally, given the bony anatomical characteristics in this region with more narrow, sagitally oriented facet joints, smaller spinal canal and shorter width of the pars interarticularis, decompressive procedures geared toward the removal of central and large paracentral herniated disk fragments in the upper lumbar spine tend to be destabilizing with twice as many patients than at lower lumbar levels requiring additional fusion procedures.[42] Not surprisingly, the outcomes following surgical intervention for upper lumbar disk herniations tend to be less favorable than are those for lower lumbar disk pathologies.[42]

We recently described a minimally invasive, lateral retroperitoneal, transpsoas, direct transforaminal approach to central and paracentral disk herniation at L1–L2. The approach combines the principles of the extreme or direct lateral retroperitoneal, transpsoas approach targeting the anterior third of the disk space and the posterior, transforaminal approach through the neural foramen utilized in percutaneous endoscopic lumbar discectomy (PELD) with iCT navigational assistance playing a crucial role in the feasibility of the approach.[45]

Endoscopic Applications

The field of spine surgery has seen a resurgence in the utilization of endoscopic approaches in the last decade. Percutaneous endoscopic approaches to the lumbar, thoracolumbar, and thoracic spine utilize a posterolateral, percutaneous trajectory under fluoroscopic guidance to gain access to the spinal canal through a transforaminal approach. As with other MIS approaches, accurate anatomical localization and targeting are critical to the success of the approach. iCT navigational assistance allows for more precise anatomical localization without the increased radiation exposure to the OR staff and surgeon while also increasing the comfort level of the surgeon.[46] However, the challenge here is how to perform the mounting of the DRA and registration in an awake patient given that in most MIS navigated spine cases, the DRA is mounted into the iliac crest. We utilize a technique in which the DRA is either sutured to the skin under local anesthetic or affixed in place with Ioban. The patient is asked to hold their breath during the scan. The accuracy is confirmed by touching the navigation probe to the skin. A trajectory is then planned for access to the neural foramen of interest. Under local anesthetic, the skin is incised and a navigated Jamshidi needle is inserted along the plotted trajectory and docked on the lateral facet at the foramen. A guide wire is inserted through the Jamshidi needle which is removed and over the guide wire are inserted, serial dilators for the endoscopic tools and endoscope (Joimax). A foraminoplasty is performed with a rimming drill, a port is placed and the endoscope is inserted through this. The endoscope itself may be rendered navigable by attaching a DRA.

Tumor Resection Surgery

Perhaps, the greatest progress and widespread adaption of spinal navigation technology in non-instrumented spine cases has been in the field of spinal oncology with the resection of metastatic and primary spinal tumors.

Primary Spinal Tumors

En bloc resection of primary spinal tumor has been shown to result in lower recurrence rates and improved survival.[47] In certain lesions, such as tumors confined within a single thoracic segment, en bloc spondylectomy may not be as challenging, given that the anatomical elements and the tumor are reasonably well defined. However, it may be a challenge where the tumor extends significantly outside of the normal anatomical confines of the bony elements or in sacral or other anatomical lesions. In these instances, the ability to perform en bloc tumor resection may be greatly enhanced by 3D intraoperative anatomical definition with iCT for bony lesions or iCT-fused MRI for soft tissue lesions. Recent case reports have demonstrated that 3D computer navigation systems and intraoperative stereotactic navigation to construct and identify spinal cord tumors significantly enhanced en bloc resection of primary lesions.[48,49]

Metastatic Spinal Tumors

Recent advances in technology have led to a paradigm shift in the treatment of metastatic spinal lesions. Until two decades ago, the mainstay treatment was either radiation therapy or laminectomy followed by radiation therapy.[50–54] As techniques emerged for performing circumferential decompression and stabilization procedures, spine surgeons developed the ability to address both the complex neurological and biomechanical issues that arose in the setting of metastatic spinal pathology.[55,56] Patchell et al. demonstrated that circumferential surgical decompression and stabilization followed by radiation therapy was superior to radiation therapy alone and even to radiation therapy followed by surgical intervention.[57] Further technological advancements in stereotactic body radiotherapy allowed for the delivery of higher-dose, precise, and conformal tumoricidal radiation therapy, with the limitation being the dose exposure of the spinal cord. The goal of surgical intervention could then be seen as addressing any need to stabilize the spine while decompressing the thecal sac sufficiently to allow effective dose delivery to the metastatic focus.[58,59] In these cases, iCT-MRI fusion navigation assistance allows not only for the precise placement of instrumentation but also allows for the precise decompression of the thecal sac.[58,59]

Intradural and Intramedullary Cases

As with extradural tumors, fused iCT-MRI navigational assistance has proved a powerful adjunct in the localization and resection of intradural,[1,5,60] and more recently, intramedullary spinal lesions.[6,60,61] Previous techniques in the resection of intradural lesions have utilized intraoperative ultrasound for localization.[62] However, this imaging modality is most useful following laminectomy or bony removal and is limited in its utility in pre-decompression localization and skin incision planning. In contrast, fused iCT-MRI navigation assistance may be used for incision planning, for tumor localization prior to laminectomy, and for defining the extent of bony removal with laminectomy. This potentially reduces the risk of wrong-level surgery and iatrogenic instability from excessive bone removal.

Recent reports have illustrated the utility of this technology in the localization and resection of intramedullary spinal lesions.[6,60,61] Zhang et al. describe their experience with five patients.[6] Fused iCT-MRI navigation has also been used by our group in the resection of intramedullary spinal cavernoma.[61] We describe the details of this published case in further detail below in the Clinical Case Studies section. A more recent account describes combining fused iCT-MRI with tractography in the resection of intramedullary spinal cord tumors including an ependymoma where the tractography showed the tumor displacing fiber tracts and a glioblastoma where the tumor invaded the fiber tracts.[63] In both instances, the fused iCT-MRI-tractography was essential to the safe total and subtotal resection of the two tumors respectively.

Laser Interstitial Thermal Therapy

Laser interstitial thermal therapy (LITT) first described in 2015, combines laser ablative technology with MRI stereotactic image guidance to deliver ablative thermal treatment to spinal metastatic lesions as a means of achieving epidural decompression and as an alternative to separation surgery.[64] In the operating suite, skin fiducial markers and an MRI-compatible spinous process clamp are placed and an intraoperative MRI scan is obtained with thin slice T2 weighted sequences. The images are then transferred to the image guidance console where surface matching registration is performed. Axial, sagittal, and coronal reconstructions are used to plan trajectories for ideal laser catheter placement targeting the epidural tumor. Using multiple catheters with different trajectories and ablation zones of 10 to 20 mm per catheter, a treatment plan is designed targeting the epidural metastatic disease. Stereotactic radiosurgery may then be used to target the remainder of the vertebral body disease.

CLINICAL CASE STUDIES

Posterior Cervical Discectomy Case

History/Clinical Presentation

A 52-year-old man with a past medical history of asthma presented with left-hand weakness. One year prior he was moving a refrigerator when the refrigerator slipped pulling his arms forward rapidly. The patient noted that since then he has had pain in the back of his neck that radiated down the left upper extremity. He subsequently developed left upper extremity paresthesias with numbness and associated weakness that was most notable in the left fourth and fifth digits. He later began to develop cramping and weakness in the first three digits of the left upper extremity that worsened with use throughout the day. The physical examination was notable for left-hand grasp weakness, and diminished sensation to light touch in the left upper extremity in an ulnar distribution. The patient underwent electrodiagnostic testing which showed no evidence of ulnar neuropathy and was suggestive of C8 radiculopathy.

Preoperative Imaging

The initial MRI revealed a significant loss of lordosis in the cervical spine with left-sided disk herniation at the C7–T1 spinal levels causing significant nerve impingement. The CT scan of the cervical spine showed no calcification of the herniated disks (Fig. 7.1A–D).

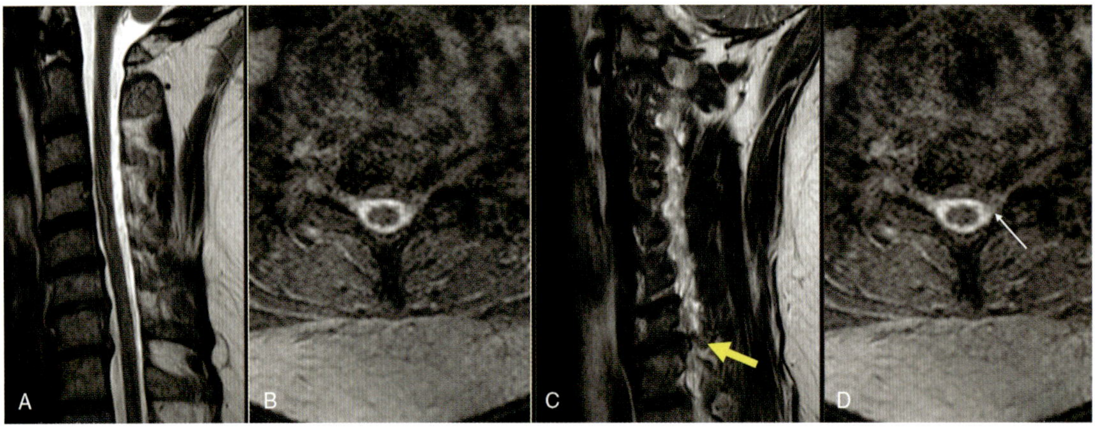

FIG. 7.1 Preoperative midsagittal (A), axial (B, D), and left parasagittal (D) T2-weighted MRI scan of the cervical spine showing a left C7–T1 disk herniation causing impingement on the left C8 nerve root (*arrows* in C and D).

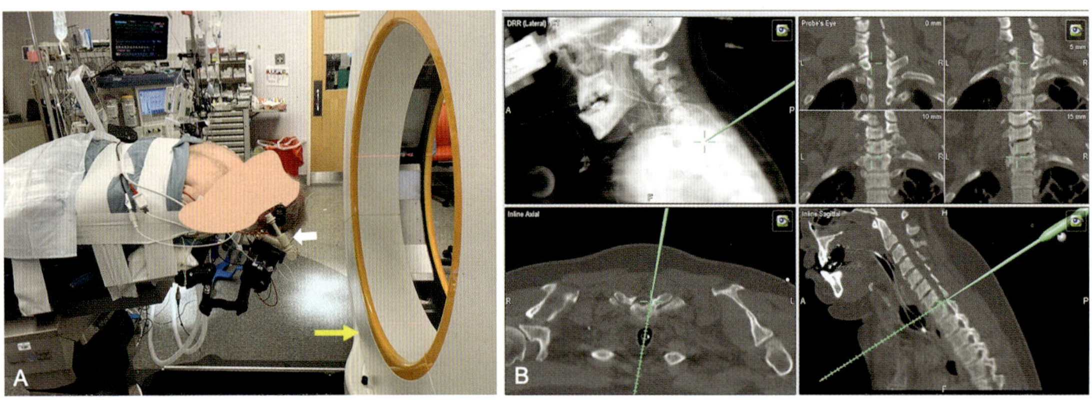

FIG. 7.2 Intraoperative setup (A) with iCT gantry (*yellow arrow*) shown. The patient is prone with his head in a radiolucent Mayfield frame and secured with 4-inch tape. The clamp for the Brainlab reference array (*white arrow*) is attached to the Mayfield frame. The actual array is attached in a sterile fashion after the patient is draped. (B) A screenshot from the Brainlab Curve navigation system showing the localization of the left C7–T1 interspace.

Surgical Plan

The patient is placed prone, with the head fixated using a three-point radiolucent Mayfield fixation device (Fig. 7.2A). The skin is prepared and draped widely in the standard surgical fashion. A digital reference array (DRA) is mounted onto the radiolucent Mayfield fixation device. An iCT scan is then obtained spanning the sacrum for localization and the operative level of interest. Respirations are suspended by anesthesia for the scan to avoid motion that may introduce errors in the registration process. The auto-registration of the iCT scan to the reference array is performed by the Brainlab Curve navigation system. Accuracy is checked by touching the navigated probe lightly on the skin following which trajectories are selected for access to the disk level of interest and used to plan the skin incision. The skin incision was planned based upon the autofused imaging and navigation to optimally target the C7–T1 disk space on the left side (see Fig. 7.2B). We also mounted a DRA onto the slimmest dilator and registered it on the Curve system to render it navigable (Fig. 7.3A). Similarly, we rendered the MIS drill navigable by attaching a DRA to the back end (see Fig. 7.3A).

The skin and thoracodorsal fascia were incised. The navigable dilator was inserted docking on the lamina at the level of interest and medial to the lamino-facet junction. Blunt dissection was performed with the dilator to strip the muscle off the bone revealing the C7–T1 facet and lamina. For the cannulated dilator, a guide wire was inserted through it to place the next-sized dilator. Alternatively, if the dilator is not cannulated, the dilator can be removed and re-inserted along with the next-sized dilator following which the navigable dilator can be removed to allow insertion of the remaining dilators. The tubular retractor was inserted, and the navigable dilator re-inserted to check for anatomical localization. Following the ideal positioning of the tubular retractor, the dilators were removed, the retractor was secured with a fixed arm, and the light source was attached. The operating microscope was brought into the field for further magnification and illumination to perform microscopic dissection. The navigable MIS drill was used to perform a hemilaminotomy at C7–T1 being careful to ensure that only a limited partial facetectomy is performed. Of note, the navigable probes may be used to confirm the surgical level of interest and to ensure adequate decompression and for localization when performing bilateral decompressions via a unilateral approach. Once decompression was completed the wound was irrigated and closed after achieving appropriate hemostasis

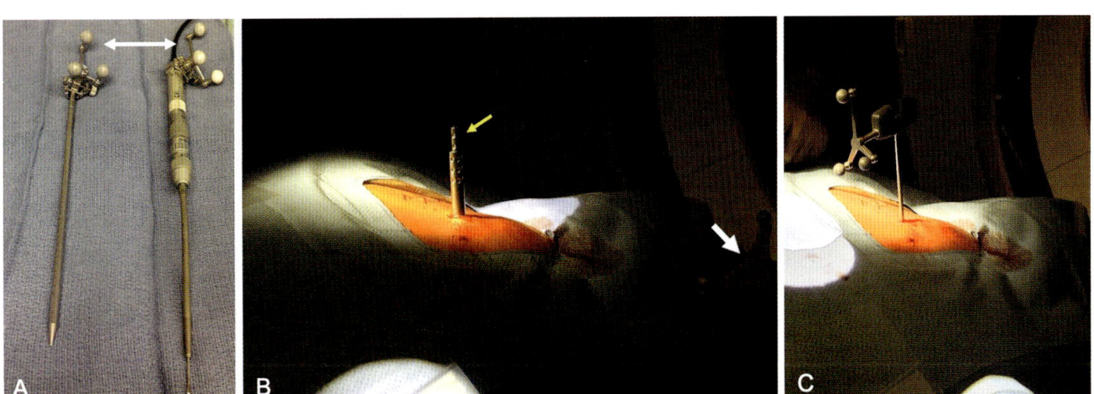

FIG. 7.3 Minimally invasive spine (MIS) dilator (A; left) and MIS drill (A; right) rendered navigable by the attachment of a digital reference array (DRA; *double arrows*) and used for targeting of the C7–T1 interspace on the left. (B) DRA (*large white arrow*) and dilators following insertion (*yellow arrow*) in a similar patient to that described in the case example. In this patient, a navigable Jamshidi needle and a guide wire (C) were used for the initial localization.

Intraoperative Imaging

Intraoperative imaging was utilized primarily for surgical planning. The intraoperative imaging was consistent with presurgical imaging and demonstrated degenerative disk disease in the lower cervical spine.

Postoperative Recovery and Follow-up

Three weeks postoperatively, the patient was recovering well from the surgery with minimal postoperative pain. The patient noted a significant reduction in the posterior neck pain that radiated to the left arm.

Overall this case of a posterior cervical discectomy utilizing a tubular MIS approach for a patient with C8 radiculopathy is an example of how spinal navigation in non-instrumented spine surgery can be utilized to optimize the precision and safety of the given procedure. Intraoperative spinal navigation based on the autofused imaging obtained with the iCT and preoperative imaging proved useful from the outset of the procedure in determining the optimal initial incision. The surgical team continued to benefit from and utilize the intraoperative navigation system to verify the spinal level and precise anatomic localization of the surgical level which would be challenging at the cervicothoracic junction in a patient with a BMI > 40. Additionally, the surgical equipment used in the procedure, such as the dilators, were developed to register with the spinal navigation system providing the surgeon with visual feedback on precise anatomic location in real-time while performing a critical component of the operation. Spinal navigation in cervical spine procedures can be especially useful given the relatively small anatomic landmarks in the cervical spine and the importance of precise navigation needed to complete safe and effective procedures.[16] The MIS approach taken in the posterior cervical discectomy is significantly enhanced by intraoperative spinal navigation.

Transthoracic Discectomy

History/Clinical Presentation

A 55-year-old woman with a past medical history notable for chronic back pain, arthritis, and carpal tunnel syndrome presented with mid-back pain and bilateral lower extremity paresthesia. This patient's symptoms began after a diving accident that took place several years prior to presentation. She had non-radiating mid-back pain that worsened with standing and walking for prolonged periods. the concurrent symptoms included mild bilateral tingling and numbness in the feet. The patient denied any weakness in the upper or lower extremities, changes in bowel or bladder function, or other neurologic symptoms. On physical examination, the patient presented with hyperreflexia in the lower extremities bilaterally and a positive Romberg sign, with an otherwise normal physical examination.

Preoperative Imaging

MRI and CT of the thoracic spine revealed T10–T11 disk herniation with extrusion causing central canal stenosis and spinal cord deformity. MRI imaging of the spinal cord was suggestive of signal changes at this level (Fig. 7.4A–D). At the segments rostral to the T10–T11 disk space, numerous partially calcified thoracic disk herniations were also causing spinal cord compression.

The patient presentation, physical examination findings, and imaging together suggest thoracic myelopathy secondary to the T10–11 disk herniation.

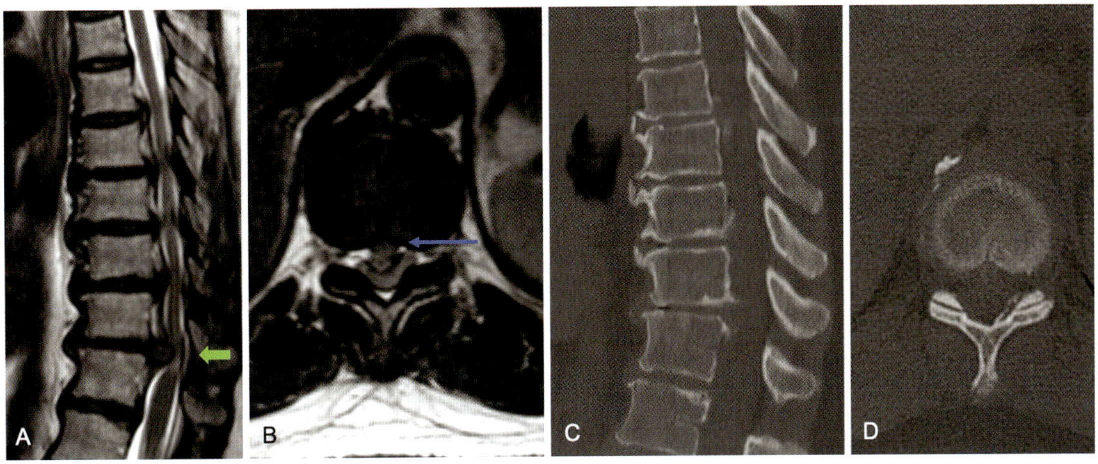

FIG. 7.4 Preoperative sagittal (A) and axial (B) MRI. Sagittal (C) and axial (D) CT scan of the thoracic spine in a 55-year-old female patient presenting with myelopathy. Although she had multilevel thoracic disk herniations, the non-calcified T10–T11 (*arrows* in A and B) causing marked cord compression with signal change was felt to be the most severe and in need of surgical intervention.

Surgical Plan

The decision to undergo thoracic spine decompression and discectomy was made by the patient after a thorough discussion of multiple treatment options. It was determined that a minimally invasive, transthoracic decompression and partial corpectomy was the best approach. Given the location of the disease, we planned on using navigational assistance and electrophysiologic monitoring for a right-sided approach. Preoperatively pedicle markers were placed percutaneously by interventional radiology at the T10 and T11 pedicles to facilitate intraoperative localization (Fig. 7.5A–D).

The patient was placed in the right lateral decubitus position with appropriate support while maintaining the spine parallel to the floor. Intraoperative 2D fluoroscopy was used to localize the previously placed pedicle markers to mark the planned incision directly over the T10 rib (see Fig. 7.5D). The skin was prepared and draped in the standard surgical fashion. We then attached a digital reference frame for intraoperative navigation directly sutured to the patient and obtained a 3D iCT scan. The skin overlying the 10th rib was then incised and intercostal musculature dissected (Fig. 7.6A). The T10 rib was identified and undermined along with the underlying neurovascular bundle from the inferior aspect of the rib. A 5-cm piece of the rib was removed with the rib cutter. The pleura was identified and blunt dissection performed toward the thoracic spine with care to remain in the retropleural space.

The T10–T11 rib heads were identified and the dissection was continued anteriorly to the respective vertebral bodies dissected. The level of interest was confirmed with the navigation probe (see Fig. 7.6B). The T11 pedicle and T10 neural foramen were identified with the navigation probe (see Fig. 7.6C), exposed, and the T10 segmental artery and sympathetic chain were identified and bluntly dissected away from the T10–T11 disk. A partial corpectomy trough was created in the posterior third of the T10 and T11 vertebral bodies adjacent to the disk space with navigable ultrasonic bone scalpel and osteotomes. The posterior cortex was removed exposing the PLL with a navigable large-diamond tipped drill, with the bony removal carried to the contralateral T11 pedicle (see Fig. 7.6C and D).

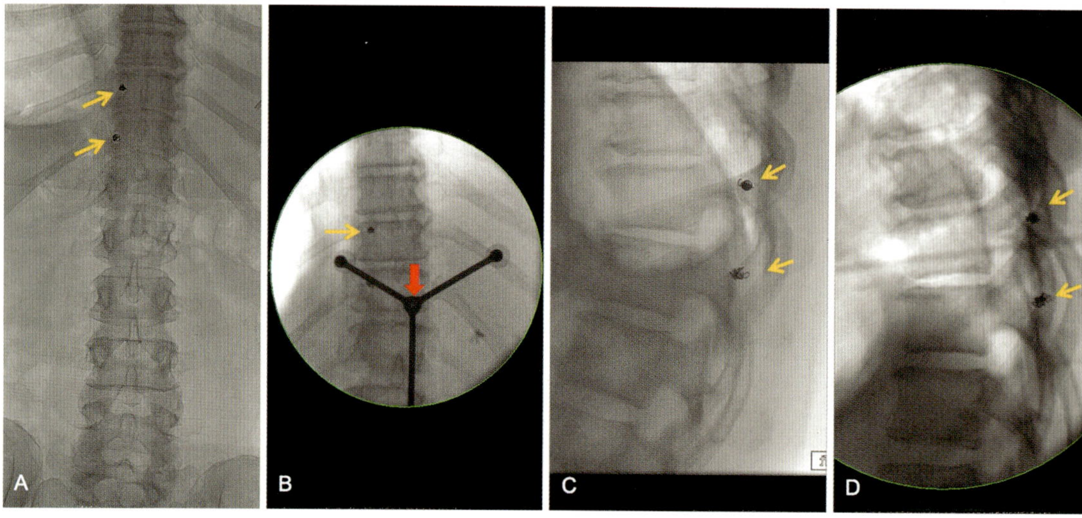

FIG. 7.5 (A–D) Marking coils (*yellow arrows*) placed percutaneously by interventional radiology preoperatively for localization of the right T10 and T11 pedicles. Note the overlapping reference array on intraoperative imaging (B; *red arrow*). (D) Radiopaque stylet (*white arrow*) used to localize the T10–T11 disk space and plan the skin incision intraoperatively.

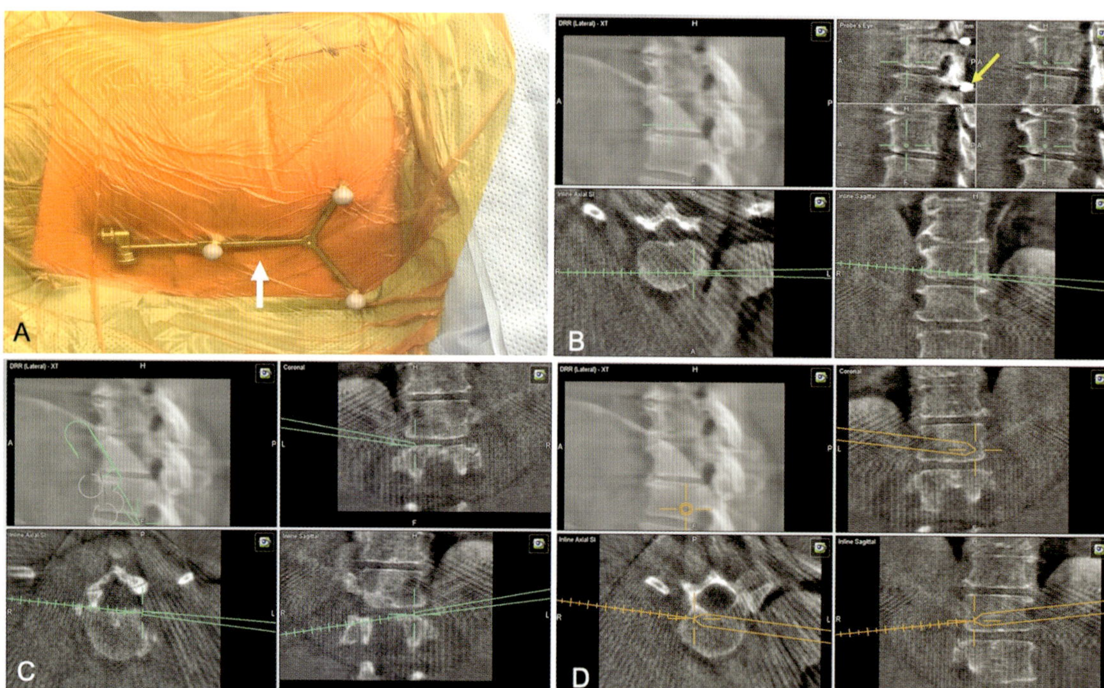

FIG. 7.6 A patient in the right lateral decubitus position (A) with the *white arrow* showing reference array sutured to the back prior to the iCT scan and auto-registration on the Brainlab Curve navigation system. A screenshot from the Curve navigation system showing localization of the T10–T11 interspace after a transthoracic, retropleural approach (B). Note the localizing pedicle markers (B, *yellow arrow*). Localization of the left T10 neural foramen with the Brainlab pointer (C) and screenshot showing the navigated drill position reaching across the canal to the contralateral pedicle (D).

The exposed PLL was then dissected away from the dura and thecal sac rostral and caudal to the disk herniation. A large partially calcified disk herniation was visualized invading into the thecal sac. Pituitary rongeurs and microdissectors were used to dissect the disk herniation from the thecal sac without placing traction on the spinal cord. The disk herniation was removed and the decompression extending to the contralateral pedicle at T10 was verified. Decompression of the thecal sac was verified using microinstruments. No anterior reconstruction was necessary as the bony removal was not deemed destabilizing. The wound was then irrigated and closed after achieving hemostasis and applying an antibiotic, saline solution.

Intraoperative Imaging

The intraoperative imaging in this case included fluoroscopy, iCT, and intraoperative x-ray (see Figs. 7.5 and 7.6). Intraoperative imaging was utilized for navigation during the procedure, as described above.

Postoperative Imaging

MRI taken one day after the procedure demonstrated a successfully decompressed T10–T11, evidenced by a widely patent central canal at T10–T11 (Fig. 7.7A–D). The postoperative MRI also demonstrated persistent cord deformity and an intermediate central high cord signal in the thoracic spine at the surgical level. The postoperative MRI also revealed additional areas of degenerative disease including right paracentral protrusion at T6–T7, central extrusion at T7–T8, right paracentral protrusion at T8–T9, central extrusion at T9–T10, and a broad-based bulge at T11–T12.

Postoperative Recovery and Follow-up

This patient's immediate postoperative recovery was without complications. At the four-month postoperative follow-up, this patient reported a significant reduction in back pain, noting that the pain was now occasional and mild. This patient noted left-sided flank

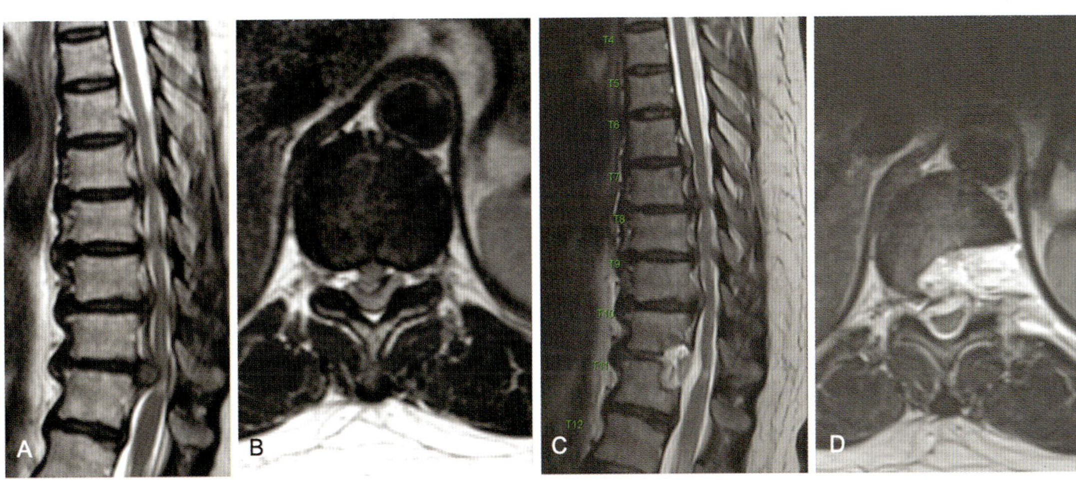

FIG. 7.7 Pre- and postoperative sagittal (A, C) and axial (B, D) T2-weighted MRI scans showing resection of the large T10–T11 disk herniation.

numbness as well as continued bilateral lower extremity numbness. The patient denied any weakness or other neurologic issues. Her physical examination was within normal limits except for hyperreflexia in the bilateral lower extremities.

As described previously, iCT and 3D fluoroscopy are highly valuable tools when performing a discectomy using a transthoracic approach. By using the fluoroscopic markers and intraoperative navigation to verify and re-verify the surgical area of interest in planning helped ensure that the operation is performed at the correct vertebral level while minimizing the size of the incision and dissection required to operate safely and effectively. This approach, which makes extensive use of spinal navigation systems and surgical equipment, allowed for the targeted and safe and successful treatment of this patient's lower thoracic disk disease.

Intramedullary Spinal Cord Cavernoma

The following case description and images have been published by our team separately in Moldovan et al.[61]

History/Clinical Presentation

A 54-year-old man came in with primary symptoms of back pain, bilateral lower extremity weakness, numbness, and saddle parasthesias. This patient also rapidly developed bowel and bladder incontinence. The reported bilateral lower extremity weakness and numbness were recapitulated on physical examination.

Preoperative Imaging

MRI of the spine demonstrated a T1-hyperintense and mixed T2-hyperintense intramedullary lesion at the level of T11 (Fig. 7.8.1). On T2 the mass also demonstrated a hypointense rim along its periphery that did not extend to the pial surface. There was marked edema within the distal spinal cord and conus medullaris as demonstrated by T2 hyperintensity.

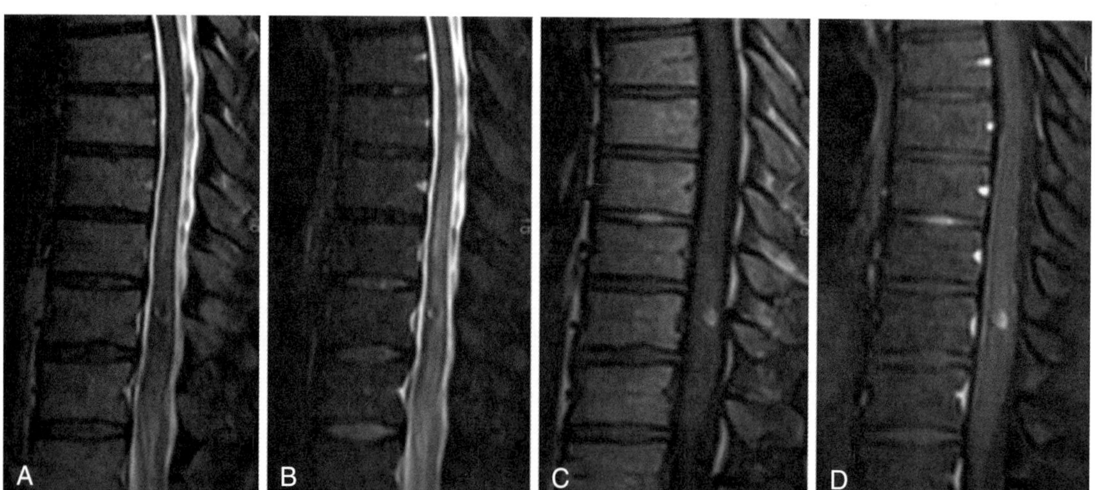

FIG. 7.8-1 Preoperative sagittal spine images demonstrating the intermedullary lesion at T11. MRI images shown include a T2-weighted image (A), Short Tau Inversion Recovery sequence (B), T1-weighted image prior to contrast (C), and a T1-weighted postcontrast image (D) of the thoracic spine in the sagittal plane.

High-resolution spinal magnetic resonance angiography revelaed no evidence of arteriovenous malformation or fistula. Taken together the radiologic imaging was suggestive of an intramedullary cavernoma, hemorrhagic metastatic lesion, or a hemorrhagic primary spinal cord neoplasm.

Surgical Plan

After careful discussion with the patient and their family about surgical and non-surgical options to treat the progressive neurologic symptoms, the decision was made to undergo surgical resection of the intramedullary lesion. Given the location of the presumed cavernoma that did not present to the pial surface, the decision was made to utilize fused MRI-iCT with navigation assistance to localize the intramedullary lesion intraoperatively for resection.

For the procedure, the patient was induced under general endotracheal anesthesia in the standard fashion, and electrodes were placed to monitor somatosensory-evoked potentials, motor-evoked potentials, and D-wave spinal cord monitoring proximal to the lesion. A high-resolution MRI scan, obtained preoperatively, was uploaded onto the Brainlab Curve navigation system (Brainlab AG, Munich, Germany), where the lesion was outlined on the MRI scan in the coronal, saggittal, and axial planes using the software's "Smartbrush" application. The patient was then placed prone on the radiolucent iCT operating table. A percutaneous pedicle marker had been placed preoperatively to localize the T11 rib and pedicle with intraoperative fluoroscopy for planning the incision (illustrated in Fig. 7.8.2).

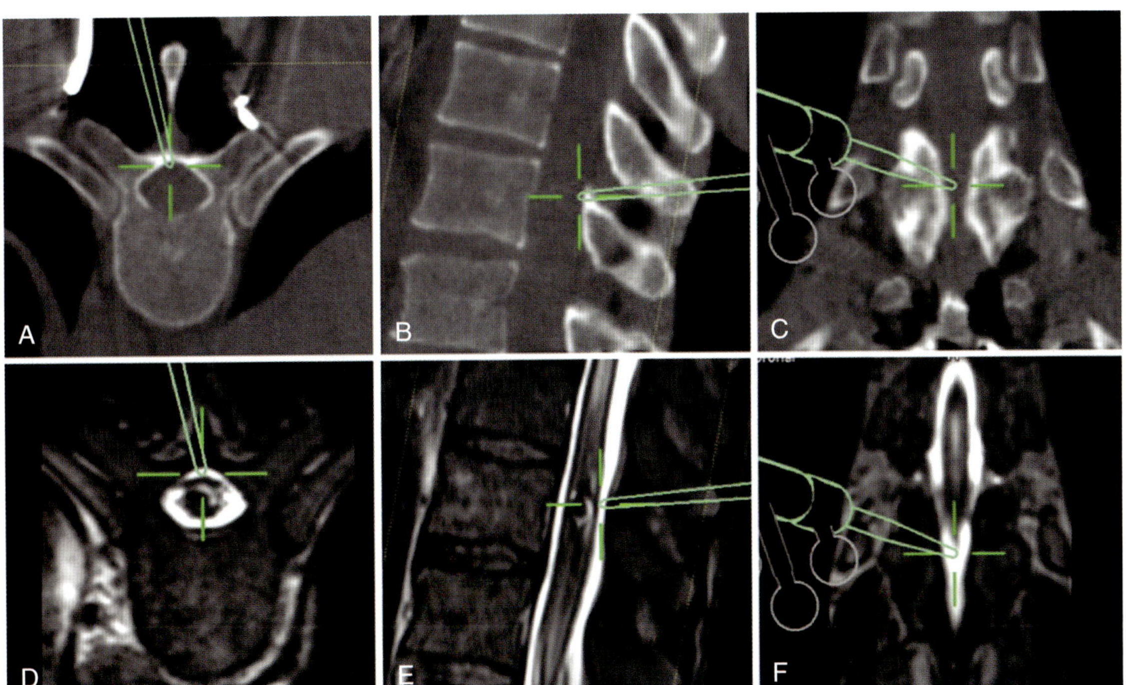

FIG. 7.8-2 This figure demonstrates CT images in the axial (A), sagittal (B), and coronal planes (C) obtained intraoperatively. (D–F) Shows fused, preoperative T2-weighted magnetic resonance imaging with the intraoperative CT imaging showing the corresponding anatomy in identical sequences for navigation purposes.

The T10–T12 dorsal spinal elements were exposed and a difital reference array for the Brainlab system was mounted onto the T12 spinous process, after which an iCT scan (Airo iCT) was obtained. The iCT scan was autofused with the MRI using bony anatomic landmarks, which allows for the navigation screen to display navigable images taken using MRI, iCT, or both in the saggittal, coronal, axial, and in-line planes. The high-resolution fused MRI-iCT image with navigation assistance was used to complete the bony opening and plan dural opening safely and adequately.

A microscope was used to perform an arachnoid-sparing dural opening, after which a proximal subarachnoid electrode was placed for monitoring spinal cord D-waves proximal to the lesion. No distal electrode was placed given the caudal position of the lesion. The arachnoid was then carefully opened and the intrameduallry lesion visualized without extension on the pial surface. Prominent vessels were noted on the surface of the spinal cord and the navigation probe was used for precise intramedullary lesion localization. Navigation proved useful to plan the myelotomy that voided the large pial veins. Somatosensory Evoked Potentials or Motor Evoked Potentials were absent during the myelotomy which was made off the midline on the left side. Careful microdissection was performed with microforceps and microdissectors to remove the hematoma and resect the lesion. The removed lesions were sent for pathologic evaluation. Afterward, adequate hemostasis was ensured prior to re-approximation of the dura and replacement of the lamina using Synthes laminoplasty plates and screws (Raynham, MA, USA).

Intraoperative Imaging

iCT and fluoroscopy were used intraoperatively and fused with the preoperative MRI of the spinal cord as described above.

Postoperative Imaging, Recovery, and Follow-up

The postoperative MRI completed with gadolinium revealed no residual lesion (see Fig. 7.8.3). Surgical pathologic evaluation showed a hypercellular, gliotic neuropil with hemorrhage, hemosiderin deposition, and hemosiderin-laden macrophages consistent with a cavernous angioma. The patient's neurologic examination and symptoms were unchanged immediately in the postoperative period. Postoperative MRI demonstrated complete resection, which supported the decision to not pursue subsequent adjuvant treatment. Follow-up examination in 6 weeks revealed improved motor function postoperatively in the left lower extremity with the return of bladder function. After 4 months this patient demonstrated improved strength in the bilateral extremity, with some persistent scattered sensory loss.

FUTURE DIRECTIONS

Spinal navigation technology offers an important opportunity for innovative approaches with existing surgical technology. Two broad areas in spine surgery that show promise to grow significantly with the integration and further development of spinal navigation technology are the use of augmented reality in spine surgery and robotic surgery.

Augmented Reality in Spinal Navigation

Virtual Augmented Reality (AR) systems represent a promising form of developing technology that allows for computer-generated data to be superimposed on the real world by projecting images and video onto lenses or monitors, thereby augmenting or enhancing

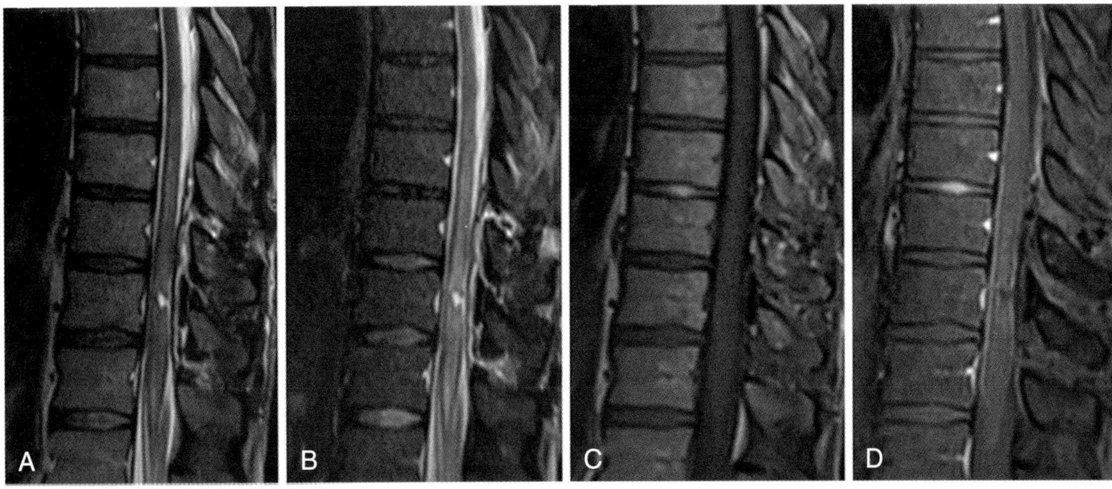

FIG. 7.8-3 Postoperative sagittal spine images obtained 48 hours after surgery demonstrating the resected intermedullary lesion at T11. The MRI images shown include a T2-weighted image (A), Short Tau Inversion Recovery sequence (B), T1-weighted image prior to contrast (C), and a T1-weighted postcontrast image (D) of the thoracic spine in the sagittal plane.

the real-time visual data available to the viewer, and, in the case of neurosurgery, providing surgeons with real-time visualization of key anatomic structures.[65] AR systems can be designed to provide guided 2D and 3D rendering of the spine and relevant structures based on CT or other imaging, and have demonstrated utility and enhanced efficacy in some preliminary spine procedures including pedicle placement in the thoracolumbar spine and MIS approaches for spinal tumors and degenerative disk disease.[65–69] AR may prove advantageous in spine surgery by improving workflow and reducing procedure time compared to the current spinal navigation techniques discussed in this chapter, as some preliminary studies have suggested.[66,70] AR use in spinal navigation for spine surgery is a burgeoning area of research that has demonstrated the potential for this technology in enhancing the accuracy of spine surgery by allowing surgeons to visualize the classic bony landmarks as well as in cases where the patient pathology significantly alters the patient anatomy (e.g., spinal tumors or severe scoliosis).[65,68] Continued research is critical in this area to determine whether this technology provides significant benefit and proves cost-effective for broader use.

Robotic Surgery Technology

Robotic assisted spine surgery is a recent development. The technology involves an elaborate software platform that allows for the pre-planning of pedicle screw trajectories and an automated robotic arm that allows for precise instrumentation placement along the preselected trajectories. The strengths of this technology are two-fold. The first is the ability to streamline the intraoperative workflow by performing screw trajectory planning in the preoperative phase and thus potentially allowing for shorter operative times. The second is the ability to perform "fixed trajectory pedicle screw cannulation" and thereby eliminate the errors introduced by human arm oscillations. However, there are limitations to this technology. Firstly, it does not eliminate errors introduced by patient motion and changes in the relationship between navigated instruments and trajectories and patient anatomy. Secondly, the focus on fixed trajectory pedicle cannulation means there is markedly decreased utility in non-instrumented spine cases where the aim of navigation is anatomical *localization* rather than pedicle *targeting*. Nonetheless, as the technology evolves to incorporate a more robust software and spinal instrument platform, it is not inconceivable that this technology may be used in more precise decompressive and resection indications in non-instrumented spine surgery.

In short, these advancements have allowed for more precise decompressive and lesion resection procedures, and further research is needed to fully uncover their potential to advance the field.

CONCLUSION

Spinal navigation technology has enhanced precision and may confer added safety for a host of non-instrumented surgical procedures in the spine including minimally invasive spine surgery, endoscopic approaches, and spine tumor resection surgery. While navigation technology in spine surgery developed and evolved primarily as a means for accurate targeting of pedicle anatomy for placement of spinal instrumentation, recent advancements have allowed the implementation of this technology in the anatomical localization of bony and non-bony spinal anatomical elements important in performing non-instrumented spine surgery.

REFERENCES

1. Overley SC, Cho SK, Mehta AI, Arnold PM. Navigation and robotics in spinal surgery: Where are we now? *Neurosurgery*. 2017;80(3S):S86–S99. https://doi.org/10.1093/neuros/nyw077.
2. Peters TM, Clark JA, Pike GB, et al. Stereotactic neurosurgery planning on a personal-computer-based work station. *J Digit Imaging*. 1989;2(2):75–81. https://doi.org/10.1007/BF03168023.
3. Wild AM, Xuereb JH, Marks PV, Gleave JR. Computerized tomographic stereotaxy in the management of 200 consecutive intracranial mass lesions. Analysis of indications, benefits and outcome. *Br J Neurosurg*. 1990;4(5):407–415. https://doi.org/10.3109/02688699008992763.
4. Konakondla S, Albers JA, Li X, et al. Maximizing sacral chordoma resection by precise 3-dimensional tumor modeling in the operating room using intraoperative computed tomography registration with preoperative magnetic resonance imaging fusion and intraoperative neuronavigation: a case series. *World Neurosurg*. 2019;125:e1125–e1131. https://doi.org/10.1016/j.wneu.2019.01.257.
5. Maduri R, Bobinski L, Duff JM. Image merge tailored access resection (IMTAR) of spinal intradural tumors. Technical report of 13 cases. *World Neurosurg*. 2017;98:594–602. https://doi.org/10.1016/j.wneu.2016.05.092.
6. Zhang P, Wang G, Sun Z, et al. Application of multimodal image fusion to precisely localize small intramedullary spinal cord tumors. *World Neurosurg*. 2018;118:246–249. https://doi.org/10.1016/j.wneu.2018.07.034.
7. Bandela JR, Jacob RP, Arreola M, Griglock TM, Bova F, Yang M. Use of CT-based intraoperative spinal navigation: management of radiation exposure to operator, staff, and patients. *World Neurosurg*. 2013;79(2):390–394. https://doi.org/10.1016/j.wneu.2011.05.019.
8. Oddy MJ, Aldam CH. Ionising radiation exposure to orthopaedic trainees: the effect of sub-specialty training. *Ann R Coll Surg Engl*. 2006;88(3):297–301. https://doi.org/10.1308/003588406X98702.
9. Theocharopoulos N, Perisinakis K, Damilakis J, Papadokostakis G, Hadjipavlou A, Gourtsoyiannis N. Occupational exposure from common fluoroscopic projections used in orthopaedic surgery. *J Bone Jt Surg Am*. 2003;85(9):1698–1703. https://doi.org/10.2106/00004623-200309000-00007.
10. Mendelsohn D, Strelzow J, Dea N, et al. Patient and surgeon radiation exposure during spinal instrumentation using intraoperative computed tomography-based navigation. *Spine J*. 2016;16(3):343–354. https://doi.org/10.1016/j.spinee.2015.11.020.
11. Dasenbrock HH, Juraschek SP, Schultz LR, et al. The efficacy of minimally invasive discectomy compared with open discectomy: a meta-analysis of prospective randomized controlled trials. *J Neurosurg Spine*. 2012;16(5):452–462. https://doi.org/10.3171/2012.1.SPINE11404.
12. Perez-Cruet MJ, Foley KT, Isaacs RE, et al. Microendoscopic lumbar discectomy: technical note. *Neurosurgery*. 2002;51(5 suppl):S129–S136.

13. Vaishnav AS, Othman YA, Virk SS, Gang CH, Qureshi SA. Current state of minimally invasive spine surgery. *J Spine Surg*. 2019;5(suppl 1):S2–S10. https://doi.org/10.21037/jss.2019.05.02.
14. Jordan J, Konstantinou K, O'Dowd J. Herniated lumbar disc. *BMJ Clin Evid*. 2009;2009:1118.
15. Evaniew N, Khan M, Drew B, Kwok D, Bhandari M, Ghert M. Minimally invasive versus open surgery for cervical and lumbar discectomy: a systematic review and meta-analysis. *CMAJ, (Open)*. 2014;2(4):E295–E305. https://doi.org/10.9778/cmajo.20140048.
16. Hussain I, Schmidt FA, Kirnaz S, Wipplinger C, Schwartz TH, Härtl R. MIS approaches in the cervical spine. *J Spine Surg*. 2019;5(suppl 1):S74–S83. https://doi.org/10.21037/jss.2019.04.21.
17. Henderson CM, Hennessy RG, Shuey Jr HM, Shackelford EG. Posterior-lateral foraminotomy as an exclusive operative technique for cervical radiculopathy: a review of 846 consecutively operated cases. *Neurosurgery*. 1983;13(5):504–512. https://doi.org/10.1227/00006123-198311000-00004.
18. Winder MJ, Thomas KC. Minimally invasive versus open approach for cervical laminoforaminotomy. *Can J Neurol Sci*. 2011;38(2):262–267. https://doi.org/10.1017/s0317167100011446.
19. Hur JW, Kim JS, Shin MH, Ryu KS. Minimally invasive posterior cervical decompression using tubular retractor: the technical note and early clinical outcome. *Surg Neurol Int*. 2014;5:34. https://doi.org/10.4103/2152-7806.128915.
20. Abbas SF, Spurgas MP, Szewczyk BS, Yim B, Ata A, German JW. A comparison of minimally invasive posterior cervical decompression and open anterior cervical decompression and instrumented fusion in the surgical management of degenerative cervical myelopathy. *Neurosurg Focus*. 2016;40(6):E7. https://doi.org/10.3171/2016.3.FOCUS1650.
21. Wang T, Han C, Jiang H, Tian P. The effect of obesity on clinical outcomes after minimally invasive surgery of the spine: a systematic review and meta-analysis. *World Neurosurg*. 2018;110:e438–e449. https://doi.org/10.1016/j.wneu.2017.11.010.
22. Avila MJ, Walter CM, Baaj AA. Outcomes and complications of minimally invasive surgery of the lumbar spine in the elderly. *Cureus*. 2016;8(3):e519. https://doi.org/10.7759/cureus.519.
23. Goel A. Interfacetal intra-articular spacers: emergence of a concept. *J Craniovertebr Junction Spine*. 2016;7(2):72–74. https://doi.org/10.4103/0974-8237.181825.
24. Voronov LI, Siemionow KB, Havey RM, Carandang G, Patwardhan AG. Biomechanical evaluation of DTRAX(®) posterior cervical cage stabilization with and without lateral mass fixation. *Med Devices (Auckl)*. 2016;9:285–290. https://doi.org/10.2147/MDER.S111031.
25. Siemionow K, Janusz P, Phillips FM, et al. Clinical and radiographic results of indirect decompression and posterior cervical fusion for single-level cervical radiculopathy using an expandable implant with 2-year follow-up. *J Neurol Surg A*. 2016;77(6):482–488. https://doi.org/10.1055/s-0036-1584210.
26. Abdullah AF, Wolber PG, Warfield JR, Gunadi IK. Surgical management of extreme lateral lumbar disc herniations: review of 138 cases. *Neurosurgery*. 1988;22(4):648–653. https://doi.org/10.1227/00006123-198804000-00005.
27. Darden 2nd BV, Wade JF, Alexander R, Wood KE, Rhyne AL III, Hicks JR. Far lateral disc herniations treated by microscopic fragment excision. Techniques and results. *Spine (Phila Pa 1976)*. 1995;20(13):1500–1505. https://doi.org/10.1097/00007632-199507000-00011.
28. Epstein NE, Epstein JA, Carras R, Hyman RA. Far lateral lumbar disc herniations and associated structural abnormalities. An evaluation in 60 patients of the comparative value of CT, MRI, and myelo-CT in diagnosis and management. *Spine (Phila Pa 1976)*. 1990;15(6):534–539. https://doi.org/10.1097/00007632-199006000-00019.
29. Jenis LG, An HS, Gordin R. Foraminal stenosis of the lumbar spine: a review of 65 surgical cases. *Am J Orthop Belle Mead NJ*. 2001;30(3):205–211.
30. Porchet F, Chollet-Bornand A, de Tribolet N. Long-term follow up of patients surgically treated by the far-lateral approach for foraminal and extraforaminal lumbar disc herniations. *J Neurol Surg*. 1999;90(1suppl):59–66. https://doi.org/10.3171/spi.1999.90.1.0059.
31. O'Hara LJ, Marshall RW. Far lateral lumbar disc herniation. The key to the intertransverse approach. *J Bone Jt Surg Br*. 1997;79(6):943–947. https://doi.org/10.1302/0301-620x.79b6.7876.
32. Park HW, Park KS, Park MS, Kim SM, Chung SY, Lee DS. The comparisons of surgical outcomes and clinical characteristics between the far lateral lumbar disc herniations and the paramedian lumbar disc herniations. *Korean J Spine*. 2013;10(3):155–159. https://doi.org/10.14245/kjs.2013.10.3.155.
33. Foley KT, Smith MM, Rampersaud YR. Microendoscopic approach to far-lateral lumbar disc herniation. *Neurosurg Focus*. 1999;7(5):e5. https://doi.org/10.3171/foc.1999.7.6.6.
34. Viswanathan R, Swamy NK, Tobler WD, Greiner AL, Keller JT, Dunsker SB. Extraforaminal lumbar disc herniations: microsurgical anatomy and surgical approach. *J Neurol Surg*. 2002;96(2 suppl):206–211. https://doi.org/10.3171/spi.2002.96.2.0206.
35. Kambin P, Brager MD. Percutaneous posterolateral discectomy. *Anat mechanism Clin Orthop Relat Res*. 1987;223(223):145–154.
36. Siu TL, Lin K. Microscopic tubular discectomy for far lateral lumbar disc herniation. *J Clin Neurosci*. 2016;33:129–133. https://doi.org/10.1016/j.jocn.2016.02.040.
37. Ozer AF, Suzer T, Can H, et al. Anatomic assessment of variations in Kambin's triangle: a surgical and cadaver study. *World Neurosurg*. 2017;100:498–503. https://doi.org/10.1016/j.wneu.2017.01.057.
38. Ahn Y, Kim CH, Lee JH, Lee SH, Kim JS. Radiation exposure to the surgeon during percutaneous endoscopic lumbar discectomy: a prospective study. *Spine (Phila Pa 1976)*. 2013;38(7):617–625. https://doi.org/10.1097/BRS.0b013e318275ca58.
39. Iprenburg M, Wagner R, Godschalx A, Telfeian AE. Patient radiation exposure during transforaminal lumbar

endoscopic spine surgery: a prospective study. *Neurosurg Focus*. 2016;40(2):E7. https://doi.org/10.3171/2015.11.FOCUS15485.
40. Soliman H, Fridley J, Telfeian A, et al. Minimally invasive, far lateral lumbar microdiscectomy with intra-operative CT navigational assistance and electrophysiological monitoring. *World Neurosurg*. 2018.
41. Mody MG, Nourbakhsh A, Stahl DL, Gibbs M, Alfawareh M, Garges KJ. The prevalence of wrong level surgery among spine surgeons. *Spine (Phila Pa 1976)*. 2008;33(2):194–198. https://doi.org/10.1097/BRS.0b013e31816043d1.
42. Sanderson SP, Houten J, Errico T, Forshaw D, Bauman J, Cooper PR. The unique characteristics of "upper" lumbar disc herniations. *Neurosurgery*. 2004;55(2):385–389; discussion 389. https://doi.org/10.1227/01.neu.0000129548.14898.9b.
43. Fontanesi G, Tartaglia I, Cavazzuti A, Giancecchi F. Prolapsed intervertebral disc at the upper lumbar level. Diagnostic difficulties. A report on 12 cases. *Ital J Orthop Traumatol*. 1987;13(4):501–507.
44. Gutterman P, Shenkin HA. Syndromes associated with protrusion of upper lumbar intervertebral discs. Results of surgery. *J Neurol Surg*. 1973;38(4):499–503. https://doi.org/10.3171/jns.1973.38.4.0499.
45. Oyelese AA, Fridley J, Choi DB, Telfeian A, Gokaslan ZL. Minimally invasive direct lateral, retroperitoneal transforaminal approach for large L1-2 disc herniations with intraoperative CT navigational assistance: technical note and report of 3 cases. *J Neurosurg Spine*. 2018;29(1):46–53. https://doi.org/10.3171/2017.11.SPINE17509.
46. Oyelese A, Telfeian AE, Gokaslan ZL, et al. Intraoperative computed tomography navigational assistance for transforaminal endoscopic decompression of heterotopic foraminal bone formation after oblique lumbar interbody fusion. *World Neurosurg*. 2018;115:29–34. https://doi.org/10.1016/j.wneu.2018.03.188.
47. Mukherjee D, Chaichana KL, Parker SL, Gokaslan ZL, McGirt MJ. Association of surgical resection and survival in patients with malignant primary osseous spinal neoplasms from the Surveillance, Epidemiology, and End Results (SEER) database. *Eur Spine J*. 2013;22(6):1375–1382. https://doi.org/10.1007/s00586-012-2621-4.
48. Nasser R, Drazin D, Nakhla J, et al. Resection of spinal column tumors utilizing image-guided navigation: a multicenter analysis. *Neurosurg Focus*. 2016;41(2):E15. https://doi.org/10.3171/2016.5.FOCUS16136.
49. Zhang Y, Wen L, Zhang J, Yan G, Zhou Y, Huang B. Three-dimensional printing and computer navigation assisted hemipelvectomy for en bloc resection of osteochondroma: a case report. *Med (Baltim)*. 2017;96(12):e6414. https://doi.org/10.1097/MD.0000000000006414.
50. Klimo P, Thompson CJ, Kestle JR, Schmidt MH. A meta-analysis of surgery versus conventional radiotherapy for the treatment of metastatic spinal epidural disease. *Neurooncol*. 2005;7(1):64–76. https://doi.org/10.1215/S1152851704000262.
51. Maranzano E, Latini P. Effectiveness of radiation therapy without surgery in metastatic spinal cord compression: final results from a prospective trial. *Int J Radiat Oncol Biol Phys*. 1995;32(4):959–967. https://doi.org/10.1016/0360-3016(95)00572-g.
52. Maranzano E, Latini P, Checcaglini F, et al. Radiation therapy in metastatic spinal cord compression. A prospective analysis of 105 consecutive patients. *Cancer*. 1991;67(5):1311–1317. https://doi.org/10.1002/1097-0142(19910301)67:5%3C1311::aid-cncr2820670507%3E3.0.co;2-r.
53. White WA, Patterson RH, Bergland RM. Role of surgery in the treatment of spinal cord compression by metastatic neoplasm. *Cancer*. 1971;27(3):558–561. https://doi.org/10.1002/1097-0142(197103)27:3%3C558::aid-cncr2820270307%3E3.0.co;2-e.
54. Young RF, Post EM, King GA. Treatment of spinal epidural metastases. Randomized prospective comparison of laminectomy and radiotherapy. *J Neurol Surg*. 1980;53(6):741–748. https://doi.org/10.3171/jns.1980.53.6.0741.
55. Akeyson EW, McCutcheon IE. Single-stage posterior vertebrectomy and replacement combined with posterior instrumentation for spinal metastasis. *J Neurol Surg*. 1996;85(2):211–220. https://doi.org/10.3171/jns.1996.85.2.0211.
56. Gokaslan ZL, York JE, Walsh GL, et al. Transthoracic vertebrectomy for metastatic spinal tumors. *J Neurol Surg*. 1998;89(4):599–609. https://doi.org/10.3171/jns.1998.89.4.0599.
57. Patchell RA, Tibbs PA, Regine WF, et al. Direct decompressive surgical resection in the treatment of spinal cord compression caused by metastatic cancer: a randomised trial. *Lancet*. 2005;366(9486):643–648. https://doi.org/10.1016/S0140-6736(05)66954-1.
58. Rothrock R, Pennington Z, Ehresman J, et al. Hybrid therapy for spinal metastases. *Neurosurg Clin N Am*. 2020;31(2):191–200. https://doi.org/10.1016/j.nec.2019.11.001.
59. Spratt DE, Beeler WH, de Moraes FY, et al. An integrated multidisciplinary algorithm for the management of spinal metastases: an International Spine Oncology Consortium report. *Lancet Oncol*. 2017;18(12):e720–e730. https://doi.org/10.1016/S1470-2045(17)30612-5.
60. Stefini R, Peron S, Mandelli J, Bianchini E, Roccucci P. Intraoperative spinal navigation for the removal of intradural tumors: technical notes. *Oper Neurosurg (Hagerstown)*. 2018;15(1):54–59. https://doi.org/10.1093/ons/opx179.
61. Moldovan K, Konakondla S, Barber SM, et al. Intraoperative computed tomography navigation-assisted resection of symptomatic intramedullary spinal cord cavernoma: a technical note and case report. *World Neurosurg*. 2019;129:311–317. https://doi.org/10.1016/j.wneu.2019.06.101.
62. Vasudeva VS, Abd-El-Barr M, Pompeu YA, Karhade A, Groff MW, Lu Y. Use of intraoperative ultrasound during spinal surgery. *Glob Spine J*. 2017;7(7):648–656. https://doi.org/10.1177/2192568217700100.
63. Benjamin CG, Frempong-Boadu A, Hoch M, Bruno M, Shepherd T, Pacione D. Combined use of diffusion tractography and advanced intraoperative imaging for resection of cervical intramedullary spinal cord neoplasms: a case series and technical note. *Oper Neurosurg (Hagerstown)*. 2019;17(5):525–530. https://doi.org/10.1093/ons/opz039.

64. Hadzipasic M, Giantini-Larsen AM, Tatsui CE, Shin JH. Emerging percutaneous ablative and radiosurgical techniques for treatment of spinal metastases. *Neurosurg Clin N Am*. 2020;31(1):141–150. https://doi.org/10.1016/j.nec.2019.08.017.
65. Vadalà G, De Salvatore S, Ambrosio L, Russo F, Papalia R, Denaro V. Robotic spine surgery and augmented reality systems: a state of the art. *Neurospine*. 2020;17(1):88–100. https://doi.org/10.14245/ns.2040060.030.
66. Elmi-Terander A, Burström G, Nachabe R, et al. Pedicle screw placement using augmented reality surgical navigation with intraoperative 3D imaging: a first in-human prospective cohort study. *Spine (Phila Pa 1976)*. 2019;44(7): 517–525. https://doi.org/10.1097/BRS.0000000000002876.
67. Elmi-Terander A, Nachabe R, Skulason H, et al. Feasibility and accuracy of thoracolumbar minimally invasive pedicle screw placement with augmented reality navigation technology. *Spine (Phila Pa 1976)*. 2018;43(14):1018–1023. https://doi.org/10.1097/BRS.0000000000002502.
68. Elmi-Terander A, Skulason H, Söderman M, et al. Surgical navigation technology based on augmented reality and integrated 3D intraoperative imaging: a spine cadaveric feasibility and accuracy study. *Spine (Phila Pa 1976)*. 2016;41(21):E1303–E1311. https://doi.org/10.1097/BRS.0000000000001830.
69. Molina CA, Theodore N, Ahmed AK, et al. Augmented reality-assisted pedicle screw insertion: a cadaveric proof-of-concept study. *J Neurosurg Spine*. 2019;31(1):139–146. https://doi.org/10.3171/2018.12.SPINE181142.
70. Edström E, Burström G, Nachabe R, Gerdhem P, Elmi Terander A. A novel augmented-reality-based surgical navigation system for spine surgery in a hybrid operating room: design, workflow, and clinical applications. *Oper Neurosurg (Hagerstown)*. 2020;18(5):496–502. https://doi.org/10.1093/ons/opz236.

8

Robotic-Assisted Correction of Adult Spinal Deformity

Martin Nikolaus Stienen, MD, FEBNS, and Anand Veeravagu, MD, FAANS

INTRODUCTION OF TECHNOLOGY

Adult Spinal Deformity: Present Practice and Standard of Care

Adult spinal deformity (ASD) is a heterogeneous condition of typically the elderly patient, which involves misalignment in the sagittal and/or coronal plane.[1,2] ASD can be asymptomatic or, depending on its type and severity, present with varying degrees of, and oftentimes excruciating, pain and disability typically exceeding the health impact of other chronic diseases, including those of the heart and lung.[3,4] Even though nonoperative treatment is typically recommended first in patients presenting without significant or progressively worsening pain, neurological deficit, or deformity, studies have so far been unable to detect significant improvement in the health status of ASD patients with conservative measures, whereas adequate surgical treatment consistently alleviates pain and leads to clinically meaningful decrease of disability.[2,5–7]

Over the last decades, improvements in surgical technology, including both techniques and instrumentation, have advanced ASD surgery from supportive to corrective and expanded the patient population that can now hope to regain functional ability and health-related quality of life (HRQoL) after successful treatment. Surgical treatment is challenging, however, for a number of reasons, including patient selection (risk-benefit assessment of surgery), patient optimization (e.g., increase in bone quality, prehabilitation, smoking cessation, reduction of risk factors for complications in typically elderly and frail patients), surgical planning (e.g., extent, combination of approaches, need for osteotomies), use of operative technology (e.g., intraoperative imaging, navigation, electrophysiological monitoring), technical nuances during the case, operative length, and complication management intra- and postoperatively. Besides surgical excellence, modern anesthesia and critical care management are required to deal with potentially excessive blood loss during and after ASD correction.

With complication and reoperation rates as high as 70% and 28% at the 2-year follow-up,[8] there is a need to improve safety and durability of ASD surgery. The evolving minimally invasive surgery (MIS) techniques for ASD aim to reduce morbidity, lower complication rates, and shorten postoperative recovery time.[9,10] The options of the MIS surgeon include circumferential MIS techniques with anterior or lateral discectomy (indirect decompression), followed by posterior percutaneous instrumentation or hybrid techniques, again with anterior or lateral discectomy but followed by a conventional open posterior approach for instrumentation and decompression and osteotomies, as needed. Not all ASD patients are suitable for MIS techniques, and algorithms to guide decision-making with regard to the optimal approach have been proposed.[11]

Current Use of Robotic Surgery for Adult Spinal Deformity

Robots have been the logical next step in the toolbox of MIS spine surgeons, building on the platform of navigation but optimizing critical issues in MIS surgery, including radiation exposure and precision in patients with challenging anatomy. Deformity surgery requires meticulous fine motor skills and a steady hand to exploit small working corridors and minimize collateral damage during exposure, but the arduous and long procedures predispose to mental and physical fatigue.[12] Moreover, the individual patient's segmental vertebral anatomy may not be well visualized in either the AP or lateral plane using C-arm imaging, and both 3D navigation with oblique image reconstruction and robotic guidance allow accomplishing complex screw trajectories with higher confidence. The fundamental advantages of the robot are geometric precision (allowing for exact localization of the starting point, orientation, and trajectory length), infinite reproducibility, perfect "memory," lack of physiological tremor or fatigue, and insensitivity to radiation. The synergy between those qualities and the spine surgeon's inherent judgment, experience, and adaptability are key to successful robotic procedures.[13] In general, three different levels of robotic assistance can be differentiated:

- tele-surgical systems with remote command stations from where the surgeon controls the machine (e.g., the da Vinci Surgical System [Intuitive Surgical, Inc.]);
- supervisory controlled systems with pre-programmed machines that autonomously perform certain actions; and
- co-autonomy type shared-control models where robot motion is concurrently controlled (e.g., SpineAssist/Renaissance/Mazor X).[14,15]

For application in spine and ASD surgery in particular, the available robotic systems belong in the third category.

Pedicle screw constructs are today's basis of spinal fixation, providing substantial rigidity to facilitate bony healing (fusion) and in the absence of a navigation system, their safety depends largely on the patient's anatomical landmarks and the surgeon's experience. It is well documented that even in experienced hands the rate of implant malposition ranges from 5% to >30% for cases with challenging anatomy; since ASD cases often comprise revision procedures, reliable anatomical landmarks are frequently altered.[16–19] Early robotic systems have thus focused on guiding the placement of pedicle screws by preparing optimal trajectories based on navigation, a task by which most modern systems continue to be confined.[2] Even in the latest surgical robots for the spine, surgeons are still required to place the pedicle screw manually. The combination of surgical robotics with intraoperative CT or O-arm image acquisition has greatly simplified implementation, obviating the need for patient registration based on C-arm fluoroscopy, while increasing the precision of robotic surgery even further.[20]

Beyond assisting in pedicle screw fixation, today's applications of robots for ASD cases are few. To restore lordosis and obtain solid arthrodesis across the anterior spinal column, interbody fusions including anterior and lateral trajectories are commonly used. The obstacles to anterior lumbar interbody fusion (ALIF) are the ureters and large retroperitoneal blood vessels (aorta, vena cava, and branches) overlying the lumbar spine anteriorly. The da Vinci Surgical System (Intuitive Surgical) has been used successfully in animal models and several smaller case series to mobilize aforementioned critical structures and help facilitate the approach laparoscopically.[21–24] The visualization inside and around the disk space was considered superior to conventional open or laparoscopic techniques.[21] However, the da Vinci is not yet FDA approved for spinal instrumentation and outside exploratory clinical research its use—in particular for ASD cases—cannot yet be recommended.[12] The authors are not aware of any other robotic application for anterior or lateral discectomies, osteotomies or deformity correction.

Adult Spinal Deformity—Outcomes With and Without Robotic Assistance

Accuracy of Thoraco–lumbar Screw Implantation

High-quality randomized studies comparing outcomes of ASD surgery with or without use of robotic guidance are lacking. As such, our understanding of its value is taken from critical review of pro- and retrospective cohort studies or extrapolated from meta-analyses of trials in non-ASD populations.[25,26] There are some reports on the accuracy of robotic thoracolumbar pedicle screw instrumentation (summary provided in Table 8.1), where the accuracy of pedicle screw insertion is usually graded according to the classification proposed by Gertzbein and Robbins (G&R; Box 8.1).[27]

In 2010, Devito et al. described the accuracy rates of n = 646 implants deployed with the Mazor SpineAssist robot as G&R grades A in 89.3%, B in 9.0%, C in 1.4%, and D in 0.3%, reviewing their series of robotic screw guidance in a population that included about 14% of adolescents with scoliosis and adults with spinal deformity.[30]

In 2013, Hu et al. assessed screw placement accuracy based on intraoperative biplanar fluoroscopy, postoperative radiographs, and surgeon's judgment in a retrospective review of n = 102 consecutive patients, of which the robot (Mazor Renaissance) was successfully used in n = 95, including n = 85 patients (89.5%) with ASD (kyphosis and scoliosis).[31] Of n = 1085 planned screws, n = 960 were implanted and n = 949 were considered successful and accurate (98.9%). Eleven mispositioned screws amounted to a rate of 1.1%, of which one patient with a laterally placed L4 pedicle screw and L3 radicular pain required revision surgery. A total of 110 planned screws were aborted and placed manually, mostly due to poor registration or trajectory issues in the thoracic > lumbar > sacral or iliac level. Fifteen screws were not placed, at the surgeon's discretion. The authors mentioned difficulties in cases with severe obesity (BMI 49.9 kg/m^2) and deformity, precluding adequate fluoroscopic image registration.[31,32] Even though it seems from this report that in deformity and revision cases where the normal anatomical landmarks are obscured the robot is helpful to improve screw accuracy, it must be acknowledged that in studies assessing screw accuracy based on postoperative CT scans the malposition rates are about four times higher than are the rates obtained by clinical estimation.[33]

In 2016, Macke et al. published their series of n = 50 pediatric patients (n = 662 screws) with adolescent idiopathic scoliosis (AIS).[28] The overall accuracy (G&R grades A&B) with the Mazor Renaissance was 92.8% (3% medially breached), and in cases with intraoperative prone position CT scanning, the inaccuracy rate could be reduced to 2.4% (0% medially breached).

The largest comparative study analyzing clinical and radiological outcomes after robotic (Mazor Renaissance; n = 83 patients, n = 1012 screws) versus 3D-printed patient-specific template (n = 75 patients; n = 886 screws) or CT-based navigation (n = 109 patients; n = 1276 screws) in a population of n = 267 patients diagnosed with severe adult

TABLE 8.1 Review of the current literature, summarizing articles published until 07/2019 that report on the safety and accuracy of robotic-guided thoracolumbar pedicle screw placement for ASD and related spinal disorders.

Authors, year	Study design	Number of patients/ screws/type of robot	Assessment of accuracy	Assessment of safety	Assessment of feasibility
Devito et al., 2010[28]	Retrospective multicenter study (14 hospitals); population included about 14% with AIS and ASD	N = 842 patients; n = 635 (3271 implants) available with intraoperative fluoroscopy; n = 139 (646 implants) available with postoperative CT scan; Mazor SpineAssist ®	Intraoperative x-ray and postoperative CT (when available); clinical acceptance rate 97.9%; G&R grades A in 89.3%, B in 9.0%, C in 1.4%, and D in 0.3%; 98.3% within safety zone (G&R grades A and B)	N/A	Of 682 cases in which 3912 implant insertions were planned, 83.6% (3271 implants) were fully executed under robotic guidance (the remainder initiated under robotics guidance and manually continued by the surgeon)
Macke et al., 2016[28]	Retrospective cohort study; population with AIS	N = 48 patients (662 implants); Mazor Renaissance®	Review of postoperative CT; G&R grades A & B in 92.7% (safety zone), C in 4.5%, D in 1.5%; E in 1.2%	N/A	N/A
Fan et al., 2018[29]	Retrospective cohort study; population with ASD	N = 286 patients, including n = 83 with robotic PLIF, n = 75 with template-guided PLIF, n = 109 with CT-navigated PLIF	Review of postoperative CT. Robotic cases: G&R grades A in 91.3%, B in 4.7%, C in 2.8%, and D in 0.6%; 96.0% within safety zone (G&R grades A and B)	Robotic cases: Six complications in total (7.2%), including dural tear, SSI, wound revision. No neurological complications occurred. Two revisions due to cage misplacement were necessary.	N/A

AIS, Adolescent idiopathic scoliosis; *ASD*, adult spinal deformity; *G&R*, Gertzbein and Robbins; *N/A*, not available; *PLIF*, Posterior Lumbar Interbody Fusion; *SSI*, surgical site infection.

degenerative scoliosis was published in 2018.[29] The authors found a significantly higher rate of good (G&R grades A and B) screw position in robotic (96.0%), compared with both template- (90.6%; $P < .001$) or CT-navigation-based procedures (93.0%; $P = .019$). The G&R grades for robotic-assisted screws in this challenging population were 91.3% (A), 4.7% (B), 2.8% (C), 0.6% (D), and none were labeled E. Six screws in the robotic group versus n = 30 in the template- ($P < .001$) and n = 20 in the CT-navigation groups ($P = .029$) were revised manually from the original device guidance. Pedicle encroachment was lateral in all n = 88, highlighting that "tool skiving" was likely the inciting issue with mal-positioned screws. Significant violation of the proximal facet joint was not found in any of the robotic screws.[29]

BOX 8.1 The Gertzbein-Robbin (G&R) classification is illustrated, discriminating between five grades and describing the degree of screw deviation from the "ideal" intra-pedicular trajectory.

G&R type	Degree of cortical breach	Description
A	0 mm	Intra-pedicular screw without breach of the cortical layer of the pedicle
B	<2 mm	Screw that breaches the cortical layer of the pedicle but does not exceed it laterally by 2 mm
C	2–3.9 mm	Penetration of <4 mm
D	4–6 mm	Penetration of <6 mm
E	>6 mm	Screws that do not pass through the pedicle or that, at any given point in their intended intra-pedicular course, breach the cortical layer of the pedicle in any direction by more than 6 mm

Accuracy of Spino–pelvic Screw Implantation

Achieving solid fixation and fusion across the lumbosacral junction is challenging.[34] The tri-cortical S2 alar-iliac (S2Ai) trajectory finds increasing popularity as a method of low-profile pelvic fixation to reduce strain on the S1 screws and replace classic iliac bolt fixation.[35] The path of these screws is surrounded by major neural and vascular structures and the use of robots in obtaining proper S2Ai trajectories has been reported in several publications over the last decade, providing evidence that robotic-guided S2Ai screw placement is feasible and accurate (summary provided in Table 8.2).

In 2017, Laratta et al. used the bone-mounted Mazor Renaissance system to guide S2Ai screw insertion (mean screw length, 80 ± 2.6 mm; mean diameter, 8.5 ± 0 mm).[39] In a retrospective series of 23 consecutive patients treated between January and September 2016, the authors analyzed intraoperative 3D O-arm scans to determine the severity and direction of breach. For the S2 sacral alar corridor, their blinded evaluation revealed n = 2 breaches of the iliac cortex (each one anterior and posterior), of which one was moderate-severe (G&R type E; >6 mm). The overall accuracy was 95.7% for n = 46 S2Ai screws, the robotic-assisted screw placement was safe, as no complications related to the placement occurred in their series.[39]

Also in 2017, Bederman et al., using the same system (Mazor Renaissance) to guide S2Ai screw insertion (mean screw length 80, range 65–90 mm), reported on their retrospective series of 14 consecutive patients and n = 31 screws.[36] According to the G&R scale, they found type A breach in n = 10 (32.2%), type B in n = 1 (3.2%), and type C in n = 6 (19.4%), resulting in a lower overall accuracy rate of 45.2%. Of note, none of the misplacements was intrapelvic, risked visceral or neurovascular structures or needed to be removed or revised. The authors mentioned difficulties with the screw simulation software, which was limited to 60-mm screws at that time. As such, only screws >75 mm were found to breach beyond the bone cortex. Bederson et al. needed to probe manually for all screws placed at depth, as the robotic drill capacities (28 mm) were exceeded.[36]

TABLE 8.2 Review of the current literature, summarizing articles published until 07/2019 that report on the safety and accuracy of robotic-guided S2Ai screw placement for ASD and related spinal disorders.

Authors, year	Study design	Number of patients/screws/ type of robot	Assessment of accuracy	Assessment of safety	Assessment of feasibility
Bederman et al., 2017[36]	Retrospective case review	14 consecutive patients; 31 S2Ai screws; Mazor Renaissance®	Review of postoperative radiographs and CT; 45.2% accuracy; G&R type A breach in n = 10 (32.2%), type B in n = 1 (3.2%), and type C in n = 6 (19.4%)	No complications related to S2Ai placement occurred.	Difficulties with the screw simulation software, limited to 60-mm screws. Need to probe manually for all screws placed at depth, as robotic drill capacities (28 mm) were exceeded.
Hyun et al., 2017[37]	Retrospective case review	Four patients; 8 S2Ai screws; Mazor Renaissance®	Review of postoperative CT; 100% accuracy	No complications related to S2Ai placement occurred.	No intraoperative difficulties occurred.
Hu and Lieberman, 2017[38]	Retrospective case review	18 non-consecutive patients; 35 S2Ai screws; Mazor Renaissance®	Review of postoperative CT; 100% accuracy	N/A	No intraoperative difficulties occurred.
Laratta et al., 2018[39]	Retrospective case review	23 consecutive patients; 46 S2Ai screws; Mazor Renaissance®	Review of intraoperative O-Arm (CT); 95.7% accuracy (each one breach <3 mm and >6 mm)	No complications related to S2Ai placement occurred.	All planned screws were deployed. No difficulties were reported.
Shillingford et al., 2018[40]	Retrospective matched cohort study	68 consecutive patients (105 S2Ai screws); 23 in robot (46 S2Ai screws) and 28 in free-hand group (59 S2Ai screws); Mazor Renaissance®	Review of intraoperative O-Arm (CT); 95.7% accuracy in robot (2 breaches) and 91.5% in free-hand group (5 breaches; $P = 0.463$)	No significant intraoperative neurovascular or visceral complications associated with S2AI screw placement occurred in either group.	N/A

ASD, Adult spinal deformity; *G&R*, Gertzbein and Robbins; *N/A*, not available; *S2Ai*, S2 alar-iliac.

Those difficulties were overcome in the case series of Hyun et al.,[37] who implanted eight S2Ai screws (8.5-mm diameter; 80- or 90-mm length) in four adult patients undergoing corrective surgery for spinal deformity. Those authors used the Mazor Renaissance as guidance, after a software update providing a more expansive view of the pelvis for up to 80-mm screw trajectories. Applying a guiding technique with Jamshidi needles and K-wires beyond the 28-mm pilot hole, they found all eight screws (including two of 90 mm in length) to be placed accurately without cortical violation in postoperative CT studies. No intra- or postoperative complications occurred. The net mean time of the use of the robot was 13 min for screw placement utilizing 5.3 s of fluoro per screw on average.[37]

A further article from 2017 comes from Hu and Lieberman, who summarize their experience with n = 35 Mazor Renaissance-guided S2Ai placed screws (length and diameter not provided).[38] It should be noted that the authors' series originally comprised 34 patients, but 16 of those were excluded as no postoperative CT data was available. Reviewing the postoperative CT scans in 18 patients with degenerative scoliosis (n = 12), flat back syndrome (n = 2) or other diagnoses (n = 4), the authors found no breach in any of the placed screws. The average deviations from the actual screw to the treatment plan were in the ranges of 3 mm (axial plane) and 1.8 mm (lateral plane) at the entry point and 2.1 mm (axial plane) and 1.2 mm (lateral plane) at a depth of 30 mm. The authors mentioned the possibility of slight lateral skiving of the drill at the irregular and oblique sacral surface at the typical S2Ai entrance point, a deviation they considered minimal and acceptable. No difficulties with the robotic-guided S2Ai screw placement were encountered intraoperatively.

Lastly, Shillingford et al. performed a retrospective matched cohort analysis to compare the accuracy of robotic guidance versus free-hand technique for S2Ai screw placement.[40]

Rates of Intraoperative Complications

Corrective surgeries for ASD are per se associated with extraordinarily high complications rates.[2,4,8,10,11] Any technology with the potential to lower the commonly encountered intra- and postoperative complications is of potential interest to spine surgeons.

Kantelhardt et al. found a lower rate of intraoperative complications including major hemorrhage and dural tears in robotic- compared to fluoroscopy-guided surgical procedures (4.7% vs. 9.1%, $P = .04$) in their retrospective series of n = 112 consecutive patients undergoing spinal fusion for a wide range of indications.[41] The differences in postoperative complications, including wound healing disturbances (13.5% vs. 21.4%), surgical site infections (SSIs; 2.7% vs. 10.7%), and cerebrospinal fluid fistulas (0.0 vs. 6.1%) were in favor of robotic-assisted procedures but insignificant.[41]

Even more impressive interim findings with a five-fold decrease in surgical complications ($P < .001$) and a seven-fold decrease in revision surgery ($P = .012$) were announced for the robotic arm of the MIS ReFRESH, a prospective controlled multicenter study assessing the clinical impact of robotic guidance compared to fluoroscopic guidance.[42] For now, the final results of this study have not been announced, but it should be considered that the trial enrolled patients undergoing short (<4 segments) spinal fusion procedures and the results might therefore not be applicable 1:1 to the typical ASD population.

In a large, comparative analysis of n = 276 ASD patients, no marked differences between robotic- and both template- and CT-navigation-guided procedures were found with regard to estimated blood loss; length of postoperative stay; revision surgeries; and intra- and postoperative complications including dural tears, SSIs, wound revisions, and neurological complications.[29]

Proximal Facet Violation

The exact planning and execution of the pedicle screw trajectory on the uppermost instrumented vertebrae (UIV) included in long fusion constructs theoretically permits the surgeon to spare the proximal facet joint from mechanical damage.[25,29] This may result in biomechanically superior results, with the possibility to translate into lower rates of adjacent segment disease and failure in the long term after ASD correction.[43] So far, no major differences between robotic versus other sophisticated guiding tools were found in a comparative study on ASD patients.[29] More patient data with long-term follow-up is required to shed light on this potentially valuable benefit of robotic surgery.

Postoperative Pain, Disability, and Health-Related Quality of Life

One report indicates lower postoperative pain levels and a decrease in postoperative opioid use for robotic-assisted procedures,[41] potentially translating into reduced opioid-associated morbidity.[44] However, the added benefit of the robotic technique could be biased by a higher proportion of percutaneous MIS versus open cases in the non-robotic group.[41] So far, the authors are unaware of comparative studies comparing subjective or objective disability or HRQoL outcomes after robotic versus non-robotic ASD surgery; however, the VAS pain, Oswestry Disability Index (ODI), and EuroQol (EQ-5D) questionnaires were included as secondary outcome measures of the MIS ReFRESH study.[45,46]

Economical Outcomes and Cost-Effectiveness

Currently, to the best of the authors' knowledge, there is no data on the economical outcomes or cost-effectiveness of robotic-assisted spine surgery, and in particular not for ASD.[12,14,15] The high acquisition costs of robotic OR technology might be offset by a reduction in OR time, fewer revision procedures for misplaced screws, and lower rates of adjacent segment disease, but this remains to be proven by large studies with sufficiently long follow-up intervals.[14]

Radiation Exposure

Spinal deformity procedures require thorough knowledge and information about the anatomy, the orientation of the vertebrae in 3D space and their relationship to the underlying and adjacent neurovascular structures. In particular in cases with rotational deformity, many surgeons rely on either intraoperative 2D C-arm fluoroscopy or 3D CT imaging guidance to achieve optimal screw position, which can result in significant radiation exposure to both patients and surgeons alike.[32] With robotics systems, CT and/or fluoroscopy can be acquired with the surgeon and OR staff outside the OR. The procedure may then proceed without additional intraoperative scans.[15] Accordingly, savings in fluoroscopy time and radiation dose have repeatedly been demonstrated for robotic-assisted spinal fusion procedures.[25,41,47,48]

Even more than in adults, minimizing radiation exposure is paramount in the pediatric population, as a potential correlation between exposure and cancer incidence was pointed out.[15,49] With most robotic systems relying on a limited number of initial 2D or 3D images for registration,[15,41] the reduction in radiation exposure during AIS and other forms of pediatric deformity surgery is a major advantage of these systems. Even though data is currently lacking for ASD correction, it can be assumed that those savings for the surgeon and OR staff would be similarly impressive for ASD procedures that involve a higher number of spinal implants. As the thin-sliced high-resolution CT scans that most robotic systems require are generally requested as part of most deformity surgeons' preoperative assessment, the overall radiation exposure for the patient in robotic-assisted spinal ASD correction is likely also less, compared to the additional fluoroscopic radiation exposure.

Revision Rates

A limited number of studies for non-ASD populations exist and uniformly report lower revision rates for robotic comparted to conventional (free-hand) fusion procedures.

In their series of n = 72 robotic MIS fusion cases for spondylolisthesis, Schröder and Staartjes described no need for intraoperative screw reposition, conversion to open procedure using the Mazor SpineAssist system.[50] Their 1-year revision rate was n = 3 (4.2%); none of those revisions were related to screw malposition. In a meta-analysis of the existing literature, the authors found that patients undergoing free-hand fusion procedures were eight times as likely as were patients undergoing robotic fusion procedures to require revision surgery for screw malposition (OR, 8.1; 95% CI, 2–33.3; $P < .001$). Navigated fusion cases had a comparative revision profile to robotic fusion cases.[50]

In a preliminary report from the MIS ReFRESH study group after the enrollment of 250 patients in the robotic and 79 patients in the fluoro-guided study arms and a minimum of 1-year follow-up, the odds ratio for a revision surgery were 6.4 times lower in the robotic group (2 [0.8%] vs. 4 [5.1%]; $P = 0.031$).[51]

In their analysis of adult scoliosis cases, Fan et al. found similar revision rates after robotic versus CT-navigated procedures (2/83 [2.4%] vs. 4/109 [3.7%)] $P = .512$), including zero revisions due to screw malposition in the robotic group and two in the navigated group.[29] Unfortunately the follow-up time remains unclear from their publication.

OR Time

Given its relatively short time of clinical use, studies assessing the impact of robotics systems on surgical efficiency are rare for spine surgery in general and non-existent for ASD.[14,15,52] Depending on the number of instrumented spinal segments, multiple registrations will first add to the OR time. However, it can be inferred that, based on the existing literature for image guidance and navigation and considering the increased accuracy of robotics systems, there may be a positive impact on workflow and total OR time. As with the implementation of any new technology, a learning curve exists that, once overcome, may lead to greater surgical efficiency.

SURGICAL TREATMENT FOR ADULT SPINAL DEFORMITY—CASE 1 (DEGENERATIVE KYPHOSIS)

Case Description

History/Clinical Presentation

A 68-year-old obese (BMI, 35 kg/m^2) female with a prior history of L3–L5 posterior lumbar fusion in 2005 at an outside hospital presented with worsening low back pain and bilateral, right- more than left-sided, intense sciatic leg pain (VAS 8/10) in the lateral and posterior thigh, the calf, and extending to the dorsal aspect of the foot. She was only able to walk 50 to 100 yards and stand no longer than a couple of minutes due to her pain and both numbness and weakness of legs when ambulating. Lying down alleviated her pain. Her preoperative ODI was 58. The neurological examination revealed a slight (4+/5) weakness of right hip flexion and EHL, preserved sensation in all dermatomes, and generally hypoactive reflexes.

Preoperative Imaging

MRI of the lumbar spine demonstrated evidence of central disk herniation at L5–S1, worse on the right side. There was grade 1 spondylolisthesis at L5–S1 with severe facet hypertrophy. There was severe stenosis at L2–L3 and moderate stenosis at L1–L2 (Fig. 8.1A and B).

The CT studies showed prior laminectomy of L4–L5 and solid fusion between L3–L5 (see Fig. 8.1C). The scoliosis x-rays (see Fig. 8.1D and E) indicated moderate sagittal and slight coronal imbalance (SVA, 7.5 cm), a PI of 63°, and an LL of 46°, resulting in an LL–PI mismatch of 17° with partial compensation (PT 24°). Her T-score (total hip) was –0.4.

Surgical Plan

We elected for a staged revision procedure, entailing an ALIF at L5/S1 followed by a lateral discectomy at L2/3 and the placement of a lordotic extreme lateral interbody fusion (XLIF) cage in the first session. We then planned for a posterior revision, removal of previous instrumentation, decompression, and Smith-Peterson osteotomies (SPOs) at L2/3 with robotic-assisted (Mazor X®, Mazor Robotics, Caesarea, Israel) instrumentation from T10-unilateral S2Ai in a second session.

Intraoperative Imaging

No intraoperative imaging was recorded. Of note, the XLIF procedure was aborted due to unfavorable lumbosacral plexus anatomy interfering with safe docking of the retractor. The patient was flipped prone and a transforaminal lumbar interbody fusion (TLIF) with a lordotic implant was conducted at the L2/3 level instead.

Postoperative Imaging

The scoliosis x-rays at three months postoperatively (see Fig. 8.1I–J) indicate correct placement of the hardware, partial restoration of the lumbar lordosis (LL 53°, PT 28°), and no signs of proximal junctional kyphosis or failure.

Postoperative Recovery and Follow-Up

There were no intra- or immediate postoperative complications. The patient was discharged home on the sixth postoperative day. She reported feeling well at the follow-up three months postoperatively; she was still recovering from the procedure and had occasional aches, but these were of significantly lower intensity and frequency (ODI 32). She did not require pain medication and was happy with the postoperative result. There were no neurological deficits on her examination. To date, there has been no need for surgical revision over her remaining 18-month postoperative follow-up period.

Procedural Concerns in Detail (Whether Navigation, Robotics, or Both)

Due to the long segmental fusion procedure, the posterior part of the procedure was conducted in two steps. First, the preparation of all screw entry points between the T10–L2 segments was conducted and the robot was mounted to the spinous process of T12. All pedicle trajectories were drilled with robotic guidance and ball-probed without evidence of breach. After tapping and screw insertion the robot was dismounted, and the area between T10–L2 was packed with laps to obtain hemostasis. Only then was the remainder of the wound opened from L3–S2Ai and the prior hardware removed. We only re-inserted the L3 and L5 screws on the right, as well as the L4 screw on the left, manually, given that this area was fused from her prior procedure. The decompression, L2/3 TLIF, and SPOs were conducted next and then the robotic system was brought back into the operative field, mounted to the iliac crest and re-registered for the caudal part. Both the S1 screws and the left S2Ai screw were cannulated under robotic guidance and appropriately sized screws were inserted (Fig. 8.1F–H).

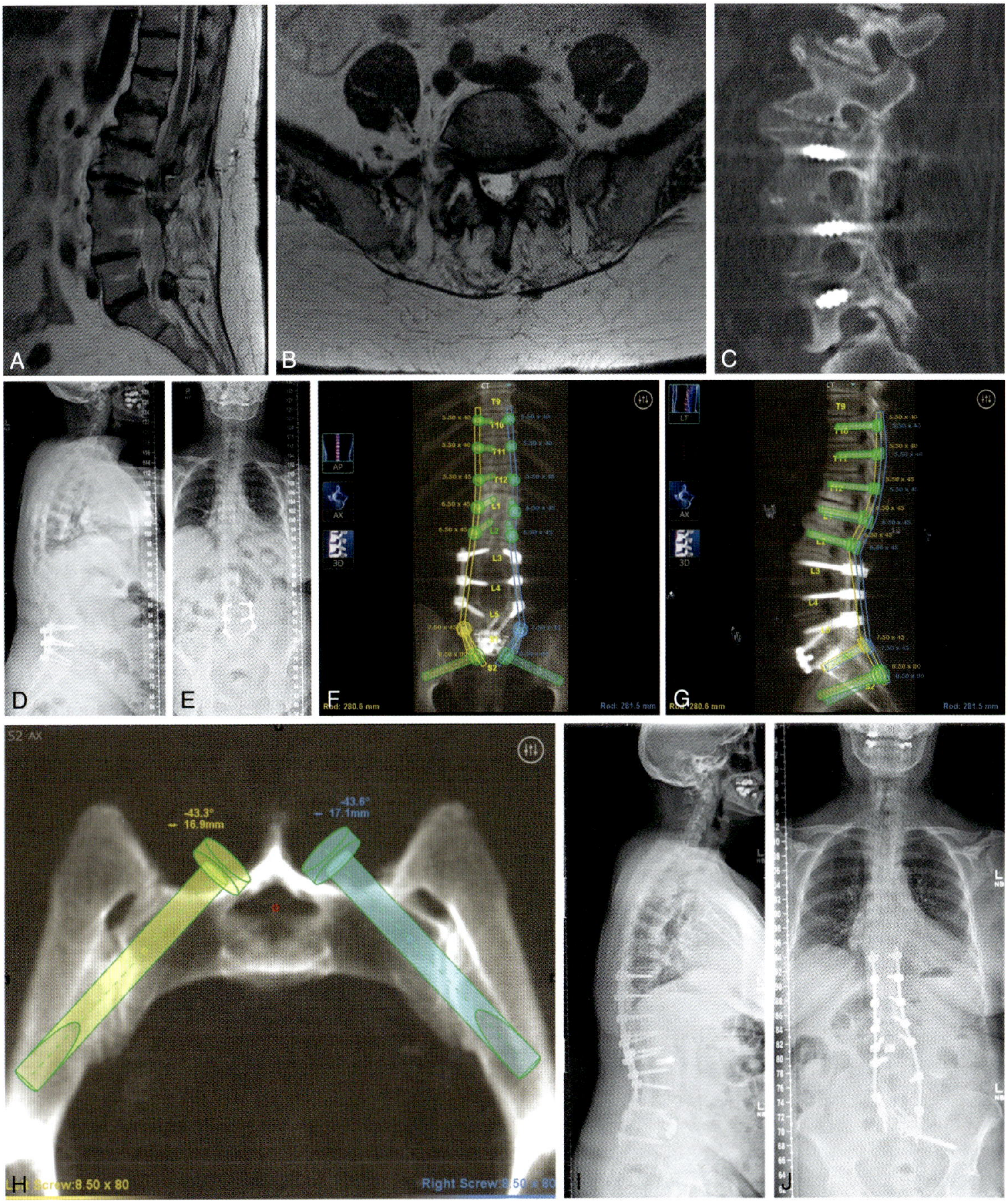

FIG. 8.1 Case vignette 1. (A) Preoperative sagittal T2-weighted MRI. (B) Preoperative axial T2-weighted MRI at the L5/S1 disk level. (C) Preoperative paramedian sagittal CT scan, illustrating the solid fusion between the previously instrumented levels of L3–L5. (D) Preoperative scoliosis x-rays, lateral view. (E) Preoperative scoliosis x-rays, anteroposterior view. (F and G) Intraoperative view on the Mazor X planning software, outlining the patient-specific screw trajectories and dimensions, as well as the rod lengths in anteroposterior (F) and lateral (G) projection. (H) Postoperative scoliosis x-rays, lateral view. (I) Postoperative scoliosis x-rays, anteroposterior view.

All screws stimulated well above the 10-mAmp threshold and a stitched long-cassette C-arm x-ray image (LessRay®, NuVasive, San Diego) provided evidence for correct screw placement and a harmonic lumbar lordosis. The rods were contoured and bent using the navigated Bendini® system (NuVasive, San Diego) and final tightened applying slight compression across the L2/3 segment.

For this procedure, we used the preoperative CT scan for robotic navigation. At the planning stage of the robotic trajectories, care was taken to avoid uneven bony structures and adequate preparation of the anatomical "landing area" for tool docking helps to circumvent tool skiving. The partial opening of the skin for long incisions can help prevent excessive blood loss during ASD cases, considering that spine robots cannot yet register more than 5 or 6 spinal segments at a time.

Treatment Side Effects

The posterior part of the procedure was associated with a 1.7-L blood loss. Cell-saver technology was used to mitigate the blood loss and no transfusion of blood products was necessary (2.5 L crystalloids and 1 L albumin).

Potential Downfalls

None.

Management of Complications

No complications were experienced, but unexpected difficulties to dock onto the psoas muscle were encountered during the procedure. A large lumbar nervous plexus spanning over the psoas muscle, which appeared quite taut in addition and was not easily mobilizable over the L2/3 disk surface, prevented us from conducting a transpsoas XLIF procedure. A prepsoas modification was not possible due to the close proximity of the large vessels. Choosing a TLIF in this situation may have prevented retraction injury of the lumbar plexus nerves. No complications with respect to the surgical robot occurred and all the planned robotic trajectories could be executed. No postoperative CT scan has so far been necessary; however, based on the intraoperative palpation and postoperative x-ray studies, there was no evidence for cortical violation of any screw.

SURGICAL TREATMENT FOR ADULT SPINAL DEFORMITY—CASE 2 (HIGH-GRADE LUMBOSACRAL SPONDYLOLISTHESIS)

Case Description

History/Clinical Presentation

A non-obese 48-year-old female patient with a history of left lower extremity deep vein thrombosis due to May-Thurner syndrome consulted us for severe low back pain when sitting or standing, as well as bilateral right > left L5-type radicular pain, localized in the buttocks, posterolateral thigh, and calf, extending to the big toes. Her complaints were unresponsive to and even worsened after L5–S1 decompression and attempted fusion at an outside hospital prior to our first encounter. Her main complaint was incapacitating axial back pain, worsened with activity such as bending over, twisting, and walking. On neurological examination, she did not reveal focal sensory or motor deficits and there was no evidence of sphincter weakness.

Preoperative Imaging

The MRI studies revealed high-grade isthmic spondylolisthesis at L5/S1 with bilateral pars defect, focal kyphosis, and hyperlordosis above L5 (Fig. 8.2A and B). The lateral-oblique reconstruction of her preoperative CT shows the almost vertical projection of the L5 pedicles (see Fig. 8.2C; a vena cava filter is in place). The scoliosis x-ray studies revealed a high PI of 78°, a LL of 56°, and a PT of 32°. Her SVA was positive at 120 mm and she was balanced in the coronal plane (see Fig. 8.2D).

Surgical Plan

Because of her young age and as her complaints seemed to originate from the pathologic mobility of the severely degenerated L5/S1 segment and not from her global imbalance, we desisted from attempting to reduce the lumbosacral kyphosis aggressively. However, we felt that a large surface area for fusion would be required for this patient, including an ALIF at L4/5 to prolong the stabilization up to L4, using the anterior approach at the same time to perform a "reverse Bohlman" technique with trans-L5/S1 placement of a fibular strut graft in a first step. This would then be followed by a percutaneous robot-guided posterior fusion including both L4 pedicles, a bilateral transdiskal L5/S1 trajectory and bilateral S2Ai screws. The three-column transdiskal fixation from the posterior approach provides additional fixation strength due to its triangular geometry and increased screw length and surface contact with cortical bone.[53] Details about the surgical plan and execution have recently been published.[54]

Intraoperative Imaging

Fig. 8.2E–G illustrate the intraoperative view on the Mazor X planning software, outlining the patient-specific screw trajectories and dimensions, as well as the rod lengths in anteroposterior and lateral projection, as well as the axial view on the S2Ai screws.

Postoperative Imaging

The standing lumbar x-ray studies reveal the correct placement of the screws in the planned trajectories (see Fig. 8.2H and I). A postoperative CT scan reveals the fibular strut graft (see Fig. 8.2J) as well as the precisely placed screws (see Fig. 8.2K–M).

Postoperative Recovery and Follow-Up

There were no intra- or immediate postoperative complications. The patient was mobilized with an LSO brace and ambulating on the second postoperative day. She was discharged home on the fourth postoperative day. In the long-term follow-up, she reported complete resolution of her lower extremity symptoms and improvement of her axial low back pain.

Procedural Concerns in Detail (Whether Navigation, Robotics, or Both)

For the unusual and complex screw trajectories of L4 (small and convergent; see Fig. 8.2K), transdiskal L5/S1 (see Fig. 8.2L), and S2Ai (see Fig. 8.2M) the robot was preferred over both 2D fluoroscopy or 3D navigation for reasons of increased efficiency, surgeon's confidence, and decreased radiation exposure.[36,37,39] Additionally, a lower revision rate for screw misplacement after robotic versus conventional fusion of spondylolisthesis was recently reported.[50] While 3D navigation might have been an alternative, we preferred the "locked" desired trajectory achieved by using the robotic arm over freely moving navigated surgical tools. Especially for the (in our hands) relatively infrequently used transdiskal L5/S1 screw

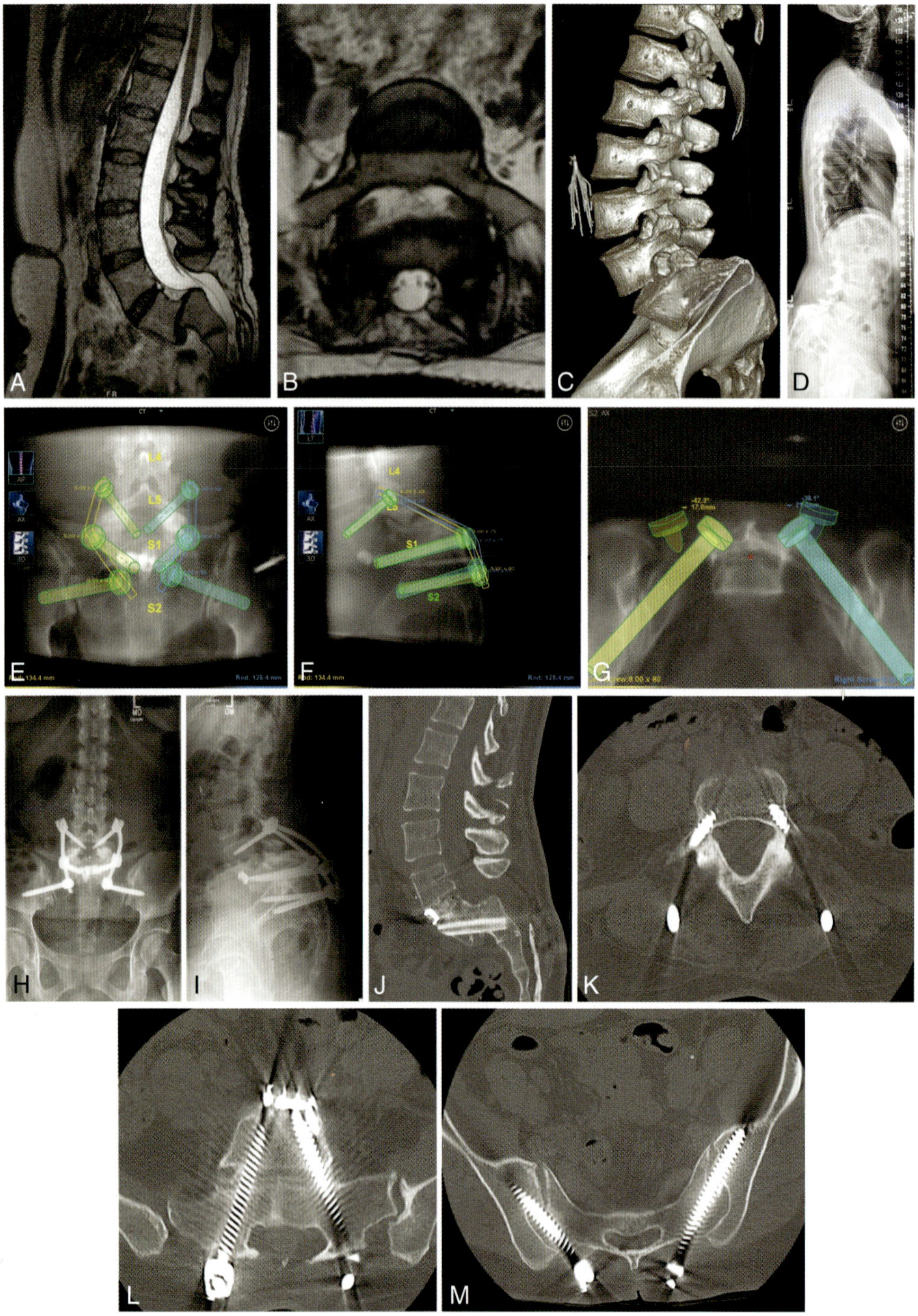

FIG. 8.2 Case vignette 2. (A) Preoperative sagittal T2-weighted MRI. (B) Preoperative axial T2-weighted MRI at the L5/S1 disk level. (C) 3D reconstruction of the preoperative lumbar CT scan, illustrating the almost vertical trajectory of the L5 pedicles. (D) Preoperative scoliosis x-rays, lateral view. (E–G) Intraoperative view on the Mazor X planning software, outlining the patient-specific screw trajectories and dimensions, as well as the rod lengths in anteroposterior (E) and lateral (F) projection, as well as the axial view on the S2Ai screws (G). (H) Postoperative x-ray studies, anteroposterior view. (I) Postoperative x-ray studies, lateral view. (J) Postoperative CT scan, lateral view on a median cut, illustrating the position of the fibular strut graft. (K–M) Postoperative CT-scan, axial views, illustrating the placement of the pedicle screws at L4 (K), transdiskcal L5/S1 screws (L), and S2Ai screws (M).

trajectory, misplacement is the main source of construct failure and robotic technology was felt optimal to ensure perfect execution of the surgical plan.[55] It allowed for the placement of screws with the optimal diameter and maximal possible length in close proximity to the L4/5 ALIF cage; however, these did not interfere with the fibular strut graft (see Fig. 8.2I–M).

The robot also allowed for conducting the posterior part of the procedure in a percutaneous, MIS-fashion. This was felt advantageous for preventing repeat muscle and soft-tissue dissection and for lowering the risk for potential dura or nerve injury inherent with scar formation from her previous surgery.

We did use navigation in parallel to the robot, to double-check accuracy of the proposed trajectories in real time. This was considered necessary due to her challenging anatomy.

Treatment Side Effects

None.

Potential Down Falls

The advantages of fixing the spondylolisthesis in situ are the lower risk for neurological complications, in particular L5 nerve root injury, resulting from a reduction maneuver.[56] Additionally, in order to reduce the spondylolisthesis an adequate decompression is required first, which in this case would have entailed dissection through the scar tissue from her previous procedure and provoked additional approach-related collateral damage.

The evident downside of operating on her in situ is that she remains sagittally imbalanced, which may lead to inferior pain and disability outcomes, a higher risk of construct failure, adjacent segment disease, and a higher risk for additional future spine surgery.

Management of Complications

No intra- or immediate postoperative complications occurred. It became evident over time that the prominent S2Ai screw heads underneath this thin patient's skin surface (very little sacral fat tissue) were the main cause of the residual low back complaints, which is why both screws were removed about one year after the index procedure, after the fusion had taken place.

SUMMARY

Current Added Value of Robotic Assistance

Currently available robotic systems provide the deformity surgeon with good to excellent accuracy for the placement of both thoracolumbar and spinopelvic implants. Moreover, they bear the potential to reduce radiation exposure (to patients and OR staff alike) and revision rates for screw misplacement. Robotic applications currently remain extremely limited regarding the treatment of cervical spine deformities. With the exception of single case reports of applications in humans,[57,58] robotic systems are currently tested on cadavers.[59] The challenges with their further application in the cervical spine relate to the higher mobility of the cervical spinal segments, resulting in greater translational and rotational errors.

For ASD, the new Mazor X Stealth Edition allows for real-time evaluation of navigation accuracy, which is helpful in cases with mobile or altered anatomy after or even before osteotomies.

Despite the added value, the downsides of this novel technology must also be considered. Decision-making during complex procedures such as ASD correction is influenced by many different factors, including both visual and tactical perception and the surgical instruments at hand. Those aspects are affected in robotic-assisted cases and surgeons must be aware of this potential "bias," which can have an impact on patient outcomes.[60] A learning curve of 25 to 30 cases until the fast and efficacious use of robot-assisted spine surgery has been appreciated; this learning curve is not unique to the surgeons but to the whole OR staff.[14,31,61] It seems reasonable to pass this learning curve first, before embarking on complex robotic-assisted deformity correction cases. Moreover, the robot cannot provide an insufficiently trained surgeon with the skillset to conduct complex ASD corrections; conversely, it can help make a well-trained surgeon even more precise and efficient.[32]

Further technical development is required to make robotic systems better applicable to ASD surgery. With the current methods of bone mounting of the robot system (e.g., insertion of a Schanz screw into the iliac crest), modern robotic systems can reach from vertebrae L3 through S2 via posterior incisions[34]; however, for longer constructs, further setups and re-registrations are required, which are time- and labor-intensive.

Future Directions

There are visionary concepts including semi-automatic robotic spine surgery devices with integrated scanners and surgical arms, even operating humanoid machines. However, machines that do not work completely independently but help the surgeon achieve the goal of safe and efficient surgery are more realistic for the decade to come.[2,26] The ways of visualization and communication between the surgeon and the robot may change over time, including augmented reality overlays of multimodal imaging beyond x-ray and CT, voice commanding, and sensor gloves.[2,26]

Currently, robots mostly function as versatile drill and screwguides, but are not yet helpful with the lengthy and tedious tasks of rod contouring and insertion, decompressing nervous elements, and conducting diskectomies and interbody fusions, even though the da Vinci has been used for some of those tasks in animal models.[24,62] Their applicability for spinal deformity procedures is moderate and even though some "early adopters" appreciate its features, the broad mass currently still relies on traditional techniques and navigation for those complex cases. It is likely, however, that ASD cases offer the most profound area of opportunity for spinal robotics to improve operative accuracy.[15] The technical challenges for the robotic industry to overcome include the extremely heterogeneous tissues of and around the spine, requiring incorporating a high degree of tactile feedback into the surgical strategy and final execution. Robotic systems currently require CT scans to identify bony elements, but for spine surgery—a field that relies heavily upon MRI—co-registration capabilities or MRI-based registration would be a valuable and potentially radiation-sparing advancement. Despite the number of robotic-guided surgeries being on the rise in the US and elsewhere, the robot industry must continue to improve surgical ergonomics and dexterity to make its utility convincingly undisputable. In consequence, for the foreseeable future, the need for spine surgeons that are trained to manually treat ASD does not appear obviated; however, untapped opportunities lie in the combination of robotics, MIS, and artificial intelligence.

REFERENCES

1. Ames CP, Smith JS, Scheer JK, et al. Impact of spinopelvic alignment on decision making in deformity surgery in adults: a review. *J Neurosurg Spine*. 2012;16(6):547–564. https://doi.org/10.3171/2012.2.SPINE11320.
2. Smith JS, Shaffrey CI, Ames CP, Lenke LG. Treatment of adult thoracolumbar spinal deformity: past, present, and future. *J Neurosurg Spine*. 2019;30(5):551–567. https://doi.org/10.3171/2019.1.SPINE181494.
3. Bess S, Line B, Fu KM, et al. The health impact of symptomatic adult spinal deformity: comparison of deformity types to United States population norms and chronic diseases. *Spine (Phila Pa 1976)*. 2016;41(3):224–233. https://doi.org/10.1097/BRS.0000000000001202.
4. Schwab F, Dubey A, Gamez L, et al. Adult scoliosis: prevalence, SF-36, and nutritional parameters in an elderly volunteer population. *Spine (Phila Pa 1976)*. 2005;30(9):1082–1085. https://doi.org/10.1097/01.brs.0000160842.43482.cd.
5. Bridwell KH, Baldus C, Berven S, et al. Changes in radiographic and clinical outcomes with primary treatment adult spinal deformity surgeries from two years to three- to five-years follow-up. *Spine (Phila Pa 1976)*. 2010;35(20):1849–1854. https://doi.org/10.1097/BRS.0b013e3181efa06a.
6. Bridwell KH, Glassman S, Horton W, et al. Does treatment (nonoperative and operative) improve the two-year quality of life in patients with adult symptomatic lumbar scoliosis: a prospective multicenter evidence-based medicine study. *Spine (Phila Pa 1976)*. 2009;34(20):2171–2178. https://doi.org/10.1097/BRS.0b013e3181a8fdc8.
7. Glassman SD, Carreon LY, Shaffrey CI, et al. The costs and benefits of nonoperative management for adult scoliosis. *Spine (Phila Pa 1976)*. 2010;35(5):578–582. https://doi.org/10.1097/BRS.0b013e3181b0f2f8.
8. Smith JS, Klineberg E, Lafage V, et al. Prospective multicenter assessment of perioperative and minimum 2-year postoperative complication rates associated with adult spinal deformity surgery. *J Neurosurg Spine*. 2016;25(1):1–14. https://doi.org/10.3171/2015.11.SPINE151036.
9. Park P, Wang MY, Lafage V, et al. Comparison of two minimally invasive surgery strategies to treat adult spinal deformity. *J Neurosurg Spine*. 2015;22(4):374–380. https://doi.org/10.3171/2014.9.SPINE131004.
10. Wang MY, Mummaneni PV, Fu KM, et al. Less invasive surgery for treating adult spinal deformities: ceiling effects for deformity correction with 3 different techniques. *Neurosurg Focus*. 2014;36(5):E12. https://doi.org/10.3171/2014.3.FOCUS1423.
11. Mummaneni PV, Shaffrey CI, Lenke LG, et al. The minimally invasive spinal deformity surgery algorithm: a reproducible rational framework for decision making in minimally invasive spinal deformity surgery. *Neurosurg Focus*. 2014;36(5):E6. https://doi.org/10.3171/2014.3.FOCUS1413.
12. Overley SC, Cho SK, Mehta AI, Arnold PM. Navigation and robotics in spinal surgery: where are we now? *Neurosurgery*. 2017;80(3S):S86–S99. https://doi.org/10.1093/neuros/nyw077.
13. Specht LM, Koval KJ. Robotics and computer-assisted orthopaedic surgery. *Bull Hosp Jt Dis*. 2001-2002;60(3-4):168–172.
14. Fiani B, Quadri SA, Farooqui M, et al. Impact of robot-assisted spine surgery on health care quality and neurosurgical economics: a systemic review. *Neurosurg Rev*. 2020;43(1):17–25. https://doi.org/10.1007/s10143-018-0971-z.
15. Kochanski RB, Lombardi JM, Laratta JL, Lehman RA, O'Toole JE. Image-guided navigation and robotics in spine surgery. *Neurosurgery*. 2019;84(6):1179–1189. https://doi.org/10.1093/neuros/nyy630.
16. Gautschi OP, Schatlo B, Schaller K, Tessitore E. Clinically relevant complications related to pedicle screw placement in thoracolumbar surgery and their management: a literature review of 35, 630 pedicle screws. *Neurosurg Focus*. 2011;31(4):E8. https://doi.org/10.3171/2011.7.FOCUS11168.
17. Gelalis ID, Paschos NK, Pakos EE, et al. Accuracy of pedicle screw placement: a systematic review of prospective in vivo studies comparing free hand, fluoroscopy guidance and navigation techniques. *Eur Spine J*. 2012;21(2):247–255. https://doi.org/10.1007/s00586-011-2011-3.
18. Kosmopoulos V, Schizas C. Pedicle screw placement accuracy: a meta-analysis. *Spine (Phila Pa 1976)*. 2007;32(3):E111–E120. https://doi.org/10.1097/01.brs.0000254048.79024.8b.
19. Shin BJ, James AR, Njoku IU, Härtl R. Pedicle screw navigation: a systematic review and meta-analysis of perforation risk for computer-navigated versus freehand insertion. *J Neurosurg Spine*. 2012;17(2):113–122. https://doi.org/10.3171/2012.5.SPINE11399.
20. Larson AN, Santos ER, Polly DW Jr, et al. Pediatric pedicle screw placement using intraoperative computed tomography and 3-dimensional image-guided navigation. *Spine (Phila Pa 1976)*. 2012;37(3):E188–E194. https://doi.org/10.1097/BRS.0b013e31822a2e0a.
21. Beutler WJ, Peppelman WC Jr, DiMarco LA. The da Vinci robotic surgical assisted anterior lumbar interbody fusion: technical development and case report. *Spine (Phila Pa 1976)*. 2013;38(4):356–363. https://doi.org/10.1097/BRS.0b013e31826b3d72.
22. Lee JY, Bhowmick DA, Eun DD, Welch WC. Minimally invasive, robot-assisted, anterior lumbar interbody fusion: a technical note. *J Neurol Surg A*. 2013;74(4):258–261. https://doi.org/10.1055/s-0032-1330121.
23. Lee Z, Lee JY, Welch WC, Eun D. Technique and surgical outcomes of robot-assisted anterior lumbar interbody fusion. *J Robot Surg*. 2013;7(2):177–185. https://doi.org/10.1007/s11701-012-0365-0.
24. Kim MJ, Ha Y, Yang MS, et al. Robot-assisted anterior lumbar interbody fusion (ALIF) using retroperitoneal approach. *Acta Neurochir (Wien)*. 2010;152(4):675–679. https://doi.org/10.1007/s00701-009-0568-y.
25. Gao S, Lv Z, Fang H. Robot-assisted and conventional freehand pedicle screw placement: a systematic review

and meta-analysis of randomized controlled trials. *Eur Spine J*. 2018;27(4):921–930. https://doi.org/10.1007/s00586-017-5333-y.

26. Madhavan K, Kolcun JPG, Chieng LO, Wang MY. Augmented-reality integrated robotics in neurosurgery: are we there yet? *Neurosurg Focus*. 2017;42(5):E3. https://doi.org/10.3171/2017.2.FOCUS177.
27. Gertzbein SD, Robbins SE. Accuracy of pedicular screw placement in vivo. *Spine (Phila Pa 1976)*. 1990;15(1):11–14. https://doi.org/10.1097/00007632-199001000-00004.
28. Macke JJ, Woo R, Varich L. Accuracy of robot-assisted pedicle screw placement for adolescent idiopathic scoliosis in the pediatric population. *J Robot Surg*. 2016;10(2):145–150. https://doi.org/10.1007/s11701-016-0587-7.
29. Fan Y, Peng Du J, Liu JJ, Zhang JN, Liu SC, Hao DJ. Radiological and clinical differences among three assisted technologies in pedicle screw fixation of adult degenerative scoliosis. *Sci Rep*. 2018;8(1):890. https://doi.org/10.1038/s41598-017-19054-7.
30. Devito DP, Kaplan L, Dietl R, et al. Clinical acceptance and accuracy assessment of spinal implants guided with SpineAssist surgical robot: retrospective study. *Spine (Phila Pa 1976)*. 2010;35(24):2109–2115. https://doi.org/10.1097/BRS.0b013e3181d323ab.
31. Hu X, Ohnmeiss DD, Lieberman IH. Robotic-assisted pedicle screw placement: lessons learned from the first 102 patients. *Eur Spine J*. 2013;22(3):661–666. https://doi.org/10.1007/s00586-012-2499-1.
32. Hu X, Lieberman IH. Robotic-assisted spine surgery. In: Phililips FM, ed. *Minimally Invasive Spine Surgery*. New York: Springer Science + Business; 2014:61–66.
33. Hicks JM, Singla A, Shen FH, Arlet V. Complications of pedicle screw fixation in scoliosis surgery: a systematic review. *Spine (Phila Pa 1976)*. 2010;35(11):E465–E470. https://doi.org/10.1097/BRS.0b013e3181d1021a.
34. Laratta JL, Shillingford JN, Meredith JS, Lenke LG, Lehman RA, Gum JL. Robotic versus freehand S2 alar iliac fixation: in-depth technical considerations. *J Spine Surg*. 2018;4(3):638–644. https://doi.org/10.21037/jss.2018.06.13.
35. Chang TL, Sponseller PD, Kebaish KM, Fishman EK. Low profile pelvic fixation: anatomic parameters for sacral alar-iliac fixation versus traditional iliac fixation. *Spine (Phila Pa 1976)*. 2009;34(5):436–440. https://doi.org/10.1097/BRS.0b013e318194128c.
36. Bederman SS, Hahn P, Colin V, Kiester PD, Bhatia NN. Robotic guidance for S2-alar-iliac screws in spinal deformity correction. *Clin Spine Surg*. 2017;30(1):E49–E53. https://doi.org/10.1097/BSD.0b013e3182a3572b.
37. Hyun SJ, Kim KJ, Jahng TA. S2 alar iliac screw placement under robotic guidance for adult spinal deformity patients: technical note. *Eur Spine J*. 2017;26(8):2198–2203. https://doi.org/10.1007/s00586-017-5012-z.
38. Hu X, Lieberman IH. Robotic-guided sacro-pelvic fixation using S2 alar-iliac screws: feasibility and accuracy. *Eur Spine J*. 2017;26(3):720–725. https://doi.org/10.1007/s00586-016-4639-5.
39. Laratta JL, Shillingford JN, Lombardi JM, et al. Accuracy of S2 alar-iliac screw placement under robotic guidance. *Spine Deform*. 2018;6(2):130–136. https://doi.org/10.1016/j.jspd.2017.08.009.
40. Shillingford JN, Laratta JL, Park PJ, et al. Human versus robot: a propensity-matched analysis of the accuracy of free hand versus robotic guidance for placement of S2 alar-iliac (S2AI) screws. *Spine (Phila Pa 1976)*. 2018;43(21):E1297–E1304. https://doi.org/10.1097/BRS.0000000000002694.
41. Kantelhardt SR, Martinez R, Baerwinkel S, Burger R, Giese A, Rohde V. Perioperative course and accuracy of screw positioning in conventional, open robotic-guided and percutaneous robotic-guided, pedicle screw placement. *Eur Spine J*. 2011;20(6):860–868. https://doi.org/10.1007/s00586-011-1729-2.
42. ODT. NASS News: Mazor robotics presents first prospective study of robotic-guided spine surgery. https://www.odtmag.com/contents/view_breaking-news/2017-10-25/nass-news-mazor-robotics-presents-first-prospective-study-of-robotic-guided-spine-surgery. Accessed July 14, 2019.
43. Kim HJ, Kang KT, Park SC, et al. Biomechanical advantages of robot-assisted pedicle screw fixation in posterior lumbar interbody fusion compared with freehand technique in a prospective randomized controlled trial-perspective for patient-specific finite element analysis. *Spine J*. 2017;17(5):671–680. https://doi.org/10.1016/j.spinee.2016.11.010.
44. Stienen MN, Smoll NR, Hildebrandt G, Schaller K, Tessitore E, Gautschi OP. Constipation after thoraco-lumbar fusion surgery. *Clin Neurol Neurosurg*. 2014;126:137–142. https://doi.org/10.1016/j.clineuro.2014.08.036.
45. MIS ReFRESH: Robotic vs. Freehand Minimally Invasive Spinal Surgeries. https://clinicaltrials.gov/ct2/show/NCT02057744. Accessed July 18, 2019.
46. Stienen MN, Ho AL, Staartjes VE, et al. Objective measures of functional impairment for degenerative diseases of the lumbar spine: a systematic review of the literature. *Spine J*. 2019;19(7):1276–1293. https://doi.org/10.1016/j.spinee.2019.02.014.
47. Hyun SJ, Kim KJ, Jahng TA, Kim HJ. Minimally invasive robotic versus open fluoroscopic-guided spinal instrumented fusions: a randomized controlled trial. *Spine (Phila Pa 1976)*. 2017;42(6):353–358. https://doi.org/10.1097/BRS.0000000000001778.
48. Keric N, Eum DJ, Afghanyar F, et al. Evaluation of surgical strategy of conventional vs. percutaneous robot-assisted spinal trans-pedicular instrumentation in spondylodiscitis. *J Robot Surg*. 2017;11(1):17–25. https://doi.org/10.1007/s11701-016-0597-5.
49. Mathews JD, Forsythe AV, Brady Z, et al. Cancer risk in 680, 000 people exposed to computed tomography scans in childhood or adolescence: data linkage study of 11 million Australians. *BMJ*. 2013;346:f2360. https://doi.org/10.1136/bmj.f2360.
50. Schröder ML, Staartjes VE. Revisions for screw malposition and clinical outcomes after robot-guided lumbar fusion for spondylolisthesis. *Neurosurg Focus*. 2017;42(5):E12. https://doi.org/10.3171/2017.3.FOCUS16534.

51. Schroerlucke SR, Wang MY, Cannestra AF, et al. Revision rate in robotic-guided vs fluoro-guided minimally invasive spinal fusion surgery: report from MIS ReFRESH prospective comparative study. *Spine J*. 2017;17(10):S255. https://doi.org/10.1016/j.spinee.2017.08.178.
52. Lieberman IH, Togawa D, Kayanja MM, et al. Bone-mounted miniature robotic guidance for pedicle screw and translaminar facet screw placement: part I—technical development and a test case result. *Neurosurgery*. 2006;59(3):641–650, discussion 641. https://doi.org/10.1227/01.NEU.0000229055.00829.5B.
53. Abdu WA, Wilber RG, Emery SE. Pedicular transvertebral screw fixation of the lumbosacral spine in spondylolisthesis. A new technique for stabilization. *Spine (Phila Pa 1976)*. 1994;19(6):710–715. https://doi.org/10.1097/00007632-199403001-00011.
54. Ho AL, Varshneya K, Medress ZA, et al. Grade II spondylolisthesis: Reverse Bohlman procedure with transdiscal S1-L5 and S2 Alar Iliac screws placed with robotic guidance. *World Neurosurg*. 2019;132:421–428.e1. https://doi:10.1016/j.wneu.2019.07.229.
55. Delgado-Fernández J, Pulido P, García-Pallero MÁ, Blasco G, Frade-Porto N, Sola RG. Image guidance in transdiscal fixation for high-grade spondylolisthesis in adults with correct spinal balance. *Neurosurg Focus*. 2018;44(1):E9. https://doi.org/10.3171/2017.10.FOCUS17557.
56. Acosta FL Jr, Ames CP, Chou D. Operative management of adult high-grade lumbosacral spondylolisthesis. *Neurosurg Clin N Am*. 2007;18(2):249–254. https://doi.org/10.1016/j.nec.2007.01.001.
57. Tian W. Robot-assisted posterior C1-2 transarticular screw fixation for atlantoaxial instability: a case report. *Spine (Phila Pa 1976)*. 2016;41(suppl 19):B2–B5. https://doi.org/10.1097/BRS.0000000000001674.
58. Molteni G, Greco MG, Presutti L. Transoral robotic-assisted surgery for the approach to anterior cervical spine lesions. *Eur Arch Otorhinolaryngol*. 2017;274(11):4011–4016. https://doi.org/10.1007/s00405-017-4731-4.
59. Kostrzewski S, Duff JM, Baur C, Olszewski M. Robotic system for cervical spine surgery. *Int J Med Robot*. 2012;8(2):184–190. https://doi.org/10.1002/rcs.446.
60. Randell R, Alvarado N, Honey S, et al. Impact of robotic surgery on decision making: perspectives of surgical teams. *AMIA Annu Symp Proc*. 2015;2015:1057–1066.
61. Schatlo B, Martinez R, Alaid A, et al. Unskilled unawareness and the learning curve in robotic spine surgery. *Acta Neurochir (Wien)*. 2015;157(10):1819–1823, discussion 23. https://doi.org/10.1007/s00701-015-2535-0.
62. Ponnusamy K, Chewning S, Mohr C. Robotic approaches to the posterior spine. *Spine (Phila Pa 1976)*. 2009;34(19):2104–2109. https://doi.org/10.1097/BRS.0b013e3181b20212.

9

Robotic-Assisted Percutaneous Fixation

Mark A. Pacult, MD, S. Harrison Farber, MD, Cyrus Elahi, MS, MD, and Juan S. Uribe, MD

INTRODUCTION OF TECHNOLOGY

Present Practice and Standard of Care

Pedicle screws have been placed to enhance spinal fusion since at least 1959. In that year, Boucher[1] published a report detailing the placement of screws into the vertebral body via the pedicle with generally excellent fusion results. These early pedicle screws passed from the lamina of the superior level through the pedicle of the inferior level, thus achieving a state of internal fixation with addition of cancellous bone graft for fusion. In 1970, Roy-Camille described the first closed system involving interpedicular screws and plates[2]; in that system, pedicle screws functioned as bone anchors for a transpedicular plate running longitudinally along the spine. Since these early days, pedicle screws have seen a remarkable array of transformations in their design, placement techniques, and compatible systems for spinal fixation. The use of robotics to place pedicle screws forms but the latest chapter in a rich and fascinating history of innovation.

Two main phenomena are responsible for the pace of innovation that has led to the introduction of robotics in spine surgery. First, the placement of pedicle screws carries a risk of neurovascular compromise while traversing the spinal canal. A persistent theme in pedicle screw literature pertains to accuracy of placement, namely avoiding breaches through cortical bone. Second, the open exposure required for pedicle screw placement historically and frequently necessitates extensive soft tissue manipulation, raising the risk for injury, perioperative morbidity, infection, and spinal destabilization. Both of these drawbacks have driven the development of computer assisted navigation and percutaneous techniques to increase accuracy and decrease the invasiveness of pedicle screw placement. Robotic-assisted pedicle screw placement relies upon and combines both of these techniques.

Percutaneous fixation was first described by Magerl[3] in 1984 via the use of intraoperative fluoroscopy. In particular, the "owl's eye" view in the oblique plane along the barrel of the pedicle was meant to aid the surgeon in the percutaneous placement of a pedicle screw without the wide exposure traditionally necessary. These percutaneously placed screws were combined with an external fixation system, because the techniques to appropriately place rods in a minimally invasive fashion were still in their infancy. It was not until Foley and Gupta[4] developed the Sextant system in 2002 (manufactured by Medtronic Sofamor Danek) that major advances were made in both virtual intraoperative navigation (via the use of the virtual fluoroscope) and percutaneous rod insertion. The adoption of three-dimensional virtual fluoroscopy (commonly referred to as computer assisted navigation) was first reported in 1997, and the validation of its accuracy in pedicle screw placement has been well reported.[5,6] Advances in percutaneous placement via accurate computer-registered intraoperative imaging allowed the entry of the robot onto the spinal fusion landscape.

A robot is a machine that can replicate certain human functions. Generally, three different robotic systems are used in surgery: tele-surgical systems (where the surgeon directly controls a robot), supervisory-controlled systems (where the surgeon plans a task, and a robot performs it), and shared-control systems (where the surgeon and robot share task completion).[7,8] The use of robots in spine surgery is unique when compared to the adoption of robotics in other surgical theaters. Robotic surgery in fields such as general surgery, urologic surgery, and gynecologic surgery has its origins in different needs, such as the visualization of previously difficult-to-reach areas. The adoption of robotic surgery in these fields relied on the successful development of the endoscope, which led to tele-surgical systems, such as the well-known da Vinci systems (Intuitive Surgical). Such systems aim to improve surgical capabilities, and the advantage of the robot is achieved by increasing manual function in an enclosed body cavity.

Robotic Systems in Spine Surgery

Modern spinal fusion involves the repetitive, minimally invasive surgical (MIS) placement of hardware that traverses sensitive neurovascular structures. The theoretical advantages of robots within this paradigm are to automate repetitive tasks, minimize surgical exposures, and increase accuracy by eliminating human error. The robotic systems used in spine surgery today generally involve shared-control systems in which an intraoperative plan is conceived by a robot's imaging software, verified and modified by a surgeon, and performed in a shared fashion by the surgeon, who creates a percutaneous exposure and places hardware positioned by a navigated robotic arm. The computer assisted navigation for image acquisition and registration allows the robot to know where its effector arm is positioned relative to desired targets both theoretically (on the preoperative image) and in real life (on the patient). Although many systems have developed unique image registration and merging software, the basic innovation of robotic systems for spine surgery is the automation of screw positioning in preparation for drilling. While the positioning of cannulas, drill guides, and screws is automated, the surgeon must still prepare the tissue via skin and fascial incisions and operate the taps, drills, and screwdrivers.

Currently, robotic systems from three manufacturers have US Food and Drug Administration (FDA) approval for use in percutaneous pedicle screw placement. A brief overview of these systems is provided below and in Table 9.1.

Mazor Systems

The first robotic system to gain FDA approval was developed by Mazor Robotics (Caesarea, Israel) and is named the SpineAssist. This system is patient-mounted by fixation to a spinous process (if an open approach is used) or to the iliac crest via Steinman pins (if a percutaneous approach is used). The basic steps involved in its operation consist of (1) attainment of preoperative computed tomography (CT); (2) preoperative planning with screw trajectories and screw size mapped out via the system's software on the preoperative image; (3) attachment of the mounting frame to the patient and placement of fiducial landmarks on the patient; (4) attainment of fluoroscopic images of the patient's spine and synchronization of

TABLE 9.1 Current generation FDA-approved robotic systems.

Robot	Manufacturer	FDA approval	Prior generations	Unique features
Mazor X Stealth Edition	Medtronic (formerly Mazor Robotics)	2018	Mazor Renaissance, Mazor SpineAssist Mazor X	Optic camera to avoid collisions between robotic arm and tools
ROSA One	Zimmer Biomet (formerly Medtech)	2019	ROSA Spine	Adaptation for orthopedic use
Excelsius	Globus	2017	–	Registration via fluoroscopy or intraoperative computed tomography

these images with the preoperative CT using the system's software; and (5) alignment of the robotic arms to planned locations and subsequent placement of Kirschner wires (K-wire), dilators, taps, and screws.

The subsequent models included the Mazor Renaissance (FDA approval in 2011) and Mazor X (FDA approval in 2016). Both of these robotic systems featured improvements to deal with reported issues of the Mazor SpineAssist, such as skiving of the drill on fascia or bone. The Mazor X also features an optic camera to register the operative field to avoid collisions between the robotic arm and intraoperative tools.

In 2018, Medtronic (Dublin, Ireland) acquired Mazor Robotics and integrated their preoperative stealth navigation software with the Mazor X robot, forming the Mazor X Stealth Edition, which received FDA clearance in 2018.

Rosa One

The ROSA spine robot was developed by Medtech SA (Montpellier, France) and received FDA clearance in 2016. It consists of a floor-mounted station with an attached flexible robotic arm and a separate floor-mounted camera for capturing patient-mounted fiducials. The system operates by obtaining an intraoperative CT scan as the robotic arm places a fiducial box overlying the area of interest on the spine.[9] The CT images are used for operative planning by the surgeon on a touchscreen attached to the robotic arm base. The robotic arm then moves into this predefined position because it recognizes spine landmarks from the overlying fiducial grid. The instruments are tracked during surgery by the fiducial system, and appropriate dilators, taps, and screws are placed. As with the Mazor system, the robotic arm moves each tool into position, but the drilling and screwing are performed by the surgeon.

In 2016, Zimmer Biomet (Warsaw, Indiana) acquired Medtech SA, and in 2019, FDA clearance was received for the ROSA One spine system. This robotic system can also be used for cranial applications under the ROSA One brain denomination. A ROSA One knee application is available for orthopedic use.

Excelsius

The Globus (Audubon, PA) Excelsius system received FDA clearance in 2017. Similar to the other systems, it consists of a mobile base with a robotic arm and screen for operative planning. A separate, mobile base involves a camera for the registration of fiducials for image merging. To operate the system, the fiducials are placed in the posterior superior iliac spine, and a grid called a dynamic reference base is overlaid above the skin attached to the iliac spine. The system can function either by taking intraoperative fluoroscopic images and merging them with a preoperative CT scan, or by registering an intraoperative CT scan. The surgeon then plans each screw trajectory and performs screw selection on the screen. The robotic arm then moves into position, and sequential dilators are placed. The steps of screw placement are performed by the surgeon, while the trajectory is maintained by the robotic arm.

Non–FDA-Approved Robots

Several robotic systems in use around the world have not been evaluated by the FDA for use in the United States. These include the Tianji Robot (Beijing Tinavi Medical Technology), which received clearance from the Chinese Food and Drug Administration in 2016.[10,11] This system consists of two bases, namely a robotic arm base and a second base that contains an optical tracking camera for instrument tracking and registration, and a planning display. To operate it, the surgeon places a reference tracker on the spinous process, and a calibration screen is held by the robotic arm over the skin as two-dimensional C-arm images are obtained. These are registered with preoperative CT images. The surgical planning then proceeds using the system's software where the surgeon views images of each level and selects screw trajectory, size, and length. The robotic arm then moves into the preselected position. Skin incisions are made, dilation is performed via sequential dilators, and cannulas are held in place by the robotic arm. Drilling and screw insertion are performed with tracked, navigated instruments that are controlled by the surgeon but guided by the guides held by the robotic arm.[12]

Current Outcomes

A wealth of literature reports on the comparison between robotic systems, free-handed approaches, and navigated approaches in the placement of pedicle screws. A summary of the pros and cons of robotic, free-handed, and CT-guided screw placement techniques is provided in Table 9.2.[12–27]

Accuracy of Pedicle Screw Placement

The most widely used system for comparing the approaches for accuracy of pedicle screw placement in the literature on robotic systems is the Gertzbein-Robbins classification, which delineates five separate grades (A–E) based on whether the screw is entirely within the pedicle (A) or breaching the medial cortical wall by less than 2 mm (B), less than 4 mm (C), less than 6 mm (D), or greater than 6 mm (E).[29] Grades A and B are generally clinically acceptable.

The safety of robotically placed pedicle screws has been well-established in a multitude of studies.[30–33] Several caveats apply when examining the literature as it pertains to accuracy for robotically assisted spine surgeries: the accuracy criteria are heterogenous, purely percutaneous approaches are rare and often combined in studies with open approaches, indications are manifold, and studies usually examine only one robotic system. However, several generalizations are possible. The reported accuracy rates for purely percutaneous robotically placed pedicle screws generally range between 97% and 98%.[17–20] An early, large, retrospective review of 3271 robotically placed pedicle screws found a "clinically safe" placement (Gertzbein-Robbins A or B) in 98.3% of screws.[32] This compares favorably to reported accuracy rates of 90.7% and 90.6%, respectively, for more than 15, 358 pedicle screws placed

TABLE 9.2 Pros and cons of robotic, free-hand, and CT-guided screw placement.

	Robotic	Free-hand	CT-guided
Pros	• Improved accuracy[13–15] • Decreased radiation exposure[12,16] • Less blood loss[12]	• Surgeon familiarity • Reliable accuracy[17–20]	• Decreased surgeon radiation exposure vs. free-hand[21]
Cons	• Steep learning curve[22,24,28] • Skiving of drill[25]	• More radiation exposure to patient and surgeon compared to robotic and CT-guided placements[26,27]	• Increased exposure to radiation vs. robotic[16]

in vivo using both nonnavigated and navigated assistance with no robotic control.[14] When compared directly in one retrospective review, 93.4% of 410 robotically placed screws were Gertzbein-Robbins A or B versus 88.9% of 397 placed in a free-handed group, a result that was statistically significant ($P = .005$).[15]

Large meta-analyses corroborate the safety and even the superiority of robotic-guided screw placement. A comparison of publications examining robotic versus free-handed techniques found that robotically placed screws were more accurate when judged as being completely within the pedicle compared to free-hand screws (OR 95% CI: 1.38–2.07, $P < .01$).[13] Another recent large meta-analysis of randomized controlled trials determined that screws placed using the Mazor Renaissance robot were no more accurate along Gertzbein-Robbins A criteria (RR = 1.00, 95% CI 0.96–1.05, $P = .95$) than were traditional free-handed techniques, but that those placed by the Tianji robot were more accurate (RR = 0.46, 95% CI 0.28–0.75, $P < .01$).[34]

In one randomized controlled trial comparing 74 robotically placed pedicle screws to 82 placed with conventional, free-handed open techniques, there was no statistically significant difference in screw placement accuracy.[35] However, robotically placed screws were less likely to violate the proximal facet joint than those placed free-handed. Another study with 30 patients each in one of two arms—a percutaneous robotic and open fluoroscopic arm—found no difference in accuracy of placement but found greater distance from the proximal facet in robotically placed screws.[36] A detailed assessment of accuracy was undertaken in one study comparing purely percutaneous robotically placed screws and standard open fluoroscopic guidance for spinal fusion in patients with metastatic spine disease. Although the rates of clinically acceptable (Gertzbein-Robbins A or B) screw placements did not differ between the two groups (84.4% of 192 screws vs. 83.6% of 214 screws), in those screws that were malpositioned, medial errors prevailed with the robot, whereas lateral errors prevailed in the free-hand group.[10]

Notably, several publications report the inferior accuracy of robotically placed screws. One early prospective randomized controlled trial found that the free-handed technique achieved superior rates of accurate screw placement compared to robotically assisted placement using the Mazor SpineAssist robot.[25] In this study, 93% of 152 free-handed screws were classified as Gertzbein-Robbins A or B, versus only 85% for 146 robotically placed screws. The authors postulated that the especially low rate of accuracy in the robotic arm was due to the use of a bed-mounted robot and a postulated high risk of skiving, as the entry point is located on the downslope of the facet.[25] One study directly compared 24 open versus 6 percutaneous robotic procedures and found a higher breach rate with percutaneous procedures, postulating that this may be due to the inability to grind down the facet at the screw entry site in percutaneous procedures.[37]

Because of their early introduction, the Mazor and ROSA systems are the most studied. However, several recent publications testify to the similarly safe and highly accurate use of the Excelsius system, with reported breach rates of 1.6% of 3.4% in two separate retrospective studies.[22,38] A summary of the prospective randomized controlled trials examining robotic placement of pedicle screws is provided in Table 9.3.[12,25,31,35,36,39–41]

Clinical Outcome Measures

Length of Stay

Reports detailing clinical outcomes of robotic-assisted percutaneous procedures are encouraging. A theoretical advantage of MIS procedures is decreased tissue manipulation, blood loss, and operative time that ideally should translate into decreased overall hospital length of stay.[42] In comparison to open free-hand procedures, length of stay for percutaneous robotically placed screws was found to be 2.6 days shorter in a prospective randomized controlled trial.[36] When directly comparing open and percutaneous robotic procedures, this advantage was maintained in a large retrospective review, with a decreased length of

TABLE 9.3 Prospective, randomized, controlled trials examining accuracy of pedicle screw placement using robotic systems.

Study, year	Robot	N (screws)	Intervention	Accuracy	Other Findings
Ringel et al., 2012[25]	Mazor SpineAssist	146 robot, 152 free-hand	Lumbar and sacral screws	Robotic 85%, free-hand 93% (GR A or B)	Free-hand: less operative time
Roser et al., 2013[31]	Mazor SpineAssist	72 robot, 40 free-hand, 36 navigation	Lumbar screws	Robotic 99%, free-hand 97.5%, navigation 92% (GR A)	
Hyun et al., 2017[36]	Mazor Renaissance	130 robot, 140 fluoro	Lumbar screws	Robotic 97.7%, fluoro 95% (GR A)	Robotic: less radiation, shorter LOS, same operative time, same VAS and ODI scores
Kim et al., 2017[35]	Mazor Renaissance	158 robot, 172 free-hand	Lumbar screws	Robotic 93.7%, free-hand 91.9% (GR A)	Robotic: longer operative time
Park et al., 2018[40]	Mazor Renaissance	37 patients robot, 41 patients free-hand	Lumbar screws	Not reported	Both groups: significant improvement in VAS back VAS leg, ODI postsurgery
Han et al., 2019[12]	Tianji TiRobot	115 robot, 119 fluoro	Thoracic and lumbar screws	Robotic 95.3%, fluoro 86.1% (GR A)	Robotic: less blood loss, less radiation exposure, same operative time, same LOS
Li et al., 2019[41]	Orthobot	32 robot, 50 free-hand	Lumbar screws	Robotic 90.6% GR A, 9.4% B; free-hand 78% A, 20% B	Robotic: shorter radiation time
Fan et al., 2020[42]	Tianji TiRobot	186 robot, 204 fluoro	Cervical screws	Robotic 87.6%, fluoro 60.8% (GR A)	Robotic: less blood loss, shorter LOS

Accuracy is defined according to specified Gertzbein-Robbins grade.

Fluoro Fluoroscopy; *GR*, Gertzbein-Robbins; *LOS*, length of stay; *ODI*, Oswestry Disability Index; *VAS*, visual analog scale.

stay of 1.5 days.[43] Compared to open free-hand placed screws, the length of stay for percutaneous robotically placed screws was 4.5 days shorter in the same study.[43]

Operative Time, Radiation Exposure, Blood Loss

Early reports on the use of robotics suggested that operative time was longer for these procedures when compared to open fluoroscopy.[22,24,25,30,31] This time difference was attributed to the steep learning curve with using robotics and associated software as well as the occasional need to revise robotically placed screws with traditional techniques during software failure. Several reports have, however, noted shorter or comparable operative times with MIS robotic procedures when compared to open free-hand ones.[10,17,36,43] Although one retrospective study did not find evidence to support a learning curve for the placement of screws, two other reports of 25 and 30 cases have shown that misplacement rates of screws in robotic surgeries seems to decline with experience.[22–24] The authors of one of these studies examined 1265 pedicle screws placed with the Mazor SpineAssist system and found a breach rate of 2.4% in the first five surgeries, a rate of 6.3% for surgeries 11 through 15, and a rate of 7.1% for surgeries 16 through 20 for each surgeon.[24] They advocate the use of supervision for new surgeons during the first 25 cases for optimal accuracy.

Another touted benefit of both CT-guided and robotic-navigated systems is the decreased radiation exposure to the surgeon. In these systems, the patient ideally undergoes one preoperative or intraoperative CT scan that the surgeon or robotic system uses to plan the screw trajectory. The intraoperatively tracked instruments display trajectory and screw placement on these images, obviating the need for intraoperative fluoroscopy under C-arm guidance. Despite conflicting evidence on operative time, evidence suggests shorter exposure time to radiation using robotic MIS techniques, with one report citing an average of 4 s for robotic MIS and 6.4 s for intraoperative CT.[16] Another prospective randomized trial confirmed this decreased radiation exposure time, with a nearly 63% reduction in per-screw radiation time, a significant decrease in radiation intensity as measured by surgeon exposure in the robotic arm, and incremental decreases in radiation exposure in robotic cases after a 15-case learning curve.[36] A theoretical advantage of the robot is decreased duration of radiation exposure to the surgeon in particular, a fact that has been validated in one study that found that, although the overall radiation times did not differ statistically between robotic and free-handed procedures, the intensity as measured by the surgeon was statistically significantly decreased in robotic procedures.[12]

The reported blood loss has also tended to be less in percutaneous robotic procedures than in open ones, either robotic or free-handed. One study found that robotic procedures resulted in less blood loss on average (186 mL) than did open free-hand procedures (217 mL), a result that was statistically significant and upheld when subdividing robotic procedures into open and percutaneous cohorts.[12]

Clinical Outcomes

In theory, MIS approaches should result in higher patient satisfaction due to the purported decreased tissue exposure, length of hospital stays, and postoperative pain. This finding has not been borne out in the research literature. In one prospective randomized controlled trial, there was no significant difference in self-reported visual analog scale back or leg pain scores between patients undergoing either robotic MIS or traditional open procedures, although patients in the robotic arm did register a greater reduction in Oswestry Disability Index scores.[36] One study found a statistically significant difference in the postoperative opioid requirement, with patients undergoing percutaneous robotic procedures requiring less opioid escalations than those undergoing open robotic procedures, and still less than those undergoing open free-handed procedures.[43]

Complications

One study examined intraoperative adverse effects and found that 4.7% of patients undergoing robotic procedures experienced an adverse event, whereas 9.1% of those undergoing open free-handed procedures experienced an event.[43] Postoperative infections were reported in the same study, with 0% of percutaneous robotic procedures, 10% of open robotic, and 10.7% of open free-handed procedure patients experiencing postoperative infections. Only the difference between the aggregate robotic procedures and conventional ones was found to be statistically significant in this study. This stratification persisted when examining the need for postoperative revision, with percutaneous procedures requiring the least and open free-hand cases the most postoperative revisions. Based on the trend of the numbers for open robotic procedures more closely resembling that for open free-hand procedures, the authors concluded that the advantage of percutaneous robotic procedures lies more in the percutaneous approach and less in the robot itself.[43]

SURGICAL TREATMENT FOR SPINAL PATHOLOGY

Minimally Invasive Extreme Lateral Interbody Fusion and Posterior Spinal Fusion: Clinical Case 1

History/Clinical Presentation

A 47-year-old woman with a longstanding history of low back pain presented to our clinic with worsening low back pain and bilateral hip pain over the previous 6 months. Conservative management, including 12 weeks of physical therapy, 5 steroid spinal injections at the L3–L4 level, and over-the-counter medications, had failed to improve her symptoms. Her physical examination findings were notable for full strength, no sensory deficits, and an antalgic gait.

Preoperative Imaging

Anteroposterior and lateral total-spine radiographs showed L3–L4 spondylosis without abnormal sagittal balance or coronal deformity (Figs. 9.1A and B). Magnetic resonance imaging (MRI) (see Fig. 9.1C) and CT (see Figs. 9.1D and E) revealed advanced L3–L4 degenerative disk disease causing severe spondylosis, loss of disk height, and moderate central canal stenosis.

Surgical Planning

We performed a minimally invasive prone retroperitoneal transpsoas lumbar interbody fusion at L3–L4 with L3–L4 percutaneous pedicle screw fixation using the ExcelsiusGPS robot (Globus Medical). First, we secured the navigation system (Fig. 9.2A), which was used to plan the pedicle screw and interbody graft placement (see Fig. 9.2B). We then placed robotic-assisted percutaneous lumbar pedicle screws with modular heads. We used a prone retroperitoneal transpsoas approach to complete the lumbar interbody fusion using a titanium interbody graft (22 × 55 × 8 mm with 10 degrees of lordosis) filled with allograft (human amniotic allograft (HAA), triphosphate calcium). We were careful to preserve the

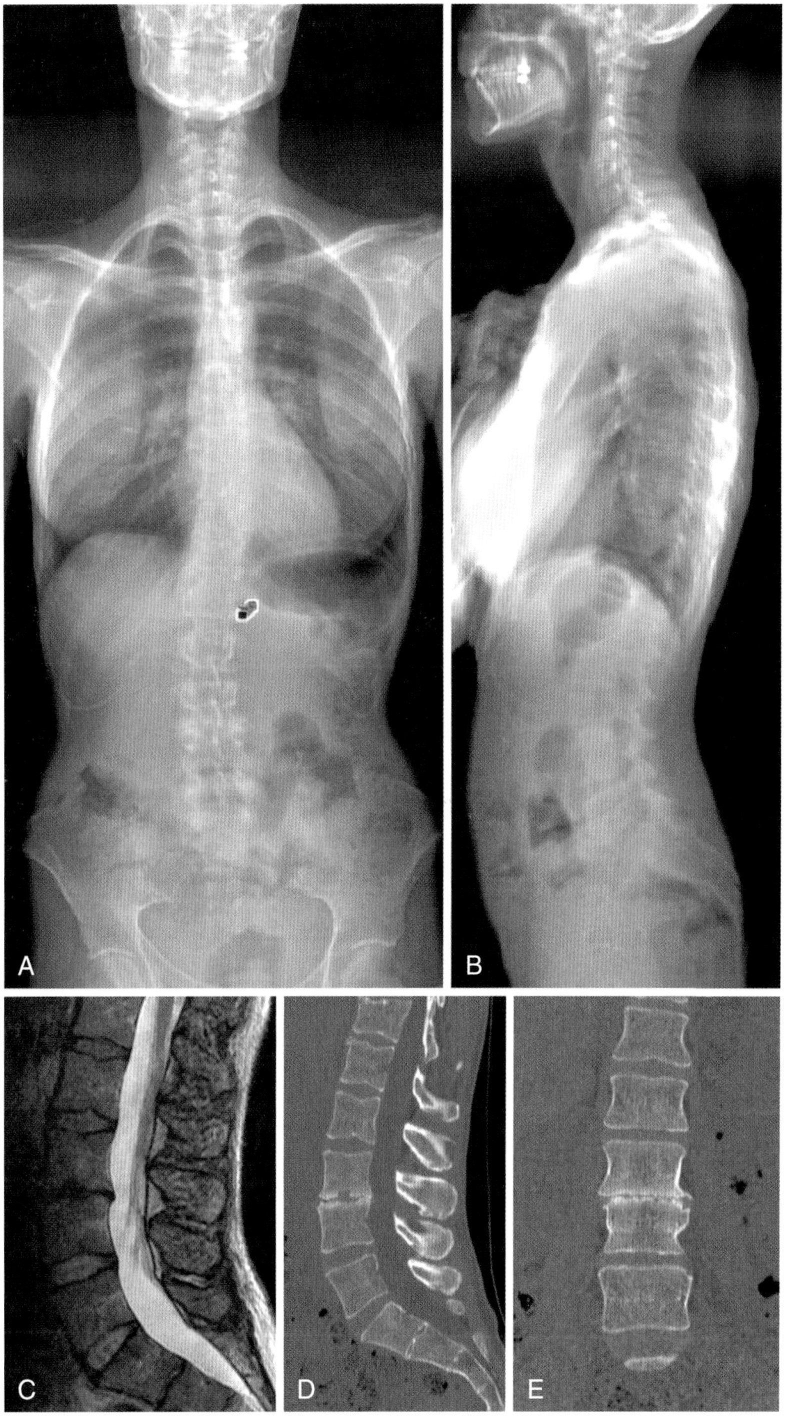

FIG. 9.1 Case 1: Preoperative images from a 47-year-old woman with a longstanding history of low back pain. L3–L4 spondylosis without abnormal sagittal balance or coronal deformity is seen on (A) anteroposterior and (B) lateral radiographs of the total spine, (C) sagittal MRI of the lumbar spine, and (D) saggital and (E) coronal CTs of the lumbar spine. (Used with permission from Barrow Neurological Institute, Phoenix, Arizona.)

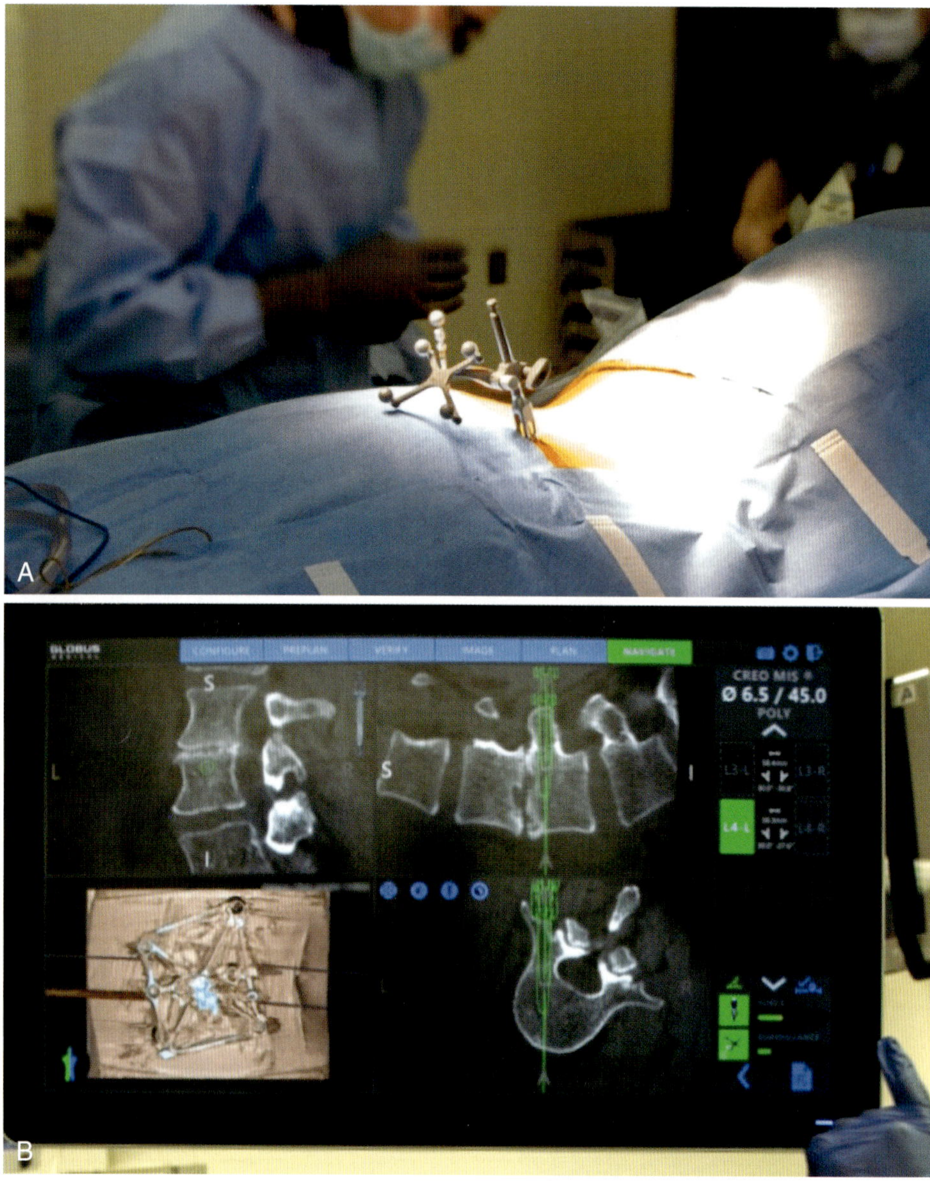

FIG. 9.2 Case 1: Surgical planning for minimally invasive extreme lateral interbody fusion and pedicle screw fixation. (A) Navigation landmarks are secured before skin incision. (B) Screw entry site and trajectory through the pedicle are planned with use of intraoperative CT. (Used with permission from Barrow Neurological Institute, Phoenix, Arizona.)

anterior longitudinal ligament. Once the implant was placed, we attached and tightened the rods to the pedicle screws.

Intraoperative Imaging

Intraoperative navigation allowed us to fine-tune pedicle screw trajectory and plan our skin entry points. Once the trajectories were confirmed, we used navigation and fluoroscopy to

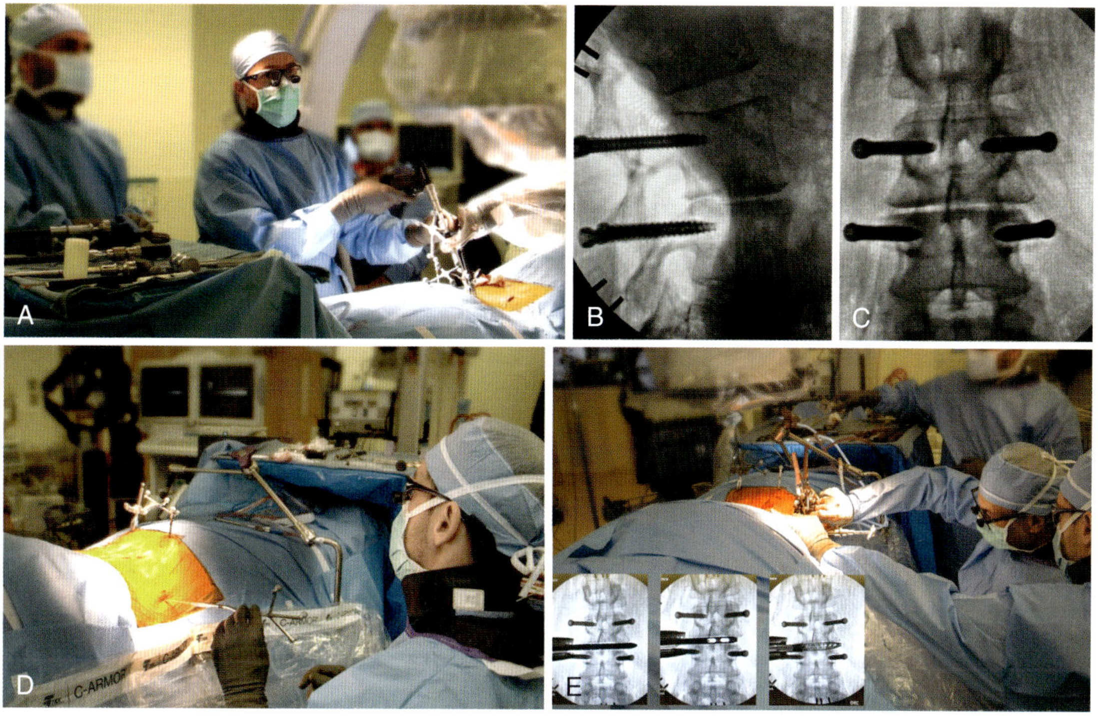

FIG. 9.3 Case 1: Intraoperative procedures and imaging during prone lateral surgery. (A) Screw placement using the robotic arm with sentinel fluoroscopy. (B) Lateral and (C) anteroposterior radiographs show the placement of percutaneous modular screws. (D) Patient and surgeon positioning during prone lateral interbody placement. (E) Intraoperative anteroposterior radiography is used to confirm the instrument and interbody positioning. (Used with permission from Barrow Neurological Institute, Phoenix, Arizona.)

place the pedicle screws (Fig. 9.3A). The lateral and anteroposterior intraoperative radiographs confirmed placement of our pedicle screws (see Figs. 9.3B and C). We then used navigation assistance to calibrate our trajectory for the lateral lumbar interbody placement (see Fig. 9.3D). Anteroposterior radiographs were used to confirm the trajectory and place the lumbar interbody at the L3–L4 disk space (see Fig. 9.3E).

Postoperative Imaging

Postoperative radiographs demonstrated satisfactory implant placement with screw fixation (Figs. 9.4A and B). Confirmatory postoperative MRI and CT confirmed ideal screw placement without a breach (see Fig. 9.4C–H).

Postoperative Recovery and Follow-Up

The patient was discharged home on postoperative day 1 and reported resolution of symptoms by the 2-month follow-up appointment.

Procedural Concerns in Detail

Important considerations for single-position surgery for extreme lateral interbody fusion (XLIF) and pedicle screw fixation include patient positioning, instrumentation, and provider comfort level. First, in the traditional lateral decubitus XLIF positioning, the patient is

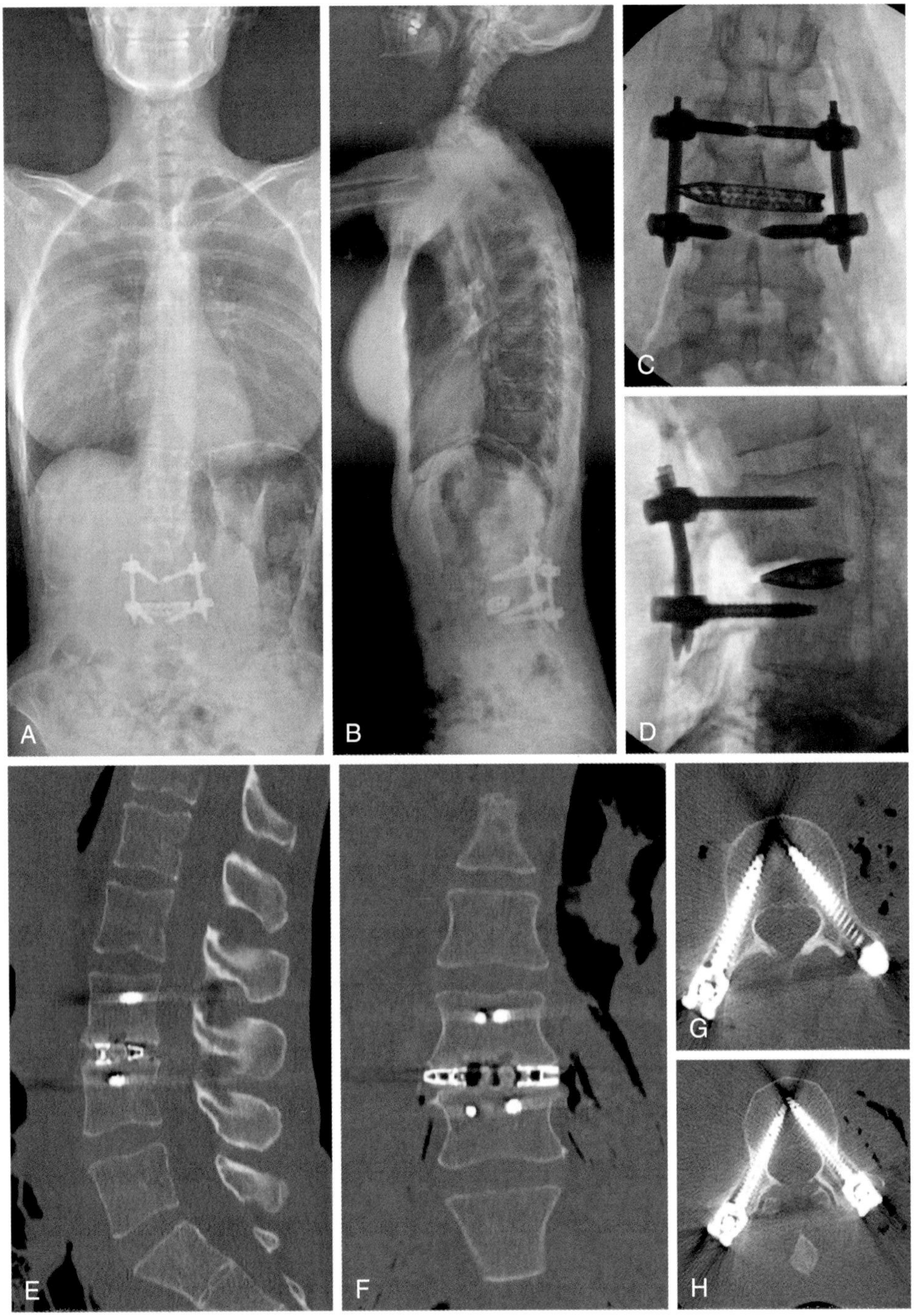

FIG. 9.4 Case 1: Postoperative imaging. (A) Anteroposterior and (B) lateral radiographs demonstrate cage and pedicle screw placement. (C) Anteroposterior and (D) saggital fluoroscopy images and (E) sagittal and (F) coronal CTs of the lumbar spine shows ideal screw placement. (G, H) Axial CTs show the ideal screw placement at L3 and L4, respectively. (Used with permission from Barrow Neurological Institute, Phoenix, Arizona.)

flexed at the hip, which is not possible in the prone position. Fortunately, the gentle lordosis found in the prone position naturally increases the rib-iliac crest distance to facilitate the lateral approach. The instrumentation is the same in both positions.

Treatment Adverse Events

Our surgical approach in case 1 had important intraoperative radiographic and efficiency considerations. First, we did require more radiographs when performing the XLIF in the prone position compared to the lateral decubitus position. One adverse effect of increased imaging is greater patient exposure to radiation. We expect the demand for radiographs to decrease as comfort with the prone positioning increases. Additionally, the use of navigation mitigated the potential for increased radiograph use. Importantly, by completing both the XLIF and pedicle screw fixation in the prone position, we decreased the total procedure time. This efficiency reduced the patient's general anesthesia time and reduced operating room space demand, which improves patient workflow.

Potential Downfalls

Patient bone density is an important consideration when determining the surgical approach. In our example case, the patient completed a preoperative dual energy x-ray absorptiometry scan that revealed poor bone density. This finding motivated us to perform a posterior spinal fusion in addition to the XLIF, rather than XLIF alone. An XLIF alone in a patient with poor bone density can cause vertebral body fracture, particularly in the coronal plane. The fracture risk must also be considered in older patients.

Management of Complications

One potential complication from an XLIF without posterior fusion is vertebral body fracture, particularly in osteoporotic patients. This complication is especially pertinent during unilateral percutaneous fusion. To mitigate this risk, we placed bilateral percutaneous pedicle screws at the L3/4 level in our patient described above.

Robotic-Assisted Minimally Invasive Transforaminal Lumbar Interbody Fusion: Clinical Case 2

History/Clinical Presentation

The patient was a 38-year-old woman with a history of years of progressive chronic low back pain and bilateral lower-extremity radiculopathy (left worse than right). The patient denied trauma or fall and described a gradual onset to her pain that intensified in the 6 months before her presentation to our clinic. The patient attempted conservative therapy for her symptoms that included 16 weeks of physical therapy, lumbar spine steroid injections, and medications (muscle relaxers, analgesics, steroids). Conservative therapy provided mild, temporary relief of her symptoms. She denied red flag symptoms, such as bowel and bladder incontinence or saddle anesthesia. On physical examination, the patient had pain-limited 4/5 weakness in bilateral hip flexion but was otherwise full strength. She noted numbness in the L5 distribution bilaterally.

Preoperative Imaging

MRI of the lumbar spine demonstrated degenerative disk disease at L5/S1 with mild central stenosis and severe bilateral neuroforaminal stenosis (Fig. 9.5A). A CT of the lumbar spine revealed hypertrophic facets with grade I spondylolisthesis of L5 over S1 (see Fig. 9.5B).

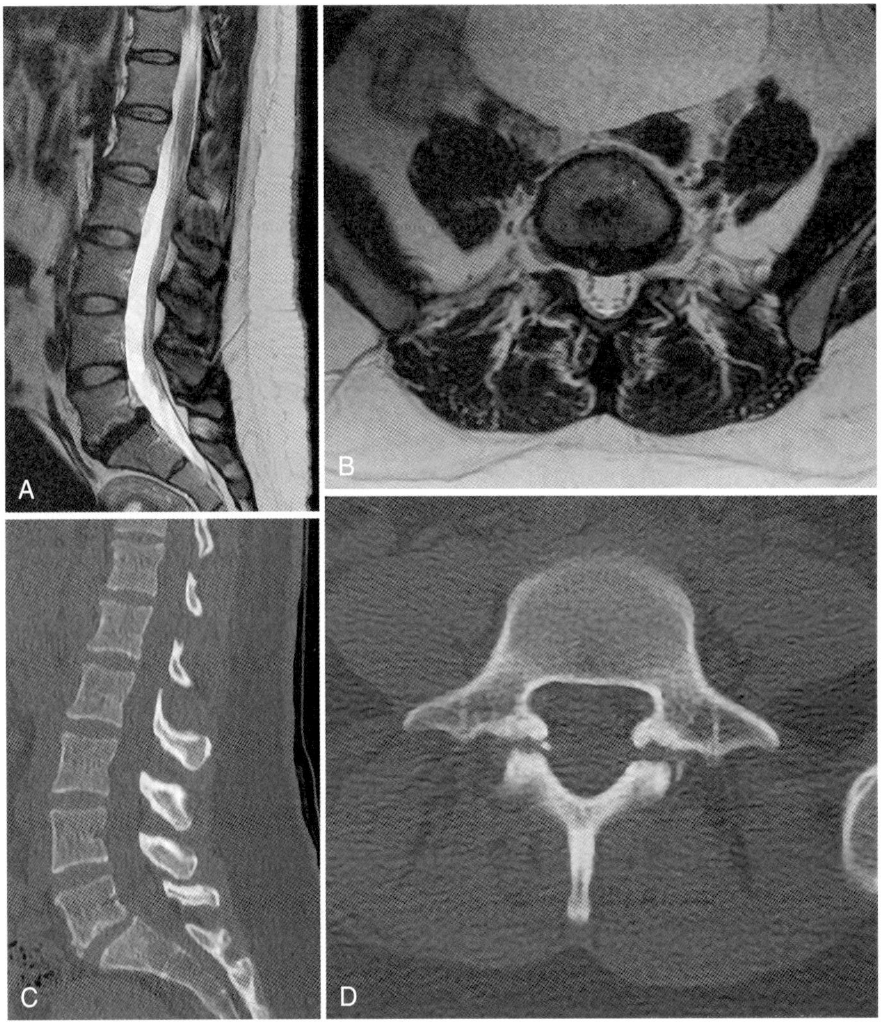

FIG. 9.5 Case 2: Preoperative images of a 38-year-old woman with a history of progressive chronic low back pain and bilateral lower-extremity radiculopathy. (A) Sagittal and (B) axial MRIs of the lumbar spine demonstrate degenerative disk disease at L5/S1. (C) Lateral and (D) axial CTs of the lumbar spine show hypertrophic facets with grade I spondylolisthesis of L5 over S1. (Used with permission from Barrow Neurological Institute, Phoenix, Arizona.)

Surgical Planning

We chose to perform a right L5/S1 MIS transforaminal lumbar interbody fusion (TLIF) with bilateral percutaneous pedicle screw fixation using CT neuronavigation and the robotic navigation platform ExcelsiusGPS (Globus Medical). The patient was in the prone position for the surgery. We used the ExcelsiusGPS for pedicle screw fixation and O-arm navigation (Medtronic) for cage placement.

Intraoperative Imaging

Intraoperative CT was obtained once we positioned the patient on the operating table and secured the stereotactic tracker (Fig. 9.6A). We then planned the trajectories of our pedicle

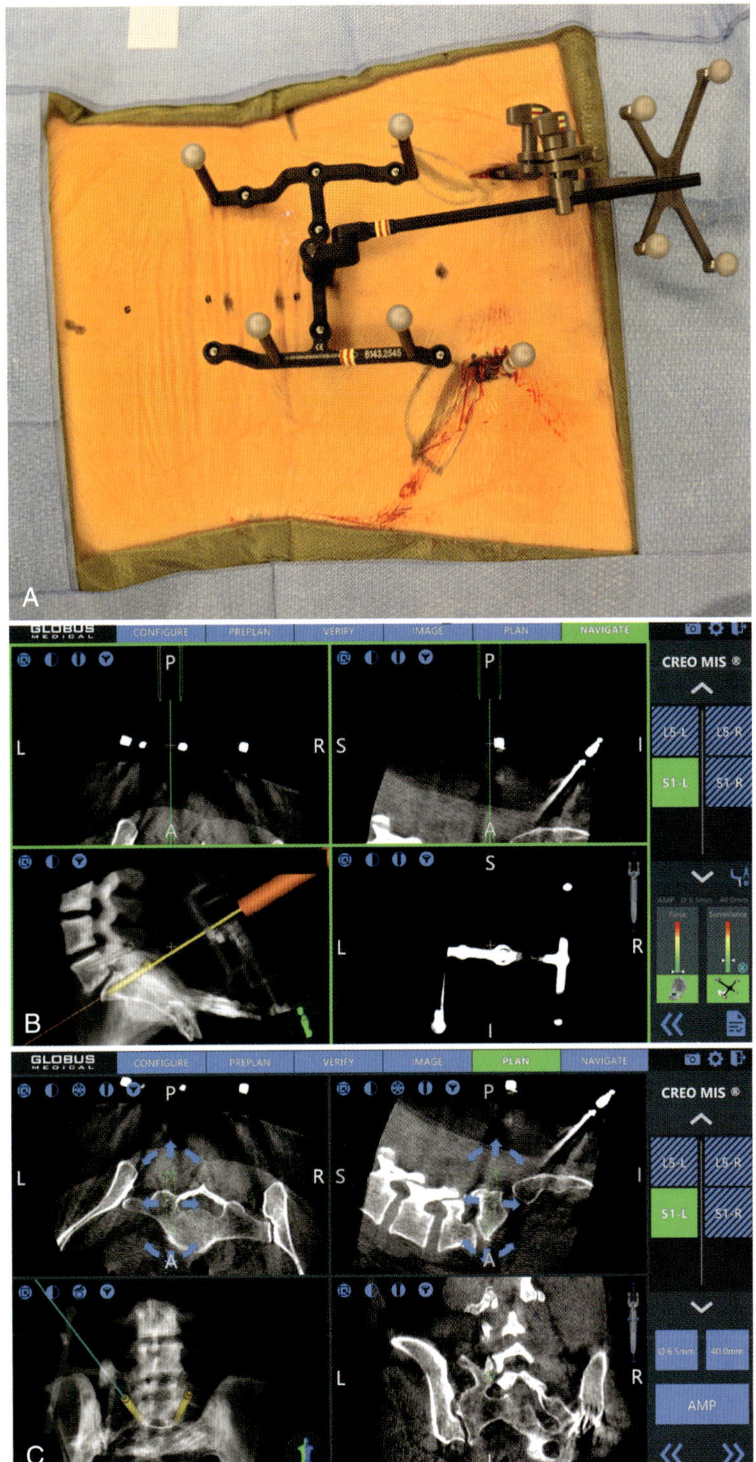

FIG. 9.6 Case 2: Intraoperative tools and planning imaging of a patient undergoing minimally invasive robotic-assisted transforaminal lumbar interbody fusion. (A) Stereotactic tracker placement. (B) Pedicle screw planning. (C) Pedicle screw navigation and incision planning.

screws using the ExcelsiusGPS software (see Fig. 9.6B and C). We used intraoperative radiographs to confirm the placement of our pedicle screws and the interbody graft (Fig. 9.7A).

Postoperative Imaging

Postoperative CT confirmed ideal L5/S1 pedicle screw placement without medial or lateral breach (see Fig. 9.7B and C).

Postoperative Recovery and Follow-Up

The patient was well with improved symptomatology at the 2-week and 6-month follow-up appointments.

Procedural Concerns in Detail

The use of MIS techniques with assistance from a robotic device can effectively decrease radiation exposure, procedure time, and postoperative infection risk. The use of robotic assistance and navigation in our case reduced the demand for intraoperative radiographs during the planning and placement of pedicle screws and the interbody fusion graft. Relatedly, the decreased use of radiographs reduced the intraoperative delays when mobilizing the imaging team and maneuvering the C-arm. Finally, the decreased surgical time, MIS approach, and reduced manual manipulation of tissue collectively reduces the patient's infection risk.

Treatment Adverse Events

As a result of our MIS approach with assistance from a robotic device, we did not use a K-wire for pedicle screw placement in the case described above. Although use of a K-wire is of low risk, there remains a small risk of K-wire fracture when placing the pedicle screws. Our technique allowed us to avoid this risk during the procedure described above.

Potential Downfalls

Despite lower risk for robotic-assisted pedicle screw placement compared to fluoroscopic-guided placement, a small risk remains for pedicle wall breach. The small risk for pedicle wall breach with robotic assistance is usually the result of provider inexperience with the technology; however, errors in navigation may also occur if movement to the navigation probe occurs after the initial O-arm CT.

Management of Complications

Fortunately, no complications were encountered during the operation or in the postoperative period. As in the previous case, complications of XLIF may include rupture of the anterior longitudinal ligament, vascular injury to the great vessels, retroperitoneal hematoma, and failure of fusion if the fusion is not accompanied by posterior fixation.

SUMMARY

The future of robotic systems in spine surgery may include further refinements and integration of the current systems with intraoperative navigation, expansion of indications for use, and emergence of surgeon-controlled systems such as the da Vinci Surgical System robot. While current systems for spinal surgery are confined to the shared-control model, whereby

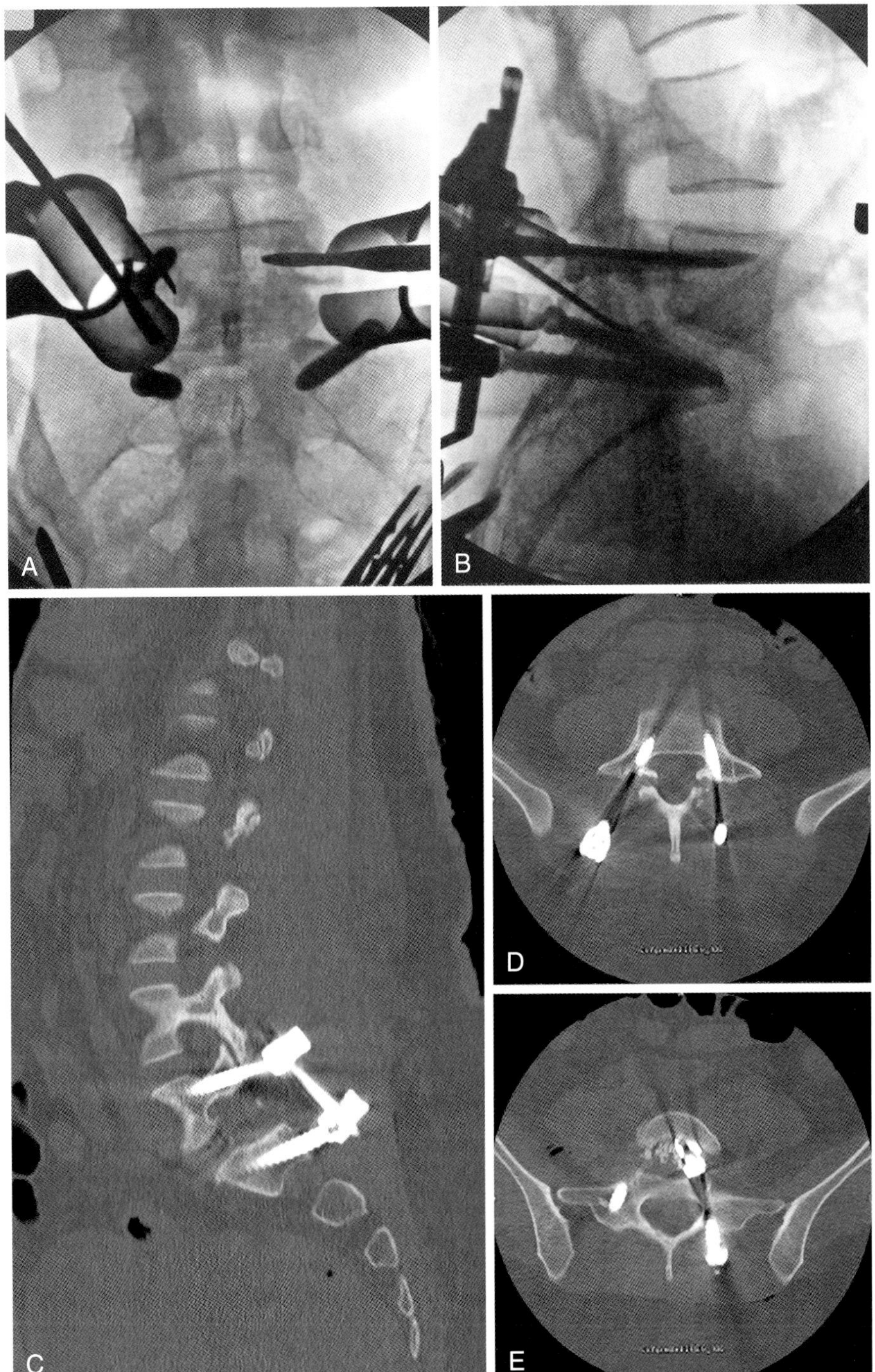

FIG. 9.7 Case 2: Intraoperative and postoperative imaging. Intraoperative (A) anteroposterior and (B) lateral radiographs confirm the placement of the instrumentation. Postoperative (C) sagittal and (D, E) axial CTs of the lumbar spine demonstrate appropriate screw placement at L5 and S1, respectively. (Used with permission from Barrow Neurological Institute, Phoenix, Arizona.)

the robot aligns screws and the surgeon places them, the use of endoscopy has been widely reported in the spine literature.[28,44] This field is ripe for the development and application of new robotic systems whereby the surgeon controls the robot, such as in the da Vinci system, which has been used in spinal procedures in retroperitoneal access and cage placement in the lumbar spine.[45] It is possible that these surgical tools will be combined with wearable technology such as gloves or heads-up displays to more seamlessly integrate the surgeon's movement with the activities of the robot.[46]

The robotic placement of pedicle screws has been demonstrated to be safe and effective, with accuracy rates comparable to free-hand and navigated techniques. Although a steep learning curve exists that necessitates familiarization and a high volume of operative cases in the initial period to gain proficiency, the result of robotically assisted MIS spinal procedures may be greater precision. Robotic systems have the disadvantage of steep costs that necessitate high case volumes to overcome. These systems will continue to improve and build upon prior generations and may see applications beyond the spine in neurosurgery.

DISCLOSURES

JSU is a consultant for NuVasive, SI-BONE, and Misonix and receives royalties from NuVasive. MAP, SHF, and CE have no disclosures.

FINANCIAL SUPPORT

No financial support was received for this publication.

ACKNOWLEDGMENTS

The authors thank the staff of Neuroscience Publications at Barrow Neurological Institute for the assistance with manuscript preparation.

REFERENCES

1. Boucher HH. A method of spinal fusion. *J Bone Joint Surg Br.* 1959;41-B(2):248–259. https://doi.org/10.1302/0301-620X.41B2.248.
2. Roy-Camille R, Berteaux D, Saillant G. Fractures instables du rachis. Les méthodes chirurgicales. Synthèse du rachis dorso-lombaire traumatique par plaques vissées dans les pédicules vertébraux. *Rev Chir Orthop Traumatol.* 2014/02;100(1): 22–24. https://doi.org/10.1016/j.rcot.2013.12.004.
3. Magerl FP. Stabilization of the lower thoracic and lumbar spine with external skeletal fixation. *Clin Orthop Relat Res.* 1984;189(189):125–141. https://doi.org/10.1097/00003086-198410000-00014.
4. Foley KT, Gupta SK. Percutaneous pedicle screw fixation of the lumbar spine: preliminary clinical results. *J Neurol Surg.* 2002;97(1 suppl):7–12. https://doi.org/10.3171/spi.2002.97.1.0007.
5. Schwarzenbach O, Berlemann U, Jost B, et al. Accuracy of computer-assisted pedicle screw placement. An in vivo computed tomography analysis. *Spine (Phila Pa 1976).* 1997;22(4):452–458. https://doi.org/10.1097/00007632-199702150-00020.
6. Verma R, Krishan S, Haendlmayer K, Mohsen A. Functional outcome of computer-assisted spinal pedicle screw placement: a systematic review and meta-analysis of 23 studies including 5, 992 pedicle screws. *Eur Spine J.* 2010;19(3):370–375. https://doi.org/10.1007/s00586-009-1258-4.
7. Galetta MS, Leider JD, Divi SN, Goyal DKC, Schroeder GD. Robotics in spinal surgery. *Ann Transl Med.* 2019;7(Suppl 5):S165. https://doi.org/10.21037/atm.2019.07.93.
8. Nathoo N, Cavuşoğlu MC, Vogelbaum MA, Barnett GH. In touch with robotics: neurosurgery for the future. *Neurosurgery.* 2005;56(3):421–433, discussion. https://doi.org/10.1227/01.neu.0000153929.68024.cf.
9. Chenin L, Peltier J, Lefranc M. Minimally invasive transforaminal lumbar interbody fusion with the ROSA(TM) Spine robot and intraoperative flat-panel CT guidance. *Acta Neurochir (Wien).* 2016;158(6):1125–1128. https://doi.org/10.1007/s00701-016-2799-z.

10. Solomiichuk V, Fleischhammer J, Molliqaj G, et al. Robotic versus fluoroscopy-guided pedicle screw insertion for metastatic spinal disease: a matched-cohort comparison. *Neurosurg Focus*. 2017;42(5):E13. https://doi.org/10.3171/2017.3.FOCUS1710.
11. Wu JY, Yuan Q, Liu YJ, Sun YQ, Zhang Y, Tian W. Robot-assisted percutaneous transfacet screw fixation supplementing oblique lateral interbody fusion procedure: accuracy and safety evaluation of this novel minimally invasive technique. *Orthop Surg*. 2019/02;11(1):25–33. https://doi.org/10.1111/os.12428.
12. Han X, Tian W, Liu Y, et al. Safety and accuracy of robot-assisted versus fluoroscopy-assisted pedicle screw insertion in thoracolumbar spinal surgery: a prospective randomized controlled trial. *J Neurosurg Spine*. 2019:1–8. https://doi.org/10.3171/2018.10.SPINE18487.
13. Fan Y, Du JP, Liu JJ, et al. Accuracy of pedicle screw placement comparing robot-assisted technology and the free-hand with fluoroscopy-guided method in spine surgery: an updated meta-analysis. *Med (Baltim)*. June 2018;97(22):e10970. https://doi.org/10.1097/MD.0000000000010970.
14. Kosmopoulos V, Schizas C. Pedicle screw placement accuracy: a meta-analysis. *Spine (Phila Pa 1976)*. 2007;32(3):E111–E120. https://doi.org/10.1097/01.brs.0000254048.79024.8b.
15. Molliqaj G, Schatlo B, Alaid A, et al. Accuracy of robot-guided versus freehand fluoroscopy-assisted pedicle screw insertion in thoracolumbar spinal surgery. *Neurosurg Focus*. 2017;42(5):E14. https://doi.org/10.3171/2017.3.FOCUS179.
16. Fan Y, Du J, Zhang J, et al. Comparison of accuracy of pedicle screw insertion among 4 guided technologies in spine surgery. *Med Sci Monit*. 2017;23:5960–5968. https://doi.org/10.12659/msm.905713.
17. Keric N, Doenitz C, Haj A, et al. Evaluation of robot-guided minimally invasive implantation of 2067 pedicle screws. *Neurosurg Focus*. 2017;42(5):E11. https://doi.org/10.3171/2017.2.FOCUS16552.
18. Kuo KL, Su YF, Wu CH, et al. Assessing the intraoperative accuracy of pedicle screw placement by using a bone-mounted miniature robot system through secondary registration. *PLoS One*. 2016;11(4):e0153235. https://doi.org/10.1371/journal.pone.0153235.
19. Tsai TH, Wu DS, Su YF, Wu CH, Lin CL. A retrospective study to validate an intraoperative robotic classification system for assessing the accuracy of Kirschner wire (K-wire) placements with postoperative computed tomography classification system for assessing the accuracy of pedicle screw placements. *Med (Baltim)*. 2016;95(38):e4834. https://doi.org/10.1097/MD.0000000000004834.
20. van Dijk JD, van den Ende RP, Stramigioli S, Köchling M, Höss N. Clinical pedicle screw accuracy and deviation from planning in robot-guided spine surgery: robot-guided pedicle screw accuracy. *Spine (Phila Pa 1976)*. 2015;40(17):E986–E991. https://doi.org/10.1097/BRS.0000000000000960.
21. Villard J, Ryang YM, Demetriades AK, et al. Radiation exposure to the surgeon and the patient during posterior lumbar spinal instrumentation: a prospective randomized comparison of navigated versus non-navigated freehand techniques. *Spine (Phila Pa 1976)*. 2014;39(13):1004–1009. https://doi.org/10.1097/BRS.0000000000000351.
22. Godzik J, Walker CT, Hartman C, et al. A quantitative assessment of the accuracy and reliability of robotically guided percutaneous pedicle screw placement: technique and application accuracy. *Oper Neurosurg*. 2019/02/06;17(4):389–395. https://doi.org/10.1093/ons/opy413.
23. Hu X, Ohnmeiss DD, Lieberman IH. Robotic-assisted pedicle screw placement: lessons learned from the first 102 patients. *Eur Spine J*. 2012;22(3):661–666. https://doi.org/10.1007/s00586-012-2499-1.
24. Schatlo B, Martinez R, Alaid A, et al. Unskilled unawareness and the learning curve in robotic spine surgery. *Acta Neurochir (Wien)*. 2015;157(10):1819–1823, discussion 1823. https://doi.org/10.1007/s00701-015-2535-0.
25. Ringel F, Stüer C, Reinke A, et al. Accuracy of robot-assisted placement of lumbar and sacral pedicle screws: a prospective randomized comparison to conventional freehand screw implantation. *Spine (Phila Pa 1976)*. 2012;37(8):E496–E501. https://doi.org/10.1097/BRS.0b013e31824b7767.
26. Urbanski W, Jurasz W, Wolanczyk M, et al. Increased radiation but no benefits in pedicle screw accuracy with navigation versus a freehand technique in scoliosis surgery. *Clin Orthop Relat Res*. 2018;476(5):1020–1027. https://doi.org/10.1007/s11999.0000000000000204.
27. Peng YN, Tsai LC, Hsu HC, Kao CH. Accuracy of robot-assisted versus conventional freehand pedicle screw placement in spine surgery: a systematic review and meta-analysis of randomized controlled trials. *Ann Transl Med*. Jul 2020;8(13):824. https://doi.org/10.21037/atm-20-1106.
28. Lippross S, Jünemann KP, Osmonov D, et al. Robot-assisted spinal surgery- A technical report on the use of DaVinci in orthopaedics. *J Orthop*. 2020;19:50–53. https://doi.org/10.1016/j.jor.2019.11.045.
29. Gertzbein SD, Robbins SE. Accuracy of pedicular screw placement in vivo. *Spine (Phila Pa 1976)*. 1990;15(1):11–14. https://doi.org/10.1097/00007632-199001000-00004.
30. Lonjon N, Chan-Seng E, Costalat V, Bonnafoux B, Vassal M, Boetto J. Robot-assisted spine surgery: feasibility study through a prospective case-matched analysis. *Eur Spine J*. 2016;25(3):947–955. https://doi.org/10.1007/s00586-015-3758-8.
31. Roser F, Tatagiba M, Maier G. Spinal robotics: current applications and future perspectives. *Neurosurgery*. 2013;72(suppl 1):12–18. https://doi.org/10.1227/NEU.0b013e318270d02c.
32. Devito DP, Kaplan L, Dietl R, et al. Clinical acceptance and accuracy assessment of spinal implants guided with SpineAssist surgical robot: retrospective study. *Spine (Phila Pa 1976)*. 2010;35(24):2109–2115. https://doi.org/10.1097/BRS.0b013e3181d323ab.
33. Pechlivanis I, Kiriyanthan G, Engelhardt M, et al. Percutaneous placement of pedicle screws in the lumbar spine using a bone mounted miniature robotic system:

first experiences and accuracy of screw placement. *Spine (Phila Pa 1976)*. 2009;34(4):392–398. https://doi.org/10.1097/BRS.0b013e318191ed32.
34. Li HM, Zhang RJ, Shen CL. Accuracy of pedicle screw placement and clinical outcomes of robot-assisted technique versus conventional freehand technique in spine surgery from nine randomized controlled trials: a meta-analysis. *Spine (Phila Pa 1976)*. 2020;45(2):E111–E119. https://doi.org/10.1097/BRS.0000000000003193.
35. Kim HJ, Jung WI, Chang BS, Lee CK, Kang KT, Yeom JS. A prospective, randomized, controlled trial of robot-assisted vs freehand pedicle screw fixation in spine surgery. *Int J Med Robot*. 2017;13(3):e1779. https://doi.org/10.1002/rcs.1779.
36. Hyun SJ, Kim KJ, Jahng TA, Kim HJ. Minimally invasive robotic versus open fluoroscopic-guided spinal instrumented fusions: A randomized controlled trial. *Spine (Phila Pa 1976)*. 2017;42(6):353–358. https://doi.org/10.1097/BRS.0000000000001778.
37. Urakov TM, Chang KH, Burks SS, Wang MY. Initial academic experience and learning curve with robotic spine instrumentation. *Neurosurg Focus*. 2017;42(5):E4. https://doi.org/10.3171/2017.2.FOCUS175.
38. Elswick CM, Strong MJ, Joseph JR, Saadeh Y, Oppenlander M, Park P. Robotic-assisted spinal surgery: current generation instrumentation and new applications. *Neurosurg Clin N Am*. 2020;31(1):103–110. https://doi.org/10.1016/j.nec.2019.08.012.
39. Park SM, Kim HJ, Lee SY, Chang BS, Lee CK, Yeom JS. Radiographic and clinical outcomes of robot-assisted posterior pedicle screw fixation: two-year results from a randomized controlled trial. *Yonsei Med J*. May 2018;59(3):438–444. https://doi.org/10.3349/ymj.2018.59.3.438.
40. Li Z, Chen J, Zhu QA, et al. A preliminary study of a novel robotic system for pedicle screw fixation: a randomised controlled trial. *J Orthop Transl*. 2020;20:73–79. https://doi.org/10.1016/j.jot.2019.09.002.
41. Fan M, Liu Y, He D, et al. Improved accuracy of cervical spinal surgery with robot-assisted screw insertion: A prospective, randomized, controlled study. *Spine (Phila Pa 1976)*. 2020;45(5):285–291. https://doi.org/10.1097/BRS.0000000000003258.
42. Lucio JC, Vanconia RB, Deluzio KJ, Lehmen JA, Rodgers JA, Rodgers W. Economics of less invasive spinal surgery: an analysis of hospital cost differences between open and minimally invasive instrumented spinal fusion procedures during the perioperative period. *Risk Manag Healthc Policy*. 2012;5:65–74. https://doi.org/10.2147/RMHP.S30974.
43. Kantelhardt SR, Martinez R, Baerwinkel S, Burger R, Giese A, Rohde V. Perioperative course and accuracy of screw positioning in conventional, open robotic-guided and percutaneous robotic-guided, pedicle screw placement. *Eur Spine J*. 2011;20(6):860–868. https://doi.org/10.1007/s00586-011-1729-2.
44. Elhadi AM, Zehri AH, Zaidi HA, et al. Surgical efficacy of minimally invasive thoracic discectomy. *J Clin Neurosci*. 2015;22(11):1708–1713. https://doi.org/10.1016/j.jocn.2015.05.013.
45. Regan JP, Cattey RP, Henry LG, Robbins S. Laparoscopically assisted retroperitoneal spinal surgery. *JSLS*. 2006;10(4):493–495.
46. Liounakos JI, Urakov T, Wang MY. Head-up display assisted endoscopic lumbar discectomy—a technical note. *Int J Med Robot*. 2020;16(3):e2089 https://doi.org/10.1002/rcs.2089.

10

Robotics in Spine Surgery: Beyond Pedicle Screw Placement

Ketan Yerneni, BA, Harsh Wadhwa, BS, Parastou Fatemi, MD, Nicholas Theodore, MD, and Corinna Clio Zygourakis, MD

Intraoperative image-guided (IG) navigation and robotic assistance in spine surgery have traditionally been used to improve pedicle screw placement accuracy, decrease radiation exposure for operating room staff and patients, help surgeon ergonomics, and improve overall surgical outcomes.[1–9] More recently, however, the application of these technologies has expanded to include the resection of spinal column and intradural tumors, evacuation of infection, revision arthrodesis surgery, and deformity surgery.[10–18]

Intraoperative IG navigation systems provide real-time image guidance via reconstruction of images to three-dimensional (3D) spine representations in addition to navigation via an anatomic reference and surgical instruments with reference points.[19] Multiple computed tomography (CT) based intraoperative IG navigation systems are in use today. For example, the StealthStation™ navigation (Medtronic©, Dublin, Ireland), which is a 360-degree CT scanner, utilizes intraoperative CT, a spinous process or iliac crest reference clamp, and surgical instruments with reference points to allow for surgeon-controlled navigated drilling, tapping, and screw placement during surgery. Another system is the Airo® Mobile Intraoperative CT platform (Brainlab©, Munich, Germany), which is similar to the StealthStation with the exception of using a 360-degree CT scanner attached to the OR table. A robust body of literature has established the advantages of 3D navigation in spine surgery including improved screw placement accuracy.[20–24] New alternative IG systems include the 7D Surgical System (7D Surgical©, Toronto, Canada), which utilizes camera-based imaging to register bony anatomy through machine vision technology.[25] Such systems reduce radiation exposure by circumventing the need for CT or fluoroscopy intraoperatively and may can help streamline intraoperative workflow, although further studies are needed to evaluate this new technology.[26,27]

Robotic-assisted spine surgery goes beyond intraoperative IG. It not only utilizes imaging for trajectory planning by the surgeon, but also provides an automated robotic arm that manipulates surgical instruments. To date, the FDA has approved three robotic systems for spine surgery: Mazor X™ (and its prior iterations Renaissance™ and Spine Assist™; Mazor Robotics©, Caesarea, Israel), ROSA® robot (Medtech Surgical©, Montpellier, France), and ExcelsiusGPS™ (Globus Medical©, Audubon, PA, USA). The Mazor X™ robot attaches to the OR table and has a surgical arm that moves to a predetermined trajectory, a camera with

3D spatial tracking, and a computer program that allows for preoperative screw trajectory planning and intraoperative trajectory verification.[28] Several studies have shown greater accuracy in pedicle screw placement using Mazor Rotobitcs© compared to conventional fluoroscopy-assisted free-hand techniques.[19,29–34] The ROSA® robot uses intraoperative planning and navigation to determine the surgical arm trajectory. Its camera system tracks a reference clamped to the patient and a reference attached to the robot; the tracking feedback is used by the robot to adjust its position if the patient moves.[35] A retrospective study has shown improved accuracy of screw placement with ROSA® compared to the free-hand technique.[36] Lastly, the ExcelsiusGPS™ provides intraoperative imaging, trajectory planning, and screw placement through a rigid external arm that allows for navigated drilling and navigated interbody cage placement without the use of K-wires.[37] The robot does not attach to the OR table or patient and tracks its dynamic reference base with a second surveillance marker for movements. Several studies have shown accurate percutaneous and open pedicle screw placement with the ExcelsiusGPS™.[38–40] In a recent meta-analysis of pedicle screw accuracy for all methods (robotic-assisted, CT-based navigation, fluoroscopy-assisted, and free-hand), CT-based navigation had the overall highest accuracy rate, although in the thoracic spine, robotic assistance showed the highest accuracy.[41]

While the short-term benefits of robotic-assisted spine surgery have been well established, its definitive long-term clinical advantages have not yet been proven.[42,43] Two recent randomized controlled trials evaluated the long-term (1- and 2-year) outcomes after robotic-assisted pedicle screw fixation with the Renaissance™ system versus the conventional free-hand technique.[42] The patients reported similar quality of life measures across the groups. In one study, two patients in the free-hand group required revision surgery while none in the robotic group did. In the other study, the free-hand group had more adjacent segment degeneration. The long-term outcomes using robotic surgery need further investigation.

As work evaluating the new generation of robotics continues to unfold, a combined approach integrating navigation and robotic assistance may prove to be superior to the current standard of care.[44] While the overwhelming majority of work done with robotics has focused on facilitating screw placement,[31] the future may in fact see robots providing a much larger role in spine procedures. Here, we present two cases demonstrating the potential use of robotics for novel methods of screw placement and navigated assistance for corpectomy and interbody cage placement.

CASE 1: TRANSVERTEBRAL SCREW PLACEMENT

Here, we present our experience performing a robotic-assisted L4–S1 fusion for grade 2 spondylolisthesis. In this case, we demonstrate how the use of navigated-robotics technology allows us to place screws in an entirely novel trajectory (transvertebral, instead of through the pedicle) that would not otherwise be feasible without navigation or robotic guidance.

History and Clinical Presentation

A 66-year-old woman with a prior history of hypertension, anxiety, and sleep apnea presented with one year of severe low back pain radiating to the right lower extremity and bilateral lower extremity numbness. The patient was neurologically intact on examination.

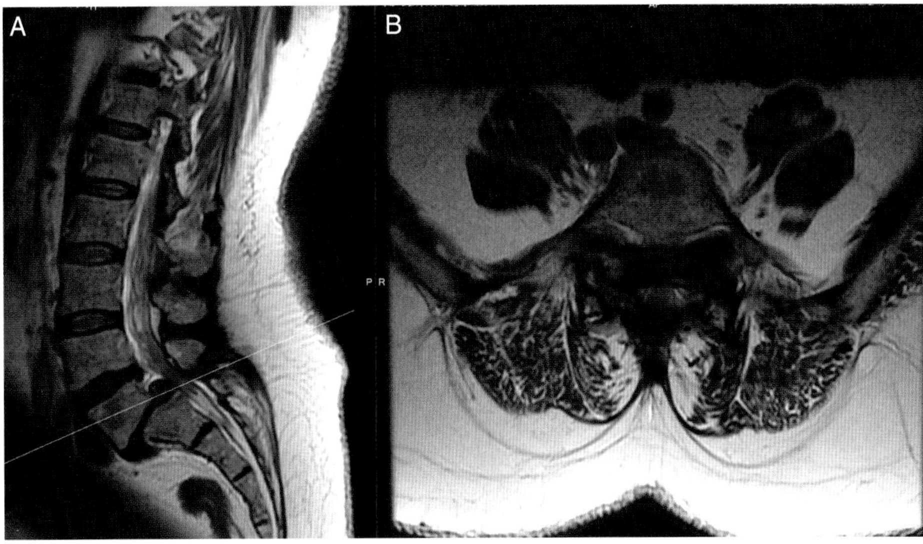

FIG. 10.1 (A) Sagittal T2-weighted magnetic resonance imaging demonstrating grade 2 L5–S1 spondylolisthesis with severe central stenosis. (B) Axial T2-weighted magnetic resonance imaging at the L5–S1 level.

Preoperative Imaging

The preoperative lumbar spine MR imaging demonstrated grade 2 L5/S1 spondylolisthesis with severe central and foraminal stenosis (Fig. 10.1).

Surgical Technique Including Intraoperative Imaging

The patient underwent an L4–S1 robotic-assisted lumbar decompression and fusion using the ExcelsiusGPS robot. After standard prone positioning on the Jackson table and sterile preparation and draping, the ExcelsiusGPS™ Dynamic Reference Base (DRB) and surveillance markers were placed on the posterior superior iliac spines. The intraoperative CT (iCT) fixture was then attached, and the O-arm was brought into use. A 3D CT scan was rendered and sent to the robotic system for screw trajectory planning.

Due to the patient's steep lumbosacral angulation and pedicle anatomy, we found that the trajectories of the L5 and S1 pedicles in this patient would overlap and the screw heads would collide. We therefore used our navigation technology to plan a more favorable transvertebral screw trajectory from the S1 vertebral body into the L5 vertebral body and crossing the disk space. This was planned bilaterally for the L5/S1 screws. We then removed the iCT fixture, exposed the spine in the routine manner, and used the ExcelsiusGPS™ robotic arm to place these screws in an open, robotic- or navigation-assisted fashion. The standard L4 pedicle screws were also placed using the ExcelsiusGPS™ robot (Fig. 10.2).

After confirming good hardware placement, a routine lumbar decompression, including full laminectomy and bilateral foraminotomies, was performed. Rods were placed, the transverse processes and lamina were decorticated, and demineralized bone matrix was placed to promote fusion. A routine, multi-layered closure was performed.

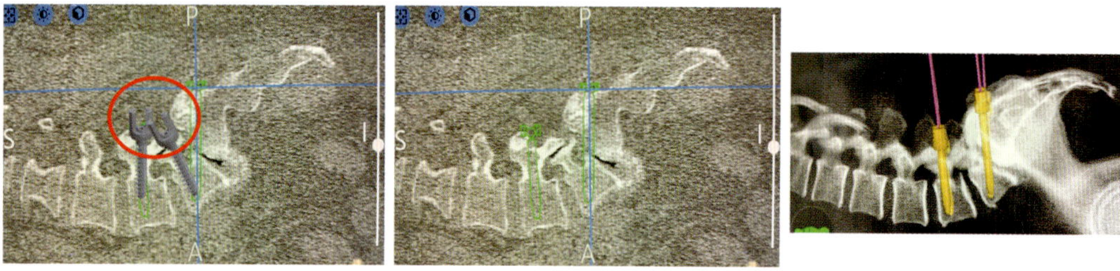

FIG. 10.2 Conventional pedicle screw placement was challenging due to the patient anatomy (*left*). Robotic-assisted trajectory planning and navigation allowed the placement of transvertebral screws (*right*).

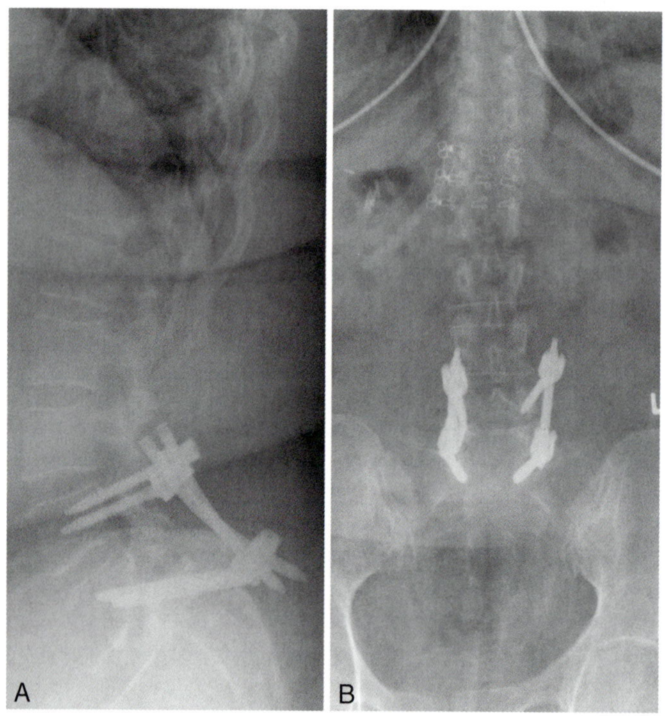

FIG. 10.3 Postoperative (A) lateral and (B) anterior-posterior views demonstrating accurate screw trajectories and intact instruments with no screw pull-out.

Postoperative Imaging

The postoperative lumbar radiographs demonstrated the L4–S1 fusion construct with the L5/S1 transvertebral screws in excellent position (Fig. 10.3).

Postoperative Recovery and Follow-up

At the two-month postoperative follow-up, the patient's lower back and right lower extremity pain had resolved. She regained full strength in all muscle groups and ambulated independently without the use of an assistive device.

Procedural Concerns in Detail (Whether Navigation, Robotics, or Both)

Transvertebral screw placement is typically not performed via a free-hand technique due to a paucity of anatomic landmarks. There is particular concern regarding the possibility of entering the foramen and causing injury to the nerve root via a free-hand technique. However, with the real-time image guidance and preoperative planning provided by ExcelsiusGPS™, this procedure can be performed with a greatly reduced risk of complications. The advantages of the transvertebral screw technique include tri-cortical purchase and placement of a much longer screw than the routine lumbar pedicle screw trajectory.

Treatment Side Effects

This case was one of the first performed with the ExcelsiusGPS™ robot. At this stage in our robotics learning curve, we were performing O-arm spins intraoperatively, instead of preoperatively with intraoperative fluoroscopy. We were also obtaining O-arm spins after the screw placement to confirm screw accuracy and for research purposes. As a result, this case provided 31.13 Gy of exposure for the patient. For his robotics cases using the ExcelsiusGPS™ robot, senior author N.T. is now routinely doing a preoperative CT scan, with intraoperative fluoroscopy and no confirmatory O-arm spin, which results in significantly less exposure to patients on average.

Potential Downfalls

Although the robotic system allowed us to place a transvertebral screw in a unique trajectory, we did not reduce the patient's grade 2 spondylolisthesis. We felt that we could obtain an adequate decompression of the nerve roots via a full laminectomy and bilateral foraminotomies in order to address the patient's radicular symptoms. Moreover, the patient's overall alignment was reasonable in terms of lumbar lordosis (LL), pelvic incidence (PI), and LL-PI mismatch, so we did not feel that a reduction was essential to improve the overall spinal global alignment.

In addition to the well-established risks of decompression and fusion lumbosacral surgery, cases involving decompression and fusion with or without the reduction of high-grade spondylolisthesis are especially technically challenging. These are associated with motor and sensory deficits. The incidence of neurologic deficit following distraction for reduction high-grade spondylolisthesis is reportedly from 10% to 31%, with the majority being transient.[45–47]

Management of Complications

In cases of lower-grade spondylolisthesis without sagittal imbalance, one may consider not performing distraction for reduction purposes. It should be noted that if a reduction is pursued for the correction of spondylolisthesis, it is generally recommended to use interbody implants and bone grafting to reduce the risk of hardware failure and nonunion.[48,49] Additionally, a study using cadaver models suggested that risk of stretch injury to the nerve root is higher in complete reduction compared to a partial reduction of high-grade spondylolisthesis.[50] Thus, if a reduction is necessary, the surgeon should consider doing so partially.

CASE 2: NAVIGATED CORPECTOMY AND SCREW PLACEMENT

Here, we present our experience performing an intraoperative image-guided L2 corpectomy and T11–L4 posterior spinal fusion for metastatic cancer. The authors contend that future updates to spine robotic technology will enable us to perform these techniques in an even safer manner by incorporating robotics with the current navigation techniques.

CASE ILLUSTRATION

History and Clinical Presentation

A 62-year-old woman with multiple medical comorbidities including congestive heart failure, recent thymic cancer (status post-chemotherapy and post-radiation), and a remote history of colon cancer presented to the hospital with a 5-month history of severe lower back pain, preventing her from being able to walk for the past month.

Preoperative Imaging

Magnetic resonance imaging (MRI) revealed a pathologic fracture at L2 with enhancing tumor involving the L1 and L2 vertebral bodies and causing severe spinal cord compression at L2 (Fig. 10.4A and B). CT scans demonstrated the bony anatomy of the L1/L2 pathologic fracture with retropulsion into the canal (Fig. 10.4C). Given the spinal instability and severe cord compression, significant pain, and only moderate radiosensitivity of the presumed metastatic thymic cancer, we elected to perform a spinal decompression and stabilization with significant tumor debulking/resection.

Surgical Technique Including Intraoperative Imaging

After standard prone positioning on a Jackson table, sterile preparation, and draping, fluoroscopy was used to identify the T10 to L4 levels. A routine exposure and sub-periosteal dissection to expose the spinous processes, lamina, and transverse processes of T10 to L4 were completed. The StealthStation™ navigation tracker was placed on the spinous process of T10 and the O-arm was used to obtain a 3D CT scan. The CT data was transferred to the StealthStation™ for anatomical accuracy, registration, and pedicle trajectory planning to enable real-time image guidance during instrumentation. The pedicles were then cannulated bilaterally at T11, T12, L3, and L4. Initially, the high-speed drill was used to drill a pilot hole before using the navigated drill guide, navigated tap, and navigated screw inserter sequentially to place the appropriately sized screws at each level (Fig. 10.5A and B).

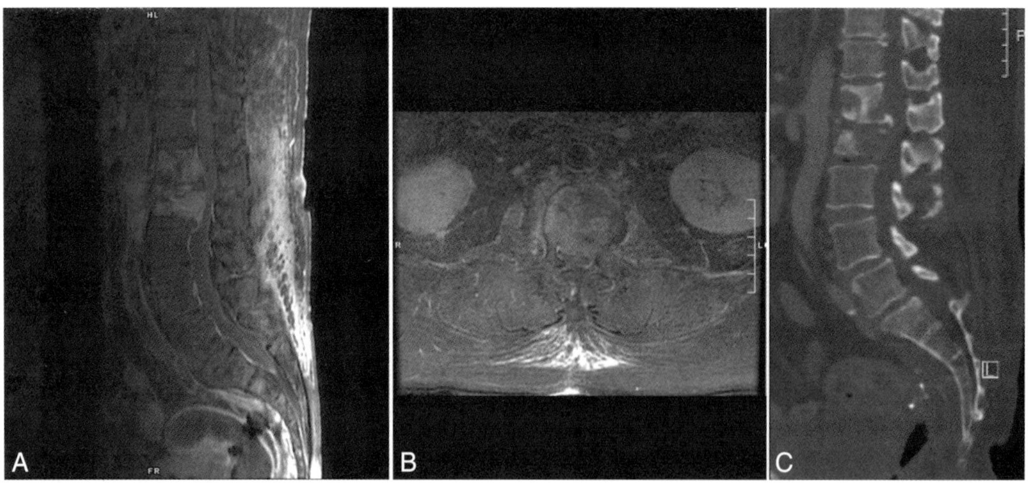

FIG. 10.4 (A) Sagittal T1-weighted magnetic resonance imaging demonstrating enhancing tumor at the L1 and L2 vertebral bodies, along with resulting severe stenosis at L1/L2. (B) Axial T1-weighted magnetic resonance imaging at L1–L2 demonstrating spinal cord compression. (C) Sagittal CT scan demonstrating pathologic fracture of L1 and L2.

The extracavitary posterolateral approach to the L2 corpectomy was accomplished using full L1 and L2 laminectomies and medial facetectomies. We began the corpectomy via the left side, using the Leksell and navigated drill to take down the facet joints, L2 transverse process, and L2 pedicle to skeletonize the left L1 and L2 nerve roots. The navigated pointer was used to indicate the superior and inferior endplate (Fig. 10.5C and D) for the corpectomy, and to determine the ventral extent (Fig. 10.5E and F). Residual tumor remained within the left L2 pedicle, which was soft. The majority of the tumor was found to be located ventrally. Using a combination of navigated drills, curettes, and pituitary rongeurs, >50% of the L2 vertebral body was removed. The soft tissue specimen was sampled and pathology was consistent with metastatic thymic cancer.

We then used the navigated drill to take down the right L2 pedicle, facet joints, and transverse process to expose the right-sided L1 and L2 nerve roots. The spinal cord was fully decompressed ventrally bilaterally using the Woodsen, curettes, and pituitary rongeurs. The Woodsen was used to ensure there was no further anterior compression on the spinal cord. Stealth navigation was used to confirm that we had reached the anterior border of the vertebral body. The bilateral L1 and L2 nerve roots were well preserved and there were no changes in motor or sensory innervation.

A sizer was used to place an expandable titanium cage, filled with demineralized bone matrix, in the space of the corpectomy. Fluoroscopy was used to ensure good placement on both the anteroposterior and lateral x-rays. Appropriately sized titanium rods were inserted into position on the screw heads on the left and right sides. The set screws were placed and locked on both sides, and we compressed across T12 to L3 to secure the corpectomy cage in place. The set screws were then tightened using appropriate torque. The wound was closed in the usual fashion with a surgical drain in place, and the patient was transferred back to the intensive care unit in a stable condition.

Postoperative Imaging

Postoperative x-rays demonstrated good hardware placement (Fig. 10.6).

Postoperative Recovery and Follow-up

The patient returned to the ICU after surgery, given her multiple medical comorbidities. She remained neurologically intact. Her postoperative course was notable for subsegmental

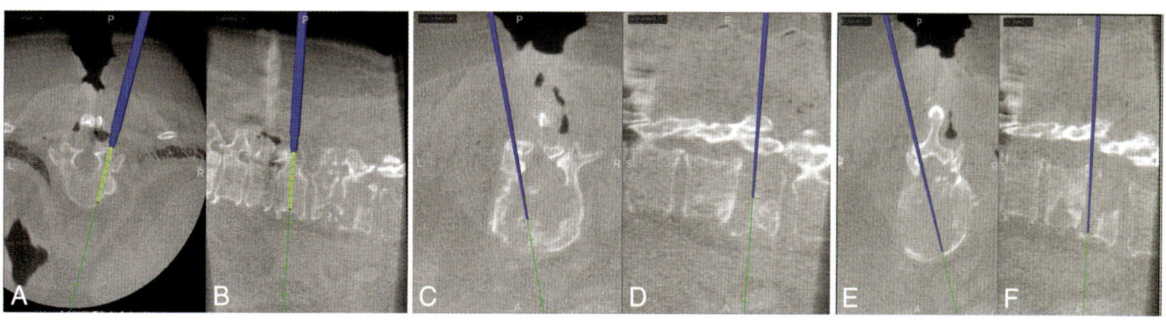

FIG. 10.5 (A and B) Pedicle screw placement at T11 using the StealthStation™ Surgical Navigation tracker. (C and D) Using the navigated probe to define the inferior endplate. (E and F) Using the navigated probe to assess ventral distance post-corpectomy at L1. Bone is visualized via incorporation of the CT taken before the corpectomy.

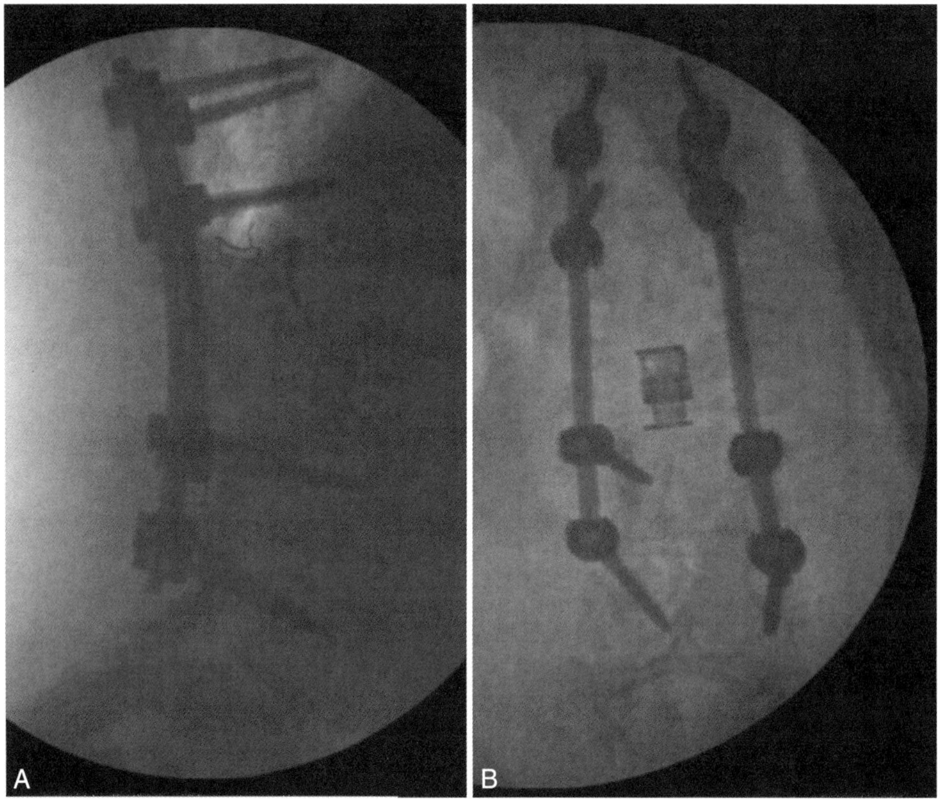

FIG. 10.6 Intraoperative fluoroscopy demonstrating successful construct placement in A) lateral and B) coronal planes.

pulmonary emboli requiring therapeutic lovenox, and she was transferred to an inpatient rehab facility 1 week after surgery. Within 5 days after surgery, she was able to stand out of bed, which she had not been able to do for a month before surgery.

Procedural Concerns in Detail (Whether Navigation, Robotics, or Both)

A major concern in performing corpectomies is properly identifying the anatomic landmarks which can be obscured in the setting of erosive, invasive tumor. First, the superior and inferior endplates should be identified so that the entire disks are resected in order to provide a good endplate upon which the corpectomy cage sits. The goal of the appropriate endplate preparation is to facilitate a solid fusion across the corpectomy site.

In addition, the nerve roots should be carefully identified and preserved, especially in the lumbar spine, where nerve roots are functionally important and cannot be sacrificed without a resulting motor deficit. Finally, it is important to identify the ventral aspect of the vertebral body, so that arterial and venous structures are not violated. At the L1/L2 level, the aorta is located ventrolateral slightly to the left side of the vertebral body and disk while the inferior vena cava is ventrolateral slightly to the right side. Farther down, the aortic bifurcation is at the L4 vertebra in a majority of patients, with possible superior migration when the patient is in the prone position.[51] The iliocaval junction if often at the L4/L5 disk or L5 vertebra; however, this too can migrate superiorly in the prone position.[51] The goal is to complete the corpectomy as far ventrally as possible so that the cage sits anteriorly, while avoiding a potentially catastrophic vascular injury.

Intraoperative navigation provides a safe and effective way to localize these anatomical landmarks to allow ideal corpectomy and cage placement. Future systems that incorporate intraoperative navigation with robotic surgery may allow for the fusion of preoperative CT scans and MR scans with angiography to establish "no-fly" zones that prevent the guided drill from going too far anteriorly and prevent it from violating the anterior vasculature or nerve roots bilaterally.

In addition, the future version of the navigated spine robotics may also establish a "no-fly" zone around the dura to help prevent a cerebrospinal fluid (CSF) leak. Perioperative CSF leaks are a known complication associated with spine surgery. Indeed, spine surgery carries a significant rate for unintended durotomies and CSF leaks, with an incidence of roughly 0.3%[52] to 35%[53] in the literature. A recent 10-year systematic review by Ghobrial et al. (2015) reported an overall 8.11% durotomy rate (range, 2%–20%) in patients undergoing lumbar degenerative spine surgery.[54] Additionally, patients undergoing surgery for spine tumors may be at increased risk of CSF leaks due to the presence of an intradural tumor requiring durotomy and reduced healing secondary to poor nutritional status and adjuvant chemotherapy and radiation. Effective protocols for preventing and treating such leakage are essential to avoiding downstream adverse outcomes, including wound infection,[55] intracranial hemorrhage,[56] and meningitis,[57] among others. Importantly, tumor seeding is a feared complication of postoperative CSF leak unique to patients undergoing resection of malignant spinal tumors.[58]

Treatment Side Effects

For patients with metastatic spinal cancer undergoing surgical intervention, pseudoarthrosis can be a painful and highly morbid complication. Postoperative radiation and chemotherapy, common in this patient population, are risk factors for a failure to fuse, or nonunion, resulting in hardware failure. Thus, cancer patients require unique considerations when undergoing fusion surgery. First, a meticulous endplate preparation should be performed at the inferior and superior endplates so that the corpectomy cage has a good bony substance to oppose. In addition, the surgeon should carefully consider the corpectomy cage material. In particular, a bony allograft (such as cadaveric fibula) or titanium expandable cage should be considered rather than polyetheretherketone (PEEK) cages. Multiple studies of mid- to low-level evidence have evaluated whether PEEK or titanium is the superior cage and have overall concluded similar fusion rates.[59–64] In a study of one-level anterior cervical discectomy and fusion, PEEK was found to have rates of pseudoarthrosis nearly five times as high as structural allograft, and twice as many revision surgeries.[65] We prefer to use titanium cages in patients with cancer due the availability of expandable configurations which offer superior fit and load-bearing, increased cell adhesion characteristics and improved osseointegration.[59,66]

Finally, careful attention must be paid to the material that is used to fill the corpectomy cage. Recombinant human bone morphogenetic protein (BMP)-2, which is being used increasingly in spinal fusion and especially in adult spinal deformity surgery (up to 61% according to studies using the ISSG dataset),[67] may encourage tumor growth and is relatively contraindicated in patients with active cancer.[68] Instead, various bone allografts, including cadaveric cancellous bone chips, and/or demineralized bone matrix (DBM), can be considered to effect an arthrodesis at the corpectomy site; the combination of allograft with DBM has been shown to have similar fusion integrity to that of iliac crest autograft.[69]

Potential Downfalls

As discussed in the preceding sections, the potential downfalls of this procedure include vascular injury with an anterior breach or nerve root damage. A potential long-term complication is nonunion resulting in hardware failure, which is more common in cancer patients whose multiple rounds of chemotherapy and radiation collectively undermine fusion.

Management of Complications

As previously mentioned, CSF leaks are a known complication of these surgeries. The most important aspect of treating CSF leak is prevention, including preoperative risk factor evaluation and excellent intraoperative technique and manipulation. For example, residual bone spikes may result in postoperative puncture of the dural sac. Primary repair of durotomies intraoperatively is the preferred means to prevent postoperative CSF leaks; however, this method is reported to have a failure rate of 5% to 9%.[70,71] A variety of dural repair techniques and materials may be used, including direct suturing, use of dural patch graft materials, and tissue sealants.[72] The authors' preferred method is primary repair with 5-0 prolene when possible, followed by Tisseel sealant. A small local muscle patch can also be used if necessary. A lumbar drain may be placed for several days for flow diversion; however, this should be avoided in patients with cancer due to risk of tumor seeding.

Summary and Future Direction

Current robotic and image-guided systems facilitate increased accuracy, precision, and consistency of pedicle screw placement in spine surgery. Such systems also provide systemic value by reducing radiation exposure to the surgical team, potentially streamlining the operative workflow,[73] enabling minimally invasive applications, and improving patient outcomes in select cases.[10]

Especially when first implemented, navigation and robotic systems can worsen workflow, due to the high learning curve,[74] and may result in increased patient morbidity during this training period. Ultimately, the onus of learning how to safely and effectively use robotic and navigation technology lies with the surgeon. All companies provide hands-on training sessions for surgeons and provide significant personnel, particularly at the beginning, to assist with cases. In addition, a major barrier to widespread robotics adoption is cost, with some robots costing over $1 million per unit. Moreover, intraoperative robotics and navigation use require restructuring and changing the OR workflow, and training all OR staff including the nurses, scrub technicians, and radiology technologists.

As the use of navigation and robotics in spine surgery expands, these systems' value in improving surgical accuracy must be considered against concerns over cost and workflow. Given the relatively recent adoption of robotics in spine surgery, studies that definitively establish the long-term benefits of such systems on clinical outcomes remain scarce. However, preliminary results are promising.[75] As demonstrated in systematic reviews and a recent meta-analysis, robotic-assisted screw placement has been shown to have more consistent accuracy compared with traditional free-hand or fluoroscopy guided approaches.[31,41,76] The additional benefits include reduction of radiation exposure.[77,78] Further clinical and cost-related benefits likely correlate with the experience of the surgeon and the institution using robotic technology. Experienced groups have shown cost savings in the forms of reduced length of stay,[78] decreased need for revision surgery, lower infection rates, and shorter operative times.[79]

The two cases presented in this chapter demonstrate what we envision for the current and next generations of spine robots. These robots do not just allow us to place pedicle screws, a procedure which many surgeons feel comfortable performing free-hand without robotic or navigation assistance and which may contribute to the low adoption rates[80] of such systems. The next generation of navigation and robotic assistance may enable us to perform surgeries that we would otherwise be unable to do, including placing screws in different trajectories that do not have good anatomic landmarks, such as the transvertebral screw. The ability to visualize the screw trajectory in multiple dimensions is important when placing transvertebral screws as the pedicle can be narrow in the axial plane and the screw must pass diagonally through the pedicle in the sagittal plane, allowing purchase of the superior vertebral body across the disk space. In our corpectomy case, we used both a navigated drill and a pointer to indicate the superior and inferior endplates for the procedure, and also to determine the ventral extent of the corpectomy. Such navigation can greatly minimize morbidity by providing surgeons with a real-time localization that helps avoid dangerous anatomy. It is easy to envision using these navigation tools to perform various types of osteotomies in spinal deformity surgery, in addition to the navigated tumor corpectomy described here.

Next-generation systems will combine the best of both robotic and navigation technologies. They will allow us to place navigated transforaminal lumbar interbody fusion (TLIF) or corpectomy cages. By fusing preoperative MRI and CT scans, the robots will generate "no-fly" zones for corpectomies or even simple TLIF cage placement, preventing the robotic arm (and hence the drill or other tool) from damaging the nerve roots, dura, or vasculature. Navigation systems can also be used to assist in planning osteotomies by modeling the resection plane and expected spinal correction.[81,82] The improved precision offered by these systems could be integrated with robotics systems to further improve procedure accuracy. Pre-planning software, which is already being used with most robotics technologies, will continue to evolve and allow us to select screw trajectories, screw lengths, rod configurations and cage sizes preoperatively to decrease the amount of sterilized hardware needed for a case and improve workflow. Additionally, improvements in engineering technology will yield fluidity of movement in robots, resulting in increasing accuracy and efficiency during mechanical tasks. This will address surgeon fatigue and minimize impact of tremor. Additionally, next-generation robotic technologies will incorporate augmented reality (AR), technology that allows visual data is overlaid onto the surgical field for direct and immediate interaction. While AR has become transformative in the world of video gaming, it has yet to gain a solid footing in the realm of surgery. While these technologies are used in surgical training and anatomical study, its applicability has only recently been evaluated in spine surgery.[83] This type of technology, when coupled to a robotic platform, has the potential to give the surgeon a much less distracting work environment and may allow them to "see through" the patient during complex percutaneous and minimally invasive procedures that will be done with robotic assistance.

Robotic spine surgery will continue to evolve, and the forefront is the application of artificial intelligence (AI) and machine learning (ML). In brief, AI is a discipline of computer science that simulates intelligent behavior in computers, while ML is a domain of AI that facilitates automatic analytical model building; that is, allowing the computer to learn patterns by studying data directly and subsequently to predict patterns of interest. Currently, AI and ML are used in diagnosis, prognosis, and outcome prediction in medicine. In the future, ML-based modeling will predict surgical candidacy by using preoperative patient demographics, comorbidities, and imaging characteristics. The era of robotic surgery, which will allow the surgeon to plan and rehearse surgery, will also benefit from complex ML algorithms that will help the operator by automatically planning best fit and alignment of screws which can be adjusted prior to surgery.[84] Eventually, by gathering outcomes from hundreds and eventually thousands of planned surgical cases, these models will be able to determine the best procedure to help a given patient, to plan the surgery in advance (including optimal fusion levels, ideal screw placement, etc.), and to guide the surgeon in performing the surgery safely.

Although the future of robotic surgery is exciting, AI-based robots are unlikely to replace the human surgeon. However, the next generation of spine surgeons will be expected to adapt to and work side-by-side with evolving navigation and robotics technologies to improve surgical efficiency and patient outcomes.

REFERENCES

1. Srinivasan D, Than KD, Wang AC, et al. Radiation safety and spine surgery: systematic review of exposure limits and methods to minimize radiation exposure. *World Neurosurg*. 2014;82(6):1337–1343. https://doi.org/10.1016/j.wneu.2014.07.041.
2. Bindal RK, Glaze S, Ognoskie M, Tunner V, Malone R, Ghosh S. Surgeon and patient radiation exposure in minimally invasive transforaminal lumbar interbody fusion. *J Neurosurg Spine*. 2008;9(6):570–573. https://doi.org/10.3171/SPI.2008.4.08182.
3. Kantelhardt SR, Martinez R, Baerwinkel S, Burger R, Giese A, Rohde V. Perioperative course and accuracy of screw positioning in conventional, open robotic-guided and percutaneous robotic-guided, pedicle screw placement. *Eur Spine J*. 2011;20(6):860–868. https://doi.org/10.1007/s00586-011-1729-2.
4. Kim CW, Lee YP, Taylor W, Oygar A, Kim WK. Use of navigation-assisted fluoroscopy to decrease radiation exposure during minimally invasive spine surgery. *Spine J*. 2008;8(4):584–590. https://doi.org/10.1016/j.spinee.2006.12.012.
5. Kraus MD, Krischak G, Keppler P, Gebhard FT, Schuetz UH. Can computer-assisted surgery reduce the effective dose for spinal fusion and sacroiliac screw insertion? *Clin Orthop Relat Res*. 2010;468(9):2419–2429. https://doi.org/10.1007/s11999-010-1393-6.
6. van der Schatte Olivier RH, Van't Hullenaar CD, Ruurda JP, Broeders IA. Ergonomics, user comfort, and performance in standard and robot-assisted laparoscopic surgery. *Surg Endosc*. 2009;23(6):1365–1371. https://doi.org/10.1007/s00464-008-0184-6.
7. Xia L, Wang X, Xu T, et al. Robotic versus open radical cystectomy: an updated systematic review and meta-analysis. *PLoS One*. 2015;10(3):e0121032. https://doi.org/10.1371/journal.pone.0121032.
8. Zihni AM, Ohu I, Cavallo JA, Cho S, Awad MM. Ergonomic analysis of robot-assisted and traditional laparoscopic procedures. *Surg Endosc*. 2014;28(12):3379–3384. https://doi.org/10.1007/s00464-014-3604-9.
9. Ponnusamy K, Chewning S, Mohr C. Robotic approaches to the posterior spine. *Spine (Phila Pa 1976)*. 2009;34(19):2104–2109. https://doi.org/10.1097/BRS.0b013e3181b20212.
10. Kochanski RB, Lombardi JM, Laratta JL, Lehman RA, O'Toole JE. Image-guided navigation and robotics in spine surgery. *Neurosurgery*. 2019;84(6):1179–1189. https://doi.org/10.1093/neuros/nyy630.
11. Park P. Three-dimensional computed tomography-based spinal navigation in minimally invasive lateral lumbar interbody fusion: feasibility, technique, and initial results. *Neurosurgery*. 2015;11(suppl 2):259–267. https://doi.org/10.1227/NEU.0000000000000726.
12. Joseph JR, Smith BW, Patel RD, Park P. Use of 3D CT-based navigation in minimally invasive lateral lumbar interbody fusion. *J Neurosurg Spine*. 2016;25(3):339–344. https://doi.org/10.3171/2016.2.SPINE151295.
13. Drazin D, Liu JC, Acosta FL. CT navigated lateral interbody fusion. *J Clin Neurosci*. 2013;20(10):1438–1441. https://doi.org/10.1016/j.jocn.2012.12.028.
14. Nagashima H, Nishi T, Yamane K, Tanida A. Case report: osteoid osteoma of the C2 pedicle: surgical technique using a navigation system. *Clin Orthop Relat Res*. 2010;468(1):283–288. https://doi.org/10.1007/s11999-009-0958-8.
15. Mori K, Neo M, Takemoto M, Nishizawa K, Imai S. Navigated pin-point approach to osteoid osteoma adjacent to the facet joint of spine. *Asian Spine J*. 2016;10(1):158–163. https://doi.org/10.4184/asj.2016.10.1.158.
16. Van Royen BJ, Baayen JC, Pijpers R, Noske DP, Schakenraad D, Wuisman PI. Osteoid osteoma of the spine: a novel technique using combined computer-assisted and gamma probe-guided high-speed intralesional drill excision. *Spine*. 2005;30(3):369–373. https://doi.org/10.1097/01.brs.0000152531.49095.34.
17. Moore T, McLain RF. Image-guided surgery in resection of benign cervicothoracic spinal tumors: a report of two

cases. *Spine J*. 2005;5(1):109–114. https://doi.org/10.1016/j.spinee.2004.06.020.
18. Fujibayashi S, Neo M, Takemoto M, et al. Computer-assisted spinal osteotomy: a technical note and report of four cases. *Spine*. 2010;35(18):E895–E903. https://doi.org/10.1097/brs.0b013e3181dc5ed1.
19. Overley SC, Cho SK, Mehta AI, Arnold PM. Navigation and robotics in spinal surgery: where are we now? *Neurosurgery*. 2017;80(3S):S86–S99. https://doi.org/10.1093/neuros/nyw077.
20. Verma R, Krishan S, Haendlmayer K, Mohsen A. Functional outcome of computer-assisted spinal pedicle screw placement: a systematic review and meta-analysis of 23 studies including 5, 992 pedicle screws. *Eur Spine J*. 2010;19(3):370–375. https://doi.org/10.1007/s00586-009-1258-4.
21. Tian NF, Xu HZ. Image-guided pedicle screw insertion accuracy: a meta-analysis. *Int Orthop*. 2009;33(4):895–903. https://doi.org/10.1007/s00264-009-0792-3.
22. Kosmopoulos V, Schizas C. Pedicle screw placement accuracy: a meta-analysis. *Spine (Phila Pa 1976)*. 2007;32(3):E111–E120. https://doi.org/10.1097/01.brs.0000254048.79024.8b.
23. Gelalis ID, Paschos NK, Pakos EE, et al. Accuracy of pedicle screw placement: a systematic review of prospective in vivo studies comparing free hand, fluoroscopy guidance and navigation techniques. *Eur Spine J*. 2012;21(2):247–255. https://doi.org/10.1007/s00586-011-2011-3.
24. Mason A, Paulsen R, Babuska JM, et al. The accuracy of pedicle screw placement using intraoperative image guidance systems. *J Neurosurg Spine*. 2014;20(2):196–203. https://doi.org/10.3171/2013.11.SPINE13413.
25. Malham GM, Wells-Quinn T. What should my hospital buy next? Guidelines for the acquisition and application of imaging, navigation, and robotics for spine surgery. *J Spine Surg*. 2019;5(1):155–165. https://doi.org/10.21037/jss.2019.02.04.
26. Brecevich AT, Dowe C, Cammisa FP, Abjornson C. 121. 2. 3D-printed titanium: a surface optimization analysis. *Spine J*. 2019;19(9):S1–S2. https://doi.org/10.1016/j.spinee.2019.05.015.
27. Jakubovic R, Guha D, Gupta S, et al. High speed, high density intraoperative 3D optical topographical imaging with efficient registration to MRI and CT for craniospinal surgical navigation. *Sci Rep*. 2018;8(1):14894. https://doi.org/10.1038/s41598-018-32424-z.
28. Lieberman IH, Togawa D, Kayanja MM, et al. Bone-mounted miniature robotic guidance for pedicle screw and translaminar facet screw placement: part I—technical development and a test case result. *Neurosurgery*. 2006;59(3):641–650. discussion 641. https://doi.org/10.1227/01.NEU.0000229055.00829.5B.
29. Roser F, Tatagiba M, Maier G. Spinal robotics: current applications and future perspectives. *Neurosurgery*. 2013;72(suppl 1):12–18. https://doi.org/10.1227/NEU.0b013e318270d02c.
30. Urakov TM, Chang KH, Burks SS, Wang MY. Initial academic experience and learning curve with robotic spine instrumentation. *Neurosurg Focus*. 2017;42(5):E4. https://doi.org/10.3171/2017.2.FOCUS175.
31. Joseph JR, Smith BW, Liu X, Park P. Current applications of robotics in spine surgery: a systematic review of the literature. *Neurosurg Focus*. 2017;42(5):E2. https://doi.org/10.3171/2017.2.FOCUS16544.
32. Devito DP, Kaplan L, Dietl R, et al. Clinical acceptance and accuracy assessment of spinal implants guided with SpineAssist surgical robot: retrospective study. *Spine (Phila Pa 1976)*. 2010;35(24):2109–2115. https://doi.org/10.1097/BRS.0b013e3181d323ab.
33. Keric N, Eum DJ, Afghanyar F, et al. Evaluation of surgical strategy of conventional vs. percutaneous robot-assisted spinal trans-pedicular instrumentation in spondylodiscitis. *J Robot Surg*. 2017;11(1):17–25. https://doi.org/10.1007/s11701-016-0597-5.
34. Fan Y, Du JP, Liu JJ, et al. Accuracy of pedicle screw placement comparing robot-assisted technology and the free-hand with fluoroscopy-guided method in spine surgery: an updated meta-analysis. *Med (Baltim)*. 2018;97(22):e10970. https://doi.org/10.1097/MD.0000000000010970.
35. Lefranc M, Peltier J. Evaluation of the ROSA™ Spine robot for minimally invasive surgical procedures. *Expert Rev Med Devices*. 2016;13(10):899–906. https://doi.org/10.1080/17434440.2016.1236680.
36. Lonjon N, Chan-Seng E, Costalat V, Bonnafoux B, Vassal M, Boetto J. Robot-assisted spine surgery: feasibility study through a prospective case-matched analysis. *Eur Spine J*. 2016;25(3):947–955. https://doi.org/10.1007/s00586-015-3758-8.
37. Orringer DA, Golby A, Jolesz F. Neuronavigation in the surgical management of brain tumors: current and future trends. *Expert Rev Med Devices*. 2012;9(5):491–500. https://doi.org/10.1586/erd.12.42.
38. Zygourakis CC, Theodore N. Primum non nocere: robots and spinal surgery. *J Spine Surg*. 2018;4(4):810–811. https://doi.org/10.21037/jss.2018.09.10.
39. Ahmed AK, Zygourakis CC, Kalb S, et al. First spine surgery utilizing real-time image-guided robotic assistance. *Comput Assist Surg*. 2019;24(1):13–17. https://doi.org/10.1080/24699322.2018.1542029.
40. Zygourakis CC, Ahmed AK, Kalb S, et al. Technique: open lumbar decompression and fusion with the Excelsius GPS robot. *Neurosurg Focus*. 2018;45(VideoSuppl1):V6 https://doi.org/10.3171/2018.7.FocusVid.18123.
41. Perdomo-Pantoja A, Ishida W, Zygourakis C, et al. Accuracy of current techniques for placement of pedicle screws in the spine: a comprehensive systematic review and meta-analysis of 51, 161 screws. *World Neurosurg*. 2019;126:664–678. https://doi.org/10.1016/j.wneu.2019.02.217.
42. Park SM, Kim HJ, Lee SY, Chang BS, Lee CK, Yeom JS. Radiographic and clinical outcomes of robot-assisted posterior pedicle screw fixation: two-year results from a randomized controlled trial. *Yonsei Med J*. 2018;59(3):438–444. https://doi.org/10.3349/ymj.2018.59.3.438.

43. Liu H, Chen W, Wang Z, Lin J, Meng B, Yang H. Comparison of the accuracy between robot-assisted and conventional freehand pedicle screw placement: a systematic review and meta-analysis. *Int J Comput Assist Radiol Surg.* 2016;11(12):2273–2281. https://doi.org/10.1007/s11548-016-1448-6.
44. Kostrzewski S, Duff JM, Baur C, Olszewski M. Robotic system for cervical spine surgery. *Int J Med Robot.* 2012;8(2):184–190. https://doi.org/10.1002/rcs.446.
45. Lamartina C, Zavatsky JM, Petruzzi M, Specchia N. Novel concepts in the evaluation and treatment of high-dysplastic spondylolisthesis. *Eur Spine J.* 2009;18(suppl 1):133–142. https://doi.org/10.1007/s00586-009-0984-y.
46. Sudarshan PK, Suthar HR, Varma VK, Krishnan A, Hegde SK. Long-term experience with reduction technique in high-grade spondylolisthesis in the young. *Int J Spine Surg.* 2018;12(3):399–407. https://doi.org/10.14444/5047.
47. Vialle R, Charosky S, Padovani JP, Rigault P, Glorion C. Surgical treatment of high-grade lumbosacral spondylolisthesis in childhood, adolescent and young adult by the "double-plate" technique: a past experience. *Eur Spine J.* 2006;15(8):1210–1218. https://doi.org/10.1007/s00586-005-0051-2.
48. Boos N, Marchesi D, Zuber K, Aebi M. Treatment of severe spondylolisthesis by reduction and pedicular fixation. A 4-6-year follow-up study. *Spine (Phila Pa 1976).* 1993;18(12):1655–1661. https://doi.org/10.1097/00007632-199309000-00014.
49. Suk SI, Lee CK, Kim WJ, Lee JH, Cho KJ, Kim HG. Adding posterior lumbar interbody fusion to pedicle screw fixation and posterolateral fusion after decompression in spondylolytic spondylolisthesis. *Spine (Phila Pa 1976).* 1997;22(2):210–219. https://doi.org/10.1097/00007632-199701150-00016.
50. Petraco DM, Spivak JM, Cappadona JG, Kummer FJ, Neuwirth MG. An anatomic evaluation of L5 nerve stretch in spondylolisthesis reduction. *Spine (Phila Pa 1976).* 1996;21(10):1133–1138. discussion 1139. https://doi.org/10.1097/00007632-199605150-00002.
51. Vaccaro AR, Kepler CK, Rihn JA, et al. Anatomical relationships of the anterior blood vessels to the lower lumbar intervertebral discs: analysis based on magnetic resonance imaging of patients in the prone position. *J Bone Jt Surg Am.* 2012;94(12):1088–1094. https://doi.org/10.2106/JBJS.K.00671.
52. Mayfield FH, Kurokawa K. Watertight closure of spinal dura mater. Technical note. *J Neurol Surg.* 1975;43(5):639–640. https://doi.org/10.3171/jns.1975.43.5.0639.
53. Rodriguez-Olaverri JC, Zimick NC, Merola A, et al. Comparing the clinical and radiological outcomes of pedicular transvertebral screw fixation of the lumbosacral spine in spondylolisthesis versus unilateral transforaminal lumbar interbody fusion (TLIF) with posterior fixation using anterior cages. *Spine.* 2008;33(18):1977–1981. https://doi.org/10.1097/BRS.0b013e31817ecc01.
54. Ghobrial GM, Theofanis T, Darden BV, Arnold P, Fehlings MG, Harrop JS. Unintended durotomy in lumbar degenerative spinal surgery: a 10-year systematic review of the literature. *Neurosurg Focus.* 2015;39(4):E8. https://doi.org/10.3171/2015.7.FOCUS15266.
55. Sun X, Sun C, Liu X, et al. The frequency and treatment of dural tears and cerebrospinal fluid leakage in 266 patients with thoracic myelopathy caused by ossification of the ligamentum flavum. *Spine.* 2012;37(12):E702–E707. https://doi.org/10.1097/BRS.0b013e31824586a8.
56. Lu CH, Ho ST, Kong SS, Cherng CH, Wong CS. Intracranial subdural hematoma after unintended durotomy during spine surgery. *Can J Anesth.* 2002;49(1):100–102. https://doi.org/10.1007/BF03020428.
57. Fourney DR, Abi-Said D, Rhines LD, et al. Simultaneous anterior-posterior approach to the thoracic and lumbar spine for the radical resection of tumors followed by reconstruction and stabilization. *J Neurosurg.* 2001;94(2)(suppl):232–244. https://doi.org/10.3171/spi.2001.94.2.0232.
58. Laufer I, Hanover A, Lis E, Yamada Y, Bilsky M. Repeat decompression surgery for recurrent spinal metastases. *J Neurosurg Spine.* 2010;13(1):109–115. https://doi.org/10.3171/2010.3.SPINE08670.
59. Seaman S, Kerezoudis P, Bydon M, Torner JC, Hitchon PW. Titanium vs. polyetheretherketone (PEEK) interbody fusion: meta-analysis and review of the literature. *J Clin Neurosci.* 2017;44:23–29. https://doi.org/10.1016/j.jocn.2017.06.062.
60. Junaid M, Rashid MU, Bukhari SS, Ahmed M. Radiological and clinical outcomes in patients undergoing anterior cervical discectomy and fusion: comparing titanium and PEEK (polyetheretherketone) cages. *Pak J Med Sci.* 2018;34(6):1412–1417. https://doi.org/10.12669/pjms.346.15833.
61. Li ZJ, Wang Y, Xu GJ, Tian P. Is PEEK cage better than titanium cage in anterior cervical discectomy and fusion surgery? A meta-analysis. *BMC Musculoskelet Disord.* 2016;17:379. https://doi.org/10.1186/s12891-016-1234-1.
62. Cabraja M, Oezdemir S, Koeppen D, Kroppenstedt S. Anterior cervical discectomy and fusion: comparison of titanium and polyetheretherketone cages. *BMC Musculoskelet Disord.* 2012;13:172. https://doi.org/10.1186/1471-2474-13-172.
63. Nemoto O, Asazuma T, Yato Y, Imabayashi H, Yasuoka H, Fujikawa A. Comparison of fusion rates following transforaminal lumbar interbody fusion using polyetheretherketone cages or titanium cages with transpedicular instrumentation. *Eur Spine J.* 2014;23(10):2150–2155. https://doi.org/10.1007/s00586-014-3466-9.
64. Chen Y, Wang X, Lu X, et al. Comparison of titanium and polyetheretherketone (PEEK) cages in the surgical treatment of multilevel cervical spondylotic myelopathy: a prospective, randomized, control study with over 7-year follow-up. *Eur Spine J.* 2013;22(7):1539–1546. https://doi.org/10.1007/s00586-013-2772-y.
65. Krause KL, Obayashi JT, Bridges KJ, Raslan AM, Than KD. Fivefold higher rate of pseudarthrosis with polyetheretherketone interbody device than with structural allograft used for 1-level anterior cervical discectomy and fusion. *J Neurosurg Spine.* 2018;30(1):46–51.

66. Chong E, Pelletier MH, Mobbs RJ, Walsh WR. The design evolution of interbody cages in anterior cervical discectomy and fusion: a systematic review. *BMC Musculoskelet Disord*. 2015;16:99. https://doi.org/10.1186/s12891-015-0546-x.
67. Bess S, Line BG, Lafage V, et al. Does recombinant human bone morphogenetic protein-2 use in adult spinal deformity increase complications and are complications associated with location of rhBMP-2 use? A prospective, multicenter study of 279 consecutive patients. *Spine (Phila Pa 1976)*. 2014;39(3):233–242. https://doi.org/10.1097/BRS.0000000000000104.
68. Skovrlj B, Koehler SM, Anderson PA, et al. Association between BMP-2 and carcinogenicity. *Spine*. 2015;40(23):1862–1871. https://doi.org/10.1097/BRS.0000000000001126.
69. Cammisa FP Jr, Lowery G, Garfin SR, et al. Two-year fusion rate equivalency between Grafton DBM gel and autograft in posterolateral spine fusion: a prospective controlled trial employing a side-by-side comparison in the same patient. *Spine (Phila Pa 1976)*. 2004;29(6):660–666. https://doi.org/10.1097/01.brs.0000116588.17129.b9.
70. Fang Z, Tian R, Jia YT, Xu TT, Liu Y. Treatment of cerebrospinal fluid leak after spine surgery. *Chin J Traumatol*. 2017;20(2):81–83. https://doi.org/10.1016/j.cjtee.2016.12.002.
71. Narotam PK, José S, Nathoo N, Taylon C, Vora Y. Collagen matrix (DuraGen) in dural repair: analysis of a new modified technique. *Spine*. 2004;29(24):2861–2867, discussion 2868-2869. https://doi.org/10.1097/01.brs.0000148049.69541.ad.
72. Barber SM, Fridley JS, Konakondla S, et al. Cerebrospinal fluid leaks after spine tumor resection: avoidance, recognition and management. *Ann Transl Med*. 2019;7(10):217. https://doi.org/10.21037/atm.2019.01.04.
73. Khanna AR, Yanamadala V, Coumans JV. Effect of intraoperative navigation on operative time in 1-level lumbar fusion surgery. *J Clin Neurosci*. 2016;32:72–76. https://doi.org/10.1016/j.jocn.2016.02.033.
74. Hu X, Lieberman IH. What is the learning curve for robotic-assisted pedicle screw placement in spine surgery? *Clin Orthop Relat Res*. 2014;472(6):1839–1844. https://doi.org/10.1007/s11999-013-3291-1.
75. Theodore N, Arnold PM, Mehta AI. Introduction: the rise of the robots in spinal surgery. *Neurosurg Focus*. 2018;45(VideoSuppl1) (Video:Intro):Intro. https://doi.org/10.3171/2018.7.FocusVid.Intro.
76. Ghasem A, Sharma A, Greif DN, Alam M, Maaieh MA. The arrival of robotics in spine surgery: a review of the literature. *Spine (Phila Pa 1976)*. 2018;43(23):1670–1677. https://doi.org/10.1097/BRS.0000000000002695.
77. Gao S, Lv Z, Fang H. Robot-assisted and conventional freehand pedicle screw placement: a systematic review and meta-analysis of randomized controlled trials. *Eur Spine J*. 2018;27(4):921–930. https://doi.org/10.1007/s00586-017-5333-y.
78. Hyun SJ, Kim KJ, Jahng TA, Kim HJ. Minimally invasive robotic versus open fluoroscopic-guided spinal instrumented fusions: a randomized controlled trial. *Spine (Phila Pa 1976)*. 2017;42(6):353–358. https://doi.org/10.1097/BRS.0000000000001778.
79. Menger RP, Savardekar AR, Farokhi F, Sin A. A cost-effectiveness analysis of the integration of robotic spine technology in spine surgery. *Neurospine*. 2018;15(3):216–224. https://doi.org/10.14245/ns.1836082.041.
80. Choo AD, Regev G, Garfin SR, Kim CW. Surgeons' perceptions of spinal navigation: analysis of key factors affecting the lack of adoption of spinal navigation technology. *SAS J*. 2008;2(4):189–194. https://doi.org/10.1016/SASJ-2008-0007-RR.
81. Kosterhon M, Gutenberg A, Kantelhardt SR, Archavlis E, Giese A. Navigation and image injection for control of bone removal and osteotomy planes in spine surgery. *Oper Neurosurg Hagerstown*. 2017;13(2):297–304. https://doi.org/10.1093/ons/opw017.
82. Faundez A, Byrne F, Sylvestre C, Lafage V, Cogniet A, Le Huec JC. Pedicle subtraction osteotomy in the thoracic spine and thoracolumbar junction: a retrospective series of 28 cases. *Eur Spine J*. 2015;24(suppl 1):S42–S48. https://doi.org/10.1007/s00586-014-3658-3.
83. Molina CA, Theodore N, Ahmed AK, et al. Augmented reality-assisted pedicle screw insertion: a cadaveric proof-of-concept study. *J Neurosurg Spine*. 2019;31(1):139–146. https://doi.org/10.3171/2018.12.SPINE181142.
84. Vijayan R, De Silva T, Han R, et al. Automatic pedicle screw planning using atlas-based registration of anatomy and reference trajectories. *Phys Med Biol*. 2019;64(16):165020. https://doi.org/10.1088/1361-6560/ab2d66.

11

Traumatic Spinal Injury and Robotic Reconstruction

Jayanidhi Kedda, BS, Ann Liu, MD, Bowen Jiang, MD, and Nicholas Theodore, MD

INTRODUCTION OF TECHNOLOGY

Traumatic spinal injury (TSI) may involve injury to the osseous structures, discoligamentous components, spinal cord, nerve roots of the spinal column, or a combination thereof. TSI can lead to a wide range of medical conditions, from minimal nondisplaced fractures to mechanically unstable fractures with associated neurological compromise. The clinical sequelae of TSI, which can include pain and/or neurological deficit, may result in severe morbidity and mortality. Although abundant literature exists on spinal cord injury (SCI), a subset of TSI, studies have only recently investigated the epidemiology of TSI. A meta-analysis of 102 studies from 32 countries by Kumar et al. found the global incidence of TSI to be 10.5 cases per 100,000 persons.[1] With the world population exceeding 7 billion people, this translates to over 750,000 new cases of TSI worldwide.[1] Men are more commonly affected than are women, with an average age of injury of 40 years old.[1] The leading causes of TSI worldwide are traffic collisions (40%) and falls (39%).[1] Although multiple older studies have reported approximately 160,000 spine fractures in North America,[2–4] Kumar et al. found an incidence of 5.1 cases of TSI per 100,000 persons for an estimated 18,220 cases (95% confidence interval: 5002–67,881) annually.[1]

Fractures of the thoracolumbar spine are common. Anatomically, the upper thoracic spine is less mobile due to articulations with the ribs that attach to the sternum. The thoracolumbar junction, located at T10–L2, represents an area of transition from the rigid thoracic spine to the more dynamic lumbar spine. Injury commonly occurs in this region because the thoracic spine lacks the flexibility of the lumbar spine, so sudden and traumatic movements often stress this area at a higher load than it can handle.[5] Katsuura et al. conducted a meta-analysis and found the rate of thoracolumbar fracture to be 6.9% in patients who have sustained blunt trauma.[6] Of patients with thoracolumbar fractures, injury at the thoracolumbar junction can be as high as 41%.[7] Trauma may concurrently occur in other locations, such as the extremities (19%), head (13%), cervical spine (11%), and abdomen (7%).[6]

Fortunately, many fractures are stable and do not involve neurologic compromise; therefore, they can be treated conservatively with pain control, bracing, or both. When TSI causes neurologic deficit or instability of the spinal column, surgery may be needed for fixation, decompression of neural elements, and/or reduction of deformity. With improvements in modern trauma care, surgery can now allow for earlier mobilization, which is thought to be important in reducing morbidity and mortality. Specifically, early surgical intervention can be beneficial in:

- Improving pulmonary function with decreased rates of pneumonia and decreased time on the ventilator,[4]
- Diminishing pain from instability,
- Reducing the incidence and severity of sepsis and respiratory failure, and
- Decreasing overall intensive care unit and hospital lengths of stay.[8]

In the TSI population, however, surgical intervention does carry certain additional risks. Trauma patients can have inadequate resuscitation, propensity for increased hemorrhage, sensitivity to hypotension, overlooked or underestimated associated injuries, or some combination of these factors.[4,8,9] Surgeons may be at an even greater disadvantage by operating in less than ideal conditions.[8] These factors must be weighed by the surgeon when deciding on the need for and timing of surgical intervention.

Pedicle screw instrumentation was first described in the 1960s and 1970s[10–12] and has since become the gold standard of spinal fusion.[13] As pedicle screws and spinal fixation procedures have become more commonplace, efforts to optimize trajectory while minimizing invasiveness and malpositioning have been heavily invested in technological solutions. Beginning in 1995, computer assisted (i.e., image-guided) navigation was applied to spinal surgical procedures to improve screw placement accuracy and decrease the risk to the patient.[14] Further developments over the past two decades have brought the use of intraoperative navigation tactics (such as the C-arm and O-arm) and robotics into everyday use for spinal fixation.

Robotic navigation combines the precision of computer based navigation with the steadiness of a machine, requiring only trajectory decisions with intraoperative confirmation and screw placement by the surgeon. Several surgical robots to improve pedicle screw placement now exist, including ExcelsiusGPS (Globus Medical, Audubon, PA), Mazor (Mazor Robotics, Caesarea, Israel), ROSA (Zimmer Biomet, Warsaw, IN), TiRobot (TINAVI Medical Technology, Beijing, China), and more.[15–18] With increasing use of these surgical robots, patient outcomes are now being analyzed more thoroughly. Most patients described in the current robotic literature are those with degenerative spinal disease; indeed, very few studies have included TSI patients.

Han et al. conducted a prospective study of 234 patients with degenerative or traumatic thoracolumbar spinal injury who underwent pedicle screw placement with either the TiRobot system or conventional fluoroscopy.[15] The patients were randomly sorted into the robotic-guided ($n = 115$) or the fluoroscopy-assisted ($n = 119$) surgical groups and the safety and accuracy of pedicle screw placement in each group was assessed and compared. 76/234 (32%) of participants had a trauma-based pathology. Of the 76 TSI patients, 41 (54%) were assigned to the robotic-guided group and 35 (46%) were assigned to the fluoroscopy-guided group. Screw placement was graded on the Gertzbein-Robbins scale with grades A (i.e., screw completely within the pedicle) and B (i.e., pedicle cortical breach < 2 mm) given to clinically acceptable screw placements. Of the robotic-guided procedures, 507/532 (95.3%) screws were considered grade A and 18/532 (3.4%) grade B, whereas in the fluoroscopy-guided surgeries, 503/584 (86.1%) screws were considered grade A and 43/584 (7.4%), grade B. The proportion of group A and B screws in the robotic-guided group was greater than that in the fluoroscopy-assisted group ($p < .01$). The robot-guided group required no revision surgery (two were required in the fluoroscopy-guided group), had significantly less blood loss, and decreased surgeon radiation exposure compared with the fluoroscopy-guided group.[15] Although subgroup analyses between the degenerative versus trauma groups were not carried out, this study demonstrates the successful use of robotic guidance in patients with trauma.

Le et al., from the same research group, performed a similar study with the TiRobot to assess the safety and accuracy of cortical bone trajectory screw placement in the lumbar spine with robot guidance compared to fluoroscopy guidance.[17] Of 58 patients included, only 4 were TSI patients, and all were sorted into the fluoroscopy-guided group. Another study by Kam et al. examined the learning curve of robotic assisted screw placement in 80 patients, in which only 4 patients underwent surgery for a traumatic etiology.[16] Neither study specifically analyzed the TSI patients.

A true paucity of literature exists pertaining to robotics and TSI; however, as the use of robotics increases in spine surgery, robotic reconstruction may become more valuable in minimally invasive procedures for patients who have sustained a traumatic injury. One of the main advantages of robotic assisted spine surgery is the potential to minimize the physiologic burden associated with open surgery. Prior research has shown that minimally invasive spine surgery lessens the extent of muscle and soft tissue dissection, resulting in decreased blood loss, length of stay, and complication rates, all while producing equivalent overall postoperative outcomes.[2,19] Robotic assistance allows the surgeon to plan the screw trajectories and the place pedicle screws without the intensive dissection needed in open surgery. In trauma patients already prone to hemorrhage and who may be hemodynamically complicated due to other injuries, minimizing blood loss and invasiveness of surgery may help minimize morbidity. Additionally, robot assistance can be useful in patients with challenging anatomy (e.g., small pedicles) or abnormal anatomy by utilizing preoperative or real-time intraoperative computed tomography (CT) or fluoroscopy.

SURGICAL TREATMENT FOR SPINAL PATHOLOGY

Clinical Case #1

History/Clinical Presentation

A 73-year-old male taxicab driver with a past medical history of coronary artery disease, diabetes, hypertension, horseshoe kidney, obstructive sleep apnea, and gout presented to the emergency department (ED) after being dragged underneath his taxi for 40 feet. Upon presentation to the ED, the patient described midline back pain and abdominal pain, but denied radicular pain in his arms or legs, numbness or tingling, saddle anesthesia, and bowel/bladder dysfunction. He was a former smoker and was on aspirin 81 mg daily.

The patient was hemodynamically stable with a temperature of 36.2°C, heart rate of 74 bpm, blood pressure of 144/52, and SpO_2 of 97% on room air. The patient was morbidly obese with a body mass index of 38.6 kg/m^2. He was awake, alert, and oriented. He had baseline weakness 4/5 strength in his left deltoid from a prior injury of his left shoulder but otherwise had full strength in all muscle groups. The examination was negative for the Hoffman sign and clonus.

CT of the spine showed an unstable burst fracture of the T8 vertebral body, with up to 6 mm of anteropulsion and approximately 25% height loss of the anterior superior endplate. The scan also demonstrated multilevel diffuse bridging ossification of the anterior vertebral bodies from T3 to T11, consistent with diffuse idiopathic skeletal hyperostosis. His labs were notable for platelets of 176, 000, creatinine of 0.98 mg/dL, INR 1.1, and aPTT 23.2.

After discussion with the attending neurosurgeon, the patient was admitted to neurosurgery floor care, with regular neurological exam checks and strict spinal precautions at all times. The patient was unable to undergo magnetic resonance imaging due to metal in his left shoulder. Given his age and medical comorbidities, medicine was consulted for preoperative risk assessment and the patient was medically optimized for surgery.

Preoperative Imaging

Unstable burst fracture of the T8 vertebral body with up to 6 mm of anteropulsion and approximately 25% height loss of the anterior superior endplate (Fig. 11.1).

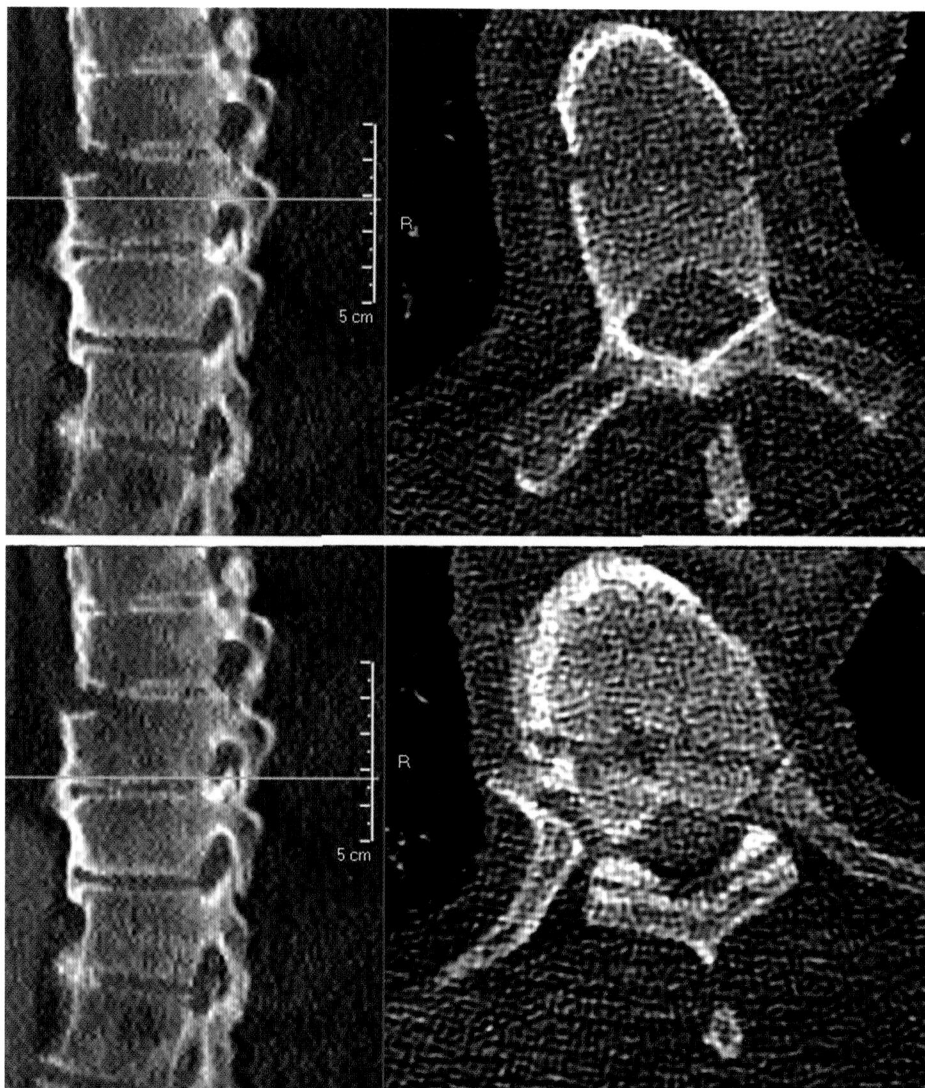

FIG. 11.1 Unstable burst fracture of the T8 vertebral body with up to 6 mm of anteropulsion and approximately 25% height loss of the anterior superior endplate.

Surgical Plan

The patient underwent T6–T10 percutaneous, minimally invasive robotic assisted fusion. Following the induction of general anesthesia, baseline intraoperative monitoring with somatosensory-evoked potentials was obtained. The patient was carefully positioned prone on the surgical table with intraoperative neuromonitoring performed throughout the entirety of the procedure. The patient was prepared and draped in the usual sterile technique. An intraoperative radiograph was used to identify T11 and a midline incision was made over the T11 spinous process. An image-guided spinal tracker and a surveillance marker were placed on the T11 spinous process. Intraoperative anteroposterior and lateral radiographs were obtained and transferred to the ExcelsiusGPS planning station. His preoperative CT was already evaluated and the screws were planned using the robot software (Fig. 11.2A and B). Once the intraoperative fluoroscopic images were merged with the preoperative CT, real-time image guidance and robotics could be used.

For screw placement, the robot was draped sterilely, wheeled into the surgical field, and stabilized. Typically, the base station, with the touchscreen monitor, robot arm, and end effector, is placed at the head of the bed while the navigation camera is placed at the foot of the bed (see Fig. 11.2C). Navigated instruments, including a position tracker, drill, and screw guide, were registered to the system. The robot foot pedal was used to move the rigid robotic arm (with a guide tube) to the planned trajectory at each level (see Fig. 11.2D). Bilateral paramedian incisions were made from T6 to T10. The navigated power drill was first placed through the guide tube to cannulate the planned trajectory (see Fig. 11.2E). The screws were then placed at each level (see Fig. 11.2F) using real-time visualization of the screw trajectory and indicators of excessive force or tip deflection (i.e., "skiving"). Shorter screws were placed in the index level of T8. Intraoperative radiographs showed excellent placement of the hardware. At this point, the facet joints bilaterally at T6–T7, T7–T8, T8–T9, and T9–T10 were decorticated with a high-speed air drill and demineralized bone matrix was packed into the interstices from T6–T10. Top-loading rods were placed with caps. The final radiographs showed excellent placement of the hardware. The incisions were irrigated and closed in the usual fashion. Neuromonitoring was stable throughout the case. The estimated blood loss was 150 mL, and the duration of the procedure from the incision to the beginning of closure was 1 h and 37 min.

Postoperative Imaging

Postoperative bilateral pedicle screw placement from T6 to T10 (Fig. 11.3).

Postoperative Recovery and Follow-Up

Postoperatively, the patient was admitted to the neurosurgical floor and, on examination, was at his neurological baseline with left deltoid weakness but otherwise full strength and sensation. On postoperative day (POD) 1, he developed atrial fibrillation with a rapid ventricular response, which was controlled with metoprolol. The postoperative CT showed excellent hardware positioning. His pain was controlled and he mobilized with physical therapy. The patient was medically and neurosurgically cleared for discharge to acute rehabilitation on POD 8.

On POD 15, the patient returned to the clinic for his follow-up appointment. At the time, he was still in an acute rehabilitation facility and was able to walk without a walker. His pain was continuing to improve and the patient noted he was only taking acetaminophen on a regular basis with occasional oxycodone. On examination, he remained at full strength and his incisions were healing well.

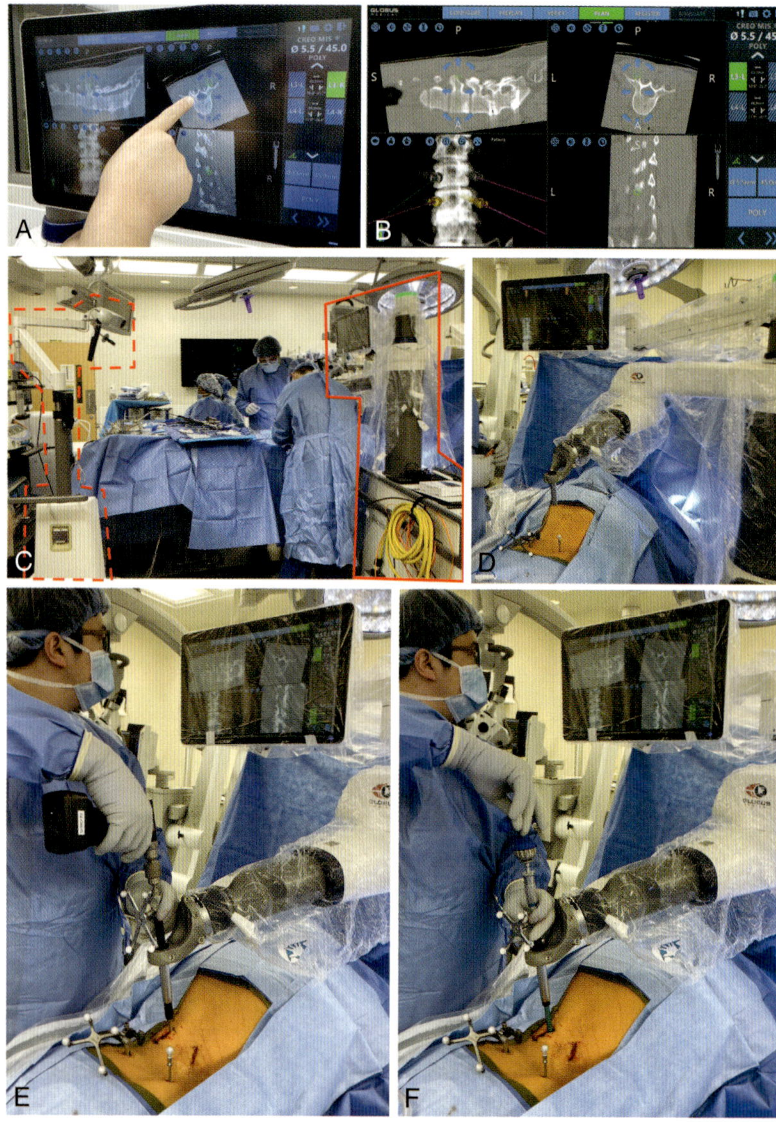

FIG. 11.2 Intraoperative use of the ExcelsiusGPS. (A, B) Screw planning. (C) Placement of the base station and navigation camera. (D) Use of the rigid robotic arm to the planned trajectory. (E) Use of the navigated power drill to cannulate the planned trajectory. (F) Screw placement.

Clinical Case #2

History/Clinical Presentation

A 63-year-old man with a past medical history of hyperlipidemia and chronic headaches presented to the ED after a fall off an 18-foot ladder. He hit his head and his right side/buttock but denied loss of consciousness. He was able to walk back to his house to call 911. In the ED, he complained of scalp, midline neck, and back pain. He denied radicular pain in

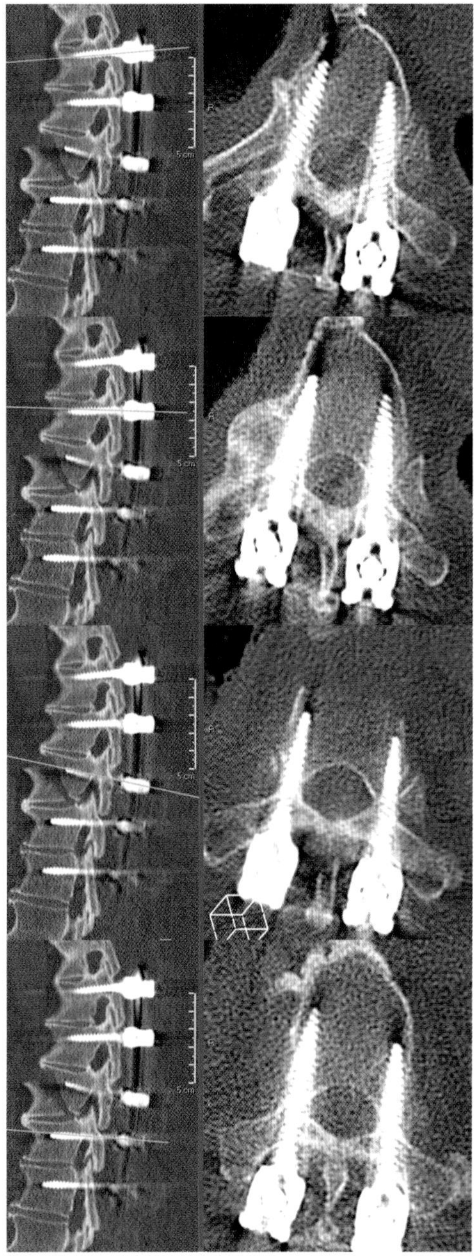

FIG. 11.3 Postoperative CT demonstrating bilateral pedicle screw placement from T6 to T10.

his arms or legs, numbness or tingling, saddle anesthesia, and bowel/bladder dysfunction. He was on aspirin 81 mg daily.

The patient was hemodynamically stable with a temperature of 36.4°C, heart rate of 119 bpm, blood pressure of 144/98, and SpO_2 of 98% on room air. The patient had a body mass index of 30.2 kg/m^2. He was awake, alert, and oriented. He was full strength in all muscle groups, and his sensation was intact throughout. The examination was negative for the Hoffman sign and clonus. The rectal tone was intact.

CT of the spine showed an unstable burst fracture of the L1 vertebral body with approximately 50% height loss anteriorly and minimal retropulsion into the spinal canal.

Preoperative Imaging

Unstable burst fracture of the L1 vertebral body with approximately 50% height loss anteriorly and minimal retropulsion into the spinal canal (Fig. 11.4).

Surgical Plan

The patient underwent T12–L2 robotic assisted fusion. Following the induction of general anesthesia, baseline intraoperative monitoring with somatosensory-evoked potentials was obtained. The patient was carefully positioned prone on the surgical table with intraoperative neuromonitoring performed throughout the entirety of the case. The patient was prepped and draped in usual sterile technique. A midline incision was made from T11 to L3 with exposure of the lamina from T12 to L2. An image-guided spinal tracker and surveillance marker were placed on the L3 spinous process. Intraoperative anteroposterior and lateral radiographs were obtained and transferred to the ExcelsiusGPS planning station. Registration and screws were placed from T12 to L2 as described in case #1. The midline incision was used for screw placement. The intraoperative radiographs showed excellent placement of the hardware. A high-speed air drill was used for decortication, and

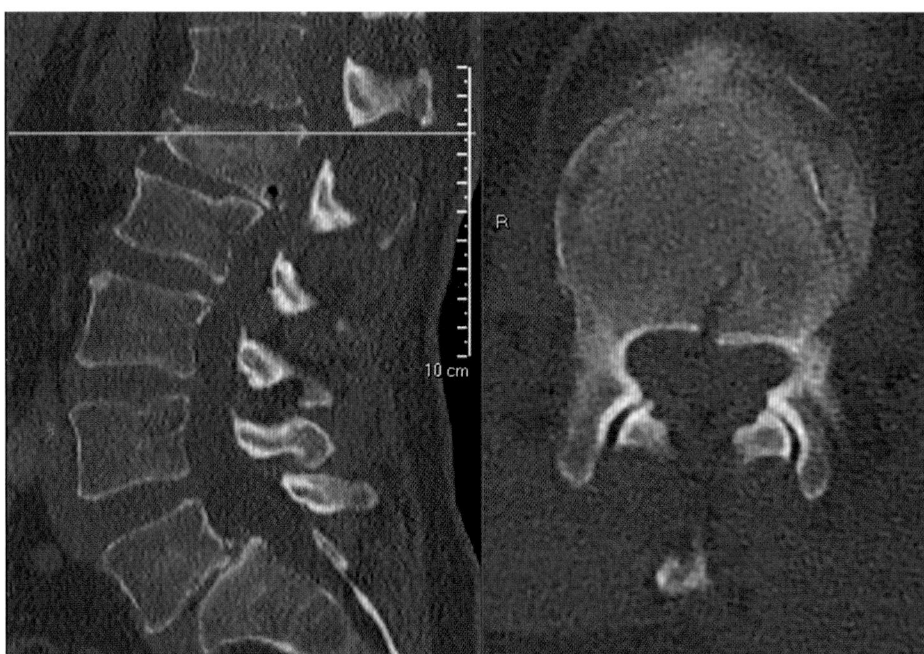

FIG. 11.4 Unstable burst fracture of the L1 vertebral body with approximately 50% height loss anteriorly and minimal retropulsion into the spinal canal.

demineralized bone matrix was packed into the interstices from T12 to L2. Top-loading rods were placed with caps. The final radiographs showed excellent placement of the hardware. The incisions were irrigated and closed in the usual fashion, and a subfascial drain was placed. Neuromonitoring was stable throughout the case. The estimated blood loss was 200 mL and the duration of the procedure from the incision to the beginning of closure was 2 h and 9 min.

Postoperative Imaging

Postoperative anteroposterior and lateral radiographs demonstrating hardware placement Fig. 11.5.

Postoperative Recovery and Follow-Up

Postoperatively, the patient was admitted to the neurosurgical floor and, on examination, was neurologically intact with full strength and sensation. On POD 1, he mobilized with physical therapy and was recommended outpatient therapy. The postoperative anteroposterior and lateral radiographs showed excellent hardware positioning. The patient was medically and neurosurgically cleared for discharge home on POD 2. He has not yet returned to the clinic for his follow-up appointment.

PROCEDURAL CONCERNS IN DETAIL

In the setting of TSI, it is imperative to evaluate the patient's other traumatic injuries and overall hemodynamic and respiratory status before proceeding with surgery. In the

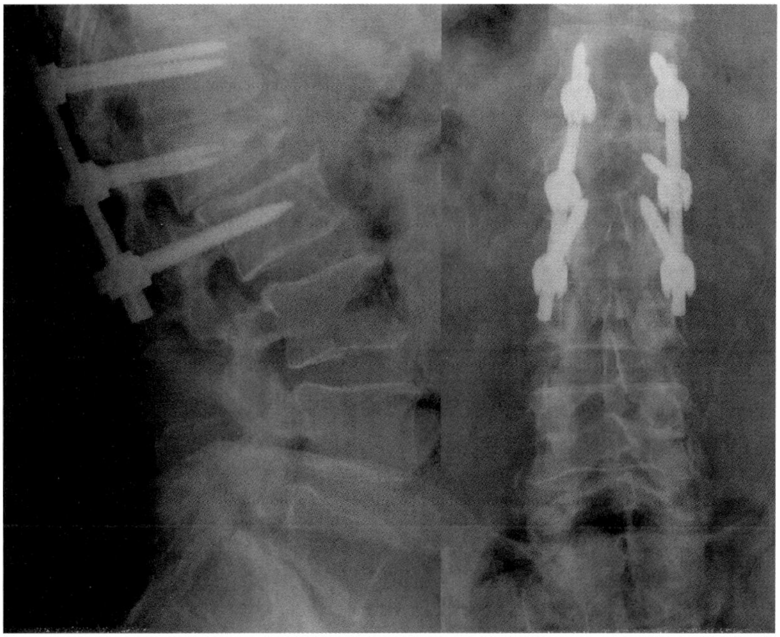

FIG. 11.5 Postoperative anteroposterior and lateral radiographs demonstrating hardware placement.

operating room, neuromonitoring is crucial and should be used for the entire duration of the case, particularly during positioning in the setting of unstable fractures. Special attention should be paid to the patient's blood pressure in the setting of elevated mean arterial pressures and continuous monitoring with an arterial line if there is concern for cord injury.

Robotic assisted surgery depends upon the accuracy of the registration and minimal movement of the spinal tracker. In the thoracic spine, initial registration can be challenging due to difficulty of obtaining high-quality fluoroscopic images to merge with the preoperative CT. Using a breath-hold during fluoroscopy may help improve the image quality. Alternatively, an intraoperative CT can be used instead of a preoperative CT if fluoroscopic registration is not accurate enough. Once registration has been completed, the ExcelsiusGPS, in particular, uses a surveillance marker that helps to ensure the accuracy of the registration throughout the case. The surgeon must also take special care to work around and not disturb the spinal tracker. In truly unstable injuries, increased mobility of the spine can increase the chances for inaccuracies due to movement of the bone in relation to the spinal tracker. Special care should be taken not to apply excessive force with the navigated power drill as this could shift the bone and spine, thus making the imaging data inaccurate. These precautions are particularly more important when placing pedicle screws in the thoracic spine given the smaller-sized pedicles. In cases of trauma causing a focal kyphosis, the angle of the end effector can be quite steep and prevent the ability of the navigation camera to see the instruments. In these cases, the camera may need to be moved to the head instead of the foot of the bed. Finally, although preoperative CT imaging was used to plan the screw trajectory in our two cases, if there is any concern regarding inaccuracy of the preoperative imaging (e.g., in cases of traumatic deformity where partial reduction may occur with patient positioning), intraoperative CT with the O-arm after the final positioning can be used for screw trajectory planning.

ADVERSE TREATMENT EFFECTS, POTENTIAL DOWNFALLS, AND MANAGEMENT OF COMPLICATIONS

The potential risks of surgery with robotic assistance are the same as a traditional surgical approach and include, but are not limited to, neurologic deficit, spinal cord or nerve root injury, bleeding, infection, cerebrospinal fluid leak, delayed spinal instability at adjacent levels, hardware failure, paralysis, coma, death, the need for additional surgery for the patient's symptoms to resolve, worsening of the patient's symptoms, and medical complications such as pneumonia, pulmonary emboli, and deep venous thrombosis. Trauma patients in particular are at higher risk of bleeding and hemodynamic instability.

One potential downfall of robotic assisted spine surgery, not specific to TSI cases, is failure of the robot during instrumentation. The reasons for aborting the use of robotics intraoperatively include failure of registration software, failure to obtain adequate fluoroscopic images, soft tissue pressure on the robotic arm leading to inaccuracy in placement, inability to obtain the necessary angles or trajectories, and skiving of the drill or screw along the bone.[20] In the event of robotic failure, the surgeon can convert to traditional open, free-handed methods. Another general downside to robotic reconstruction is the learning curve associated with the technology. While Kam et al. described no significant learning curve,[16] further studies are needed. Should complications occur, the management is no different from that of a complication that occurred using the traditional methods.

FUTURE DIRECTIONS

The benefits of robotics are obvious; they minimize invasiveness, reduce tissue dissection, and lessen blood loss. These features make robotics particularly useful as a minimally invasive technique in patients with TSI. Currently, however, very little data exists regarding the use of robotics in trauma, and further research is needed on this subset of patients needing spine surgery.

REFERENCES

1. Kumar R, Lim J, Mekary RA, et al. Traumatic spinal injury: global epidemiology and worldwide volume. *World Neurosurg*. 2018;113:e345–e363. https://doi.org/10.1016/j.wneu.2018.02.033.
2. Camacho JE, Usmani MF, Strickland AR, Banagan KE, Ludwig SC. The use of minimally invasive surgery in spine trauma: a review of concepts. *J Spinal Surg*. 2019;5(suppl 1):S91–S100. https://doi.org/10.21037/jss.2019.04.13.
3. Chang V, Holly LT. Bracing for thoracolumbar fractures. *Neurosurg Focus*. 2014;37(1):E3. https://doi.org/10.3171/2014.4.FOCUS1477.
4. O'Boynick CP, Kurd MF, Darden BV 2nd, Vaccaro AR, Fehlings MG. Timing of surgery in thoracolumbar trauma: is early intervention safe? *Neurosurg Focus*. 2014;37(1):E7. https://doi.org/10.3171/2014.5.FOCUS1473.
5. Wood KB, Li W, Lebl DR, Ploumis A. Management of thoracolumbar spine fractures. *Spine J*. 2014;14(1):145–164. https://doi.org/10.1016/j.spinee.2012.10.041.
6. Katsuura Y, Osborn JM, Cason GW. The epidemiology of thoracolumbar trauma: a meta-analysis. *J Orthop*. 2016;13(4):383–388. https://doi.org/10.1016/j.jor.2016.06.019.
7. Holmes JF, Miller PQ, Panacek EA, Lin S, Horne NS, Mower WR. Epidemiology of thoracolumbar spine injury in blunt trauma. *Acad Emerg Med*. 2001;8(9):866–872. https://doi.org/10.1111/j.1553-2712.2001.tb01146.x.
8. Bellabarba C, Fisher C, Chapman JR, Dettori JR, Norvell DC. Does early fracture fixation of thoracolumbar spine fractures decrease morbidity or mortality? *Spine*. 2010; 35(suppl 9):S138–S145. https://doi.org/10.1097/BRS.0b013e3181d830c1.
9. Kerwin AJ, Griffen MM, Tepas JJ, III Schinco MA, Devin T, Frykberg ER. Best practice determination of timing of spinal fracture fixation as defined by analysis of the National Trauma Data Bank. *J Trauma*. 2008;65(4):824–830, discussion 830. https://doi.org/10.1097/TA.0b013e318182af7b.
10. Harrington PR, Tullos HS. Reduction of severe spondylolisthesis in children. *South Med J*. 1969;62(1):1–7. https://doi.org/10.1097/00007611-196901000-00001.
11. Roy-Camille R, Saillant G, Berteaux D, Salgado V. Osteosynthesis of thoraco-lumbar spine fractures with metal plates screwed through the vertebral pedicles. *Reconstr Surg Traumatol*. 1976;15:2–16.
12. Kabins MB, Weinstein JN. The history of vertebral screw and pedicle screw fixation. *Iowa Orthop J*. 1991;11:127–136.
13. Gaines Jr. RW. The use of pedicle-screw internal fixation for the operative treatment of spinal disorders. *J Bone Joint Surg Am*. 2000;82(10):1458–1476. https://doi.org/10.2106/00004623-200010000-00013.
14. Amiot LP, Labelle H, DeGuise JA, Sati M, Brodeur P, Rivard CH. Computer-assisted pedicle screw fixation. A feasibility study. *Spine*. 1995;20(10):1208–1212. https://doi.org/10.1097/00007632-199505150-00019.
15. Han X, Tian W, Liu Y, et al. Safety and accuracy of robot-assisted versus fluoroscopy-assisted pedicle screw insertion in thoracolumbar spinal surgery: a prospective randomized controlled trial. *J Neurosurg Spine*. 2019;30(5):1–8. https://doi.org/10.3171/2018.10.SPINE18487.
16. Kam JKT, Gan C, Dimou S, et al. Learning curve for robot-assisted percutaneous pedicle screw placement in thoracolumbar surgery. *Asian Spine J*. 2019;9:920–927. https://doi.org/10.31616/asj.2019.0033.
17. Le X, Tian W, Shi Z, et al. Robot-assisted versus fluoroscopy-assisted cortical bone trajectory screw instrumentation in lumbar spinal surgery: a matched-cohort comparison. *World Neurosurg*. 2018;120:e745–e751. https://doi.org/10.1016/j.wneu.2018.08.157.
18. Tian W, Liu YJ, Liu B, et al. Guideline for thoracolumbar pedicle screw placement assisted by orthopaedic surgical robot. *Orthop Surg*. 2019;11(2):153–159. https://doi.org/10.1111/os.12453.
19. Fischer CR, Beaubrun B, Manning J, Qureshi S, Uribe J. Evidence based medicine review of posterior thoracolumbar minimally invasive technology. *Int J Spine Surg*. 2018;12(6):680–688. https://doi.org/10.14444/5085.
20. Joseph JR, Smith BW, Liu X, Park P. Current applications of robotics in spine surgery: a systematic review of the literature. *Neurosurg Focus*. 2017;42(5):E2. https://doi.org/10.3171/2017.2.FOCUS16544.

12

Cost-Effectiveness of Robotic and Navigation Systems

Mohamad Bydon, MD, Anshit Goyal, MBBS, MS, and Atiq Ur Rehman Bhatti, MD

INTRODUCTION

Substantial technological innovation has been made in spine surgery over the last few decades. This innovation has ranged from improvement in operative techniques, surgical implants, and biologics to improved accuracy with image-guided navigation and robotics. Robotic assistance is being increasingly utilized across multiple surgical specialties including urology, obstetrics and gynecology (OB/GYN), orthopedics, and neurosurgery. Although the utilization of robotics in spine surgery is still in its nascent stages, the recent literature has demonstrated that it has the potential to revolutionize safety and accuracy, not just for the placement of spinal instrumentation, but also to complete other critical operative steps while minimizing radiation exposure to the surgical team. However, while many providers and institutions are acquiring various surgical robots, there have been reports that the technology has failed to penetrate into routine practice. To demonstrate its *value* in healthcare, any new technology must demonstrate *cost-effectiveness* in addition to *quality* or improvement in outcomes. Spine providers have been hesitant to incorporate robotics and navigation into routine surgical care due to the notion of substantially higher costs associated with the acquisition of these newer guidance platforms. In today's pay-for-performance era, spine surgeons are under increasing pressure and scrutiny to develop measures that control pricing and allow increased accountability for surgical performance. The incorporation of robotic and navigation systems into routine practice might allow implementation of such value-based spinal care.

In addition to quality and safety, the cost-effectiveness of robotic surgery has been evaluated within other surgical specialties such as urology and OB/GYN.[1–5] The cumulative evidence has significantly changed practice patterns in urologic surgery.[6] Such cost-effectiveness analyses are essential to obtain a more balanced perspective of practice utility and are imperative to design and effect solutions to improve performance. However, such analyses are limited in the realm of spine surgery. In this chapter, the authors discuss the available evidence on the cost-effectiveness of robotics and navigation in spine surgery and provide an overview of the mechanisms regarding how the assimilation of such platforms into the daily surgical workflow could provide long-term cost savings.

SCOPE OF ROBOTIC AND NAVIGATED SPINE SURGERY

A variety of image-guided navigation and robotic platforms are currently available in the spine surgery market. Although navigation and robotic guidance have historically been mutually exclusive, the newer platforms allow the integration of the two modalities to facilitate real-time feedback in addition to the placement of instrumentation along pre-planned trajectories with the use of a robotic arm. Each type of platform achieves stereotaxy through some form of preoperative or intraoperative radiographic imaging such as x-ray, MRI, computer tomography (CT) or three-dimensional (3D) fluoroscopy to generate a comprehensive spinal map for precision and accuracy. Intraoperative cone-beam CT or O-arm ("computer-assisted navigation") and 3D fluoroscopy ("virtual fluoroscopy") are the most commonly utilized imaging modalities in modern surgical navigation systems. Both allow frameless stereotaxy with real-time, navigated feedback of instruments such as tubular dilators, screwdrivers, drills, and awls.[7] Examples of such systems include the Airo Mobile Intraoperative CT-based Spinal Navigation (Brainlab©, Feldkirchen, Germany), Stryker Spinal Navigation with SpineMask© Tracker, and SpineMap Software (Stryker©, Kalamazoo, Michigan), StealthStation Spine Surgery Imaging, and Surgical Navigation with O-arm (Medtronic©, Minneapolis, Minnesota), and Ziehm Vision FD Vario 3D with NaviPort integration (Ziehm Imaging©, Orlando, Florida). It is essential to note that instrument maneuvering with these systems is still entirely surgeon-dependent with the navigation system merely providing anatomic feedback.[8]

Robotic systems allow user-operated trajectory planning using radiographic guidance, following by "locking" of the robotic arm along the desired screw trajectory.[7] This can be additionally aided by intraoperative navigation to allow real-time feedback in more recent platforms. Surgical robots can be divided into three types depending on the levels of assistance: (1) supervisory controlled systems, in which the robot performs actions based on a pre-planned trajectory under close surgeon supervision; (2) tele-surgical systems (e.g., da Vinci robot, Intuitive Surgical, Sunnyvale, Calfornia), which allow the surgeon complete control over the robot remotely; and (3) shared-control models with varying levels of simultaneous control between the robot and the surgeon.[7,9] Most contemporary robotic systems utilized in spine surgery today are shared-control systems which allow the planning of stereotactic trajectories via preoperative or intraoperative imaging, which is then produced by the robotic arm followed by placement of the instrumentation by the surgeon.

In terms of volume, there remains significant potential in spine surgery for the utilization of robotic and navigation platforms that could justify the initial acquisition costs. From 2004 to 2015, the volume of elective lumbar spinal fusions increased 62.3% from 122,679 cases (60.4 per 100,000) in 2004 to 199, 140 (79.8 per 100,000) in 2015.[10,11] The first commercially available robotic platform for spine surgery, the Mazor SpineAssist system (Mazor Robotics, Caesarea, Israel), gained FDA approval in 2004. However, it did not see significant utilization until 2011 with a small number of installations; fewer than 100 were installed by 2015.[12] The number of procedures per system has been increasing steadily since then, implying greater penetration of spine robots in the operating room (OR), and, by 2015, over 3000 robotic spine procedures were performed annually in the United States. A similar trend has been noted for the da Vinci Surgical System in prostate and OB/GYN surgeries, with over 700,000 procedures performed in 2015.[12] Apart from being the first robotic system to be utilized in surgical care, the da Vinci robot also served to popularize robotic surgery both among medical professionals and the general public. Following the integration of these technologies into their daily surgical practice, if hospitals responsibly market themselves as state-of-the-art spine surgery centers, they could potentially leverage the high surgical volume to offset the initial acquisition and maintenance costs while simultaneously improving patient safety outcomes and satisfaction. Improvement of patient understanding of the surgical procedure is also essential to allow increased utilization. The patients should be informed that the surgeon would still perform the critical aspect of the procedure with the robot serving as a "guidance" mechanism for improved trajectory planning and kinetic feedback.

While most of the current literature on robotics and navigation focuses on the placement of pedicle screws, there are multiple other applications that could provide a justification for increased utilization. Several studies have demonstrated the feasibility of image guidance systems in the surgical workflow for minimally invasive lateral lumbar interbody fusion (MIS-LLIF).[13–15] Both navigation and robotics have also been investigated for the placement of S2-alar-iliac screws.[16–20] The applications for these systems have also expanded to the resection of both primary and metastatic spinal column and intradural tumors, along with cases of spinal deformity.[21–25] In addition to the surgical volume, such an expansion of scope for a wide range of clinical indications also provides an inherent basis for cost-effectiveness.

COST-EFFECTIVENESS OF IMAGE-GUIDED NAVIGATION SYSTEMS

There have been several studies that have demonstrated the costs and benefits associated with use of image guidance in the OR[26–29] Mainly, the currently available literature has been focused on the cost savings associated with the use of image guidance for the placement of pedicle screws. The proposed mechanisms of cost-effectiveness include a reduction in the rate of revision surgery due to screw malposition and a reduction in OR facility costs due to the shorter operating time as a consequence of the shorter time required for each pedicle screw placement. In an analysis of 100 patients who prospectively underwent thoracolumbar instrumentation with 3D fluoroscopic image guidance compared to a historical cohort of 100 patients who underwent instrumentation without image guidance, Watkins et al. demonstrated cost savings of $71,000 per 100 cases due to the reduction in rate of revision surgery from 3% to 0% and shortened time for screw placement (OR costs: $93/min).[28] The total cost of the navigation system itself was reported as $475,000. Each revision surgery cost the hospital as much as $23,000 for Medicare and ~$40,000 for private patients. Therefore, image guidance was deemed cost-effective in the long term with high surgical volume. Further, Costa et al. demonstrated that image guidance based on *intraoperative CT (O-Arm)* may be more cost-effective than is *preoperative CT*.[26] The authors found a shorter mean time for each pedicle screw placement using intraoperative CT-based computer guidance (16 min vs. 28 min) with fewer intraoperative radiographs needed. The mean cost of the procedure with intraoperative O-arm CT was also found to be lower than preoperative CT (€6482 vs. €6738). Hodges et al. projected that the use of intraoperative O-arm guidance could lead to total cost savings of $40,595,000 nationally, assuming a 1% rate of return to the OR due to breached pedicle screws with conventional C-arm fluoroscopy, compared to none in the O-arm group that was observed in their analysis from a single institution.[27]

COST-EFFECTIVENESS OF ROBOTICS IN SURGERY

Evidence From Other Surgical Specialties

While the literature specific to spine surgery has been sparse, there has been a mounting amount of evidence evaluating the cost-effectiveness associated with the use of robotic systems in other surgical specialties such as general surgery, OB/GYN, and urology. In a head-to-head comparison between robotic and open adrenalectomy, Probst et al. demonstrated that the total perioperative costs for the entire hospital admission were lower with robotic surgery (€7334 vs. €8625), although the immediate procedure costs were higher by €2288.[2] Similar results obtained from evaluations of robotic-assisted laparoscopic surgery (RALS) for prostatectomy and hysterectomy have demonstrated a higher mean cost associated with these procedures.[3,5] An important limitation of these studies is that these analyses are restricted to the direct OR and supply costs and the indirect costs and benefits associated with reduced loss of productivity, long-term treatment outcomes, etc. have not been evaluated. For instance, robotic-assisted prostatectomy has been shown to be associated with fewer positive surgical margins, lower use of androgen deprivation chemotherapy, and radiation within 2 years of surgery.[30] Similarly, robotic-assisted nephrectomy, although associated with higher procedural costs, has been linked to fewer complications and reduced length of stay.[6] It has been claimed that, on average, RALS costs 6% or $1600 more in direct costs per case performed, compared to conventional or open surgery.[31] In the literature from these surgical specialties, most authors therefore generally conclude that RALS is less cost-effective, especially when factoring in the capital investment associated with initial acquisition (estimated at $1.75 million) and subsequent maintenance. However, the cost for these procedures has also been shown to decline with increasing surgical volume.[32] Therefore, more robust cost-effectiveness analyses comprehensively taking into account all such relevant considerations are required to demonstrate a clear picture of RALS in the healthcare *value* equation. This is especially important since, if found to be less cost-effective in the absence of a clear outcome benefit, the burden of incremental cost associated with RALS may fall on the patients instead of the insurers.[33] It has been interesting to note that, despite the high procedural costs, the utilization of RALS has increased substantially in the United States, with 2862 da Vinci systems installed by 2017.[34] The global case volume also rose significantly from 2010 to 2017, from 136,000 to 877,000 cases, with a total market revenue of $3.1 billion for the manufacturer.[34]

Evidence From Spine Surgery

In contrast to other surgical specialties, robotic surgery has been claimed to be cost-effective for spine surgery. However, there is a dearth of literature directly examining the cost data associated with robotic spine surgery. The only study to date has been performed by Menger et al., who analyzed cost data from 557 cases of elective spine surgery with thoracolumbar instrumentation at a single institution over a 1-year period, out of which 58 (10.4%) were minimally invasive (MIS) fusions.[35] Although the authors did not perform any robotic cases, they attempted to analyze the projected impact on procedural distribution and costs, had robotic surgery been adopted using previously published national data. Upon review of the individual cases, it was found that the utilization of robotic assistance would allow the conversion of an additional 50 cases of open procedures (10%) to be performed as MIS; it would also be feasible to utilize robotic assistance in 337 cases (68% of open procedures). The authors used nationally available data to estimate the cost savings based on the incidence of screw malposition, operative time, reoperation rate, and length of stay. It was found that the utilization of robotic technology in the busy academic practice could have allowed annual cost savings of $608,546, with the majority of those savings attributed to the avoidance of revision surgery ($314,661) and the conversion of open procedures to MIS ($251,860), with consequent shortening of length of stay. We individually discuss below the possible reasons for the cost-effectiveness of robotic spine surgery.

Revision Rate

Reoperations are a significant cost contributor to the overall cost of spine surgery. Revision surgery within 30 days of an index operation may not be covered by medical insurance and the cost incurred may have to be borne by the provider and institution.[36] The cost of a single revision surgery may be as high as ~$40,000.[28] Robotic assistance has significant potential to reduce the incidence of reoperations due to the improved accuracy and precision of screw placement. In an analysis of 960 pedicle screws performed with robotic guidance, Hu et al. demonstrated an accuracy of 98.9%.[37] In a similar fashion, Zahrawi et al. demonstrated 100% placement accuracy for percutaneous pedicle screws compared to 97% with free-hand placement.[38] There have been multiple such studies that have demonstrated superior accuracy of pedicle screw placement with robotic assistance.[39–41] It is expected that the addition of CT-based navigation to robotic guidance would further substantially improve precision and accuracy.[42] The incidence of reoperation due to inaccurate screw placement with robotic technology is estimated at 0%.[43] We have had similar experience with the first 50 cases in our institution, with no cases of thoracolumbar spinal instrumentation performed with robotic guidance requiring revision surgery due to screw breach. Studies have also shown that pedicle screw placement with robotic surgery avoids damage to the facet joint capsule, which has been associated with a higher likelihood of adjacent segment disease.[44] In addition to pedicle screw placement, robotic assistance has been demonstrated to improve the accuracy of placement of interbody implants, vertebroplasty, and vertebral body biopsies substantially.[36,45] In addition, multiple studies have validated its accuracy for the placement of S2-alar-iliac screws.[18,46–48] Complications such as wound infections necessitating revision surgery have also been found to be lower in robotic-guided MIS compared to fluoroscopy-guided surgeries.[49–53] A multicenter prospective study using the Mazor Robotics Renaissance Guidance system demonstrated a five-fold reduction in incidence of surgical complications compared to the fluoroscopic-guided arm.[52]

Radiation Exposure

A reduction in radiation exposure due to minimizing the use of intraoperative fluoroscopy could contribute to long-term cost savings. Radiation exposure is usually measured as the number of seconds of fluoroscopy exposure per screw placed. In a comparison between robot-assisted open/percutaneous surgeries to conventional free-hand procedures, Kantelhardt et al. demonstrated a fluoroscopy time of 43 seconds per screw for robotic-guided open and 27 seconds per screw for robotic-guided percutaneous screw placement compared to a mean time of 77 seconds per screw for conventional surgeries.[52] While a small number of studies[54–56] have demonstrated little to no difference in radiation exposure, the vast majority of literature currently supports the hypothesis that radiation exposure as measured by fluoroscopy time is lower with robotic surgery.[44,52,57,58] It must be noted, however, that the amount of radiation exposure is significantly dependent on the level of surgeon variability in intraoperative practices. The literature so far only covers those robotic systems that do not have real-time navigation as an adjunct. With the newer generation of robotic systems that combine CT-based navigation with the robotic arm, the use of intraoperative CT for planning would consequently increase the amount of radiation exposure for the surgical team, as a single O-arm spin can add up to 20 s of fluoroscopy time. Thus, more multicentric studies with a diverse group of spine surgeons with varying surgical practices and those that evaluate radiation exposure with newer generation of robotic guidance systems are needed.

Operating Room Time

The cost of the OR facility would be directly proportional to the total operative time. A shorter operative time is not only important for cost savings directly by reducing facility costs, but also for the indirect costs incurred due to the higher risk of surgical complications with the longer operative time. Several studies have demonstrated a much shorter time taken per screw placement with robotic assistance than with free-hand procedures, which leads to an overall shorter OR time.[37,44,54,59,60] The cost of the OR facility per minute can be highly variable between institutions and can range anywhere from $15 to $100.[35,36] In their analysis of a single-institutional spine practice, assuming an OR cost of $18/min, Menger et al. estimated that they could save $5713 on the 57 MIS cases performed at their institution over 1 year.[35] Similarly, Watkins et al. estimated that their OR cost at $93/min and a reduction in OR time of 20 to 30 min could result in cost savings of $1860–$2790 per surgery.[28]

Surgeon Ergonomics and Efficiency

Spine surgery is a physically demanding specialty as it relies upon meticulous fine motor skills. The removal of bone and placement of instrumentation not only requires physical strength on its own, but operating in the vicinity of critical neural elements simultaneously requires tremendous dexterity and precision. This becomes even more challenging while working in narrow operative corridors with MIS procedures. Given the possibility of surgeon physical and mental fatigue with long and arduous procedures, ergonomics in the OR is also an important concern. The incidence of neck pain and shoulder pain among surgeons has been shown to be as high as 40%.[61] Therefore, spine surgery may be an ideal area where the utilization of robotics and navigation can allow ergonomically efficient procedures and prevent surgeon fatigue. This has already been shown in other surgical specialties such as cardiac surgery, OB/GYN, and urology.[62,63]

FUTURE CONSIDERATIONS

A variety of measures may be taken to ensure greater clinical application and improve the cost-effectiveness of robotic and navigation platforms. Future systems should allow co-registration with different imaging modalities such as MRI (in addition to CT) to allow greater visualization of soft tissue tumor borders and adjacent anatomy, including vascular structures and neural elements.[8] This would improve the possibility of application for the resection of spinal tumors. Allowing spine robots greater capability in bony resection and handling soft tissues would further enhance clinical penetration. An improvement in cost-effectiveness would be directly dependent on further improvement in the mechanisms of cost savings already highlighted above, including a reduction in OR time and revision rate. There is little doubt that there can be a significant learning curve with the adoption of the new technologies; hence, the steps taken to bend the slope of this curve would improve OR efficiency. These steps can include comprehensive orientation and skill development sessions for surgeons before actual adoption into daily workflow. Early adoption of these technologies to the further training of residents would also allow them to be more comfortable and efficient with their use when they start independent practice. Given the variability in internal costing, it must be remembered that cost savings would be highly variable between institutions. Therefore, providers and hospitals must conduct a priori cost-effectiveness analyses before acquiring such platforms with a careful consideration of institutional surgical volume, case mix, and revision and complication rates from their own experience. Combining this with the already published data on the outcomes following robotic surgery can help estimate the projected cost savings before acquiring a new system. There is little doubt that cost-effectiveness can only be demonstrated in the long term as the upfront acquisition costs remain high. The "number needed to treat" and consequent time duration required for cost-effectiveness goals to be met would be highly dependent on institutional practices and case volume.

CONCLUSION

Despite the prohibitive upfront cost of acquiring robotic and navigation platforms for spine surgery, there remains potential for cost savings in the long term with a reduction in rate of revision surgery, operative time, radiation exposure, and improvement in surgical ergonomics. Given the lack of evidence on this important aspect, further studies that directly examine internal costing data are required to inform current spine surgical practices about cost-effectiveness and therefore estimate the *value* of incorporating these new technologies for patient care.

REFERENCES

1. Molinari M, Puttarajappa C, Wijkstrom M, Ganoza A, Lopez R, Tevar A. Robotic versus open renal transplantation in obese patients: protocol for a cost-benefit markov model analysis. *JMIR Res Protoc.* 2018;7(3):e74. https://doi.org/10.2196/resprot.8294.
2. Probst KA, Ohlmann CH, Saar M, Siemer S, Stöeckle M, Janssen M. Robot-assisted vs. open adrenalectomy: evaluation of cost-effectiveness and peri-operative outcome. *BJU Int.* 2016;118(6):952–957. https://doi.org/10.1111/bju.13529.
3. Martínez-Maestre MA, Melero-Cortés LM, Coronado PJ, et al. Long term COST-minimization analysis of robot-assisted hysterectomy versus conventional laparoscopic hysterectomy. *Health Econ Rev.* 2019;9(1):18. https://doi.org/10.1186/s13561-019-0236-8.
4. Sleeper J, Lotan Y. Cost-effectiveness of robotic-assisted laparoscopic procedures in urologic surgery in the USA. *Expert Rev Med Devices.* 2011;8(1):97–103. https://doi.org/10.1586/erd.10.67.
5. Forsmark A, Gehrman J, Angenete E, et al. Health economic analysis of open and robot-assisted laparoscopic surgery for prostate cancer within the Prospective Multicentre LAPPRO Trial. *Eur Urol.* 2018;74(6):816–824. https://doi.org/10.1016/j.eururo.2018.07.038.
6. Yu HY, Hevelone ND, Lipsitz SR, Kowalczyk KJ, Hu JC. Use, costs and comparative effectiveness of robotic assisted, laparoscopic and open urological surgery. *J Urol.* 2012;187(4):1392–1398. https://doi.org/10.1016/j.juro.2011.11.089.
7. Kochanski RB, Lombardi JM, Laratta JL, Lehman RA, O'Toole JE. Image-guided navigation and robotics in spine surgery. *Neurosurgery.* 2019;84(6):1179–1189. https://doi.org/10.1093/neuros/nyy630.
8. Overley SC, Cho SK, Mehta AI, Arnold PM. Navigation and robotics in spinal surgery: where are we now? *Neurosurgery.* 2017;80(3S):S86–S99. https://doi.org/10.1093/neuros/nyw077.
9. Nathoo N, Cavuşoğlu MC, Vogelbaum MA, Barnett GH. In touch with robotics: neurosurgery for the future. *Neurosurgery.* 2005;56(3):421–433, discussion 421–433. https://doi.org/10.1227/01.neu.0000153929.68024.cf.
10. Martin BI, Mirza SK, Spina N, Spiker WR, Lawrence B, Brodke DS. Trends in lumbar fusion procedure rates and associated hospital costs for degenerative spinal diseases in the United States, 2004 to 2015. *Spine.* 2019;44(5):369–376. https://doi.org/10.1097/BRS.0000000000002822.
11. Goz V, Rane A, Abtahi AM, Lawrence BD, Brodke DS, Spiker WR. Geographic variations in the cost of spine surgery. *Spine.* 2015;40(17):1380–1389. https://doi.org/10.1097/BRS.0000000000001022.

12. Patel V. Future of robotics in spine surgery. *Spine*. 2018;43 (7S):528. https://doi.org/10.1097/BRS.0000000000002554.
13. Park P. Three-dimensional computed tomography-based spinal navigation in minimally invasive lateral lumbar interbody fusion: feasibility, technique, and initial results. *Neurosurgery*. 2015;11(suppl 2):259–267. https://doi.org/10.1227/NEU.0000000000000726.
14. Joseph JR, Smith BW, Patel RD, Park P. Use of 3D CT-based navigation in minimally invasive lateral lumbar interbody fusion. *J Neurosurg Spine*. 2016;25(3):339–344. https://doi.org/10.3171/2016.2.SPINE151295.
15. Drazin D, Liu JC, Acosta FL. CT navigated lateral interbody fusion. *J Clin Neurosci*. 2013;20(10):1438–1441. https://doi.org/10.1016/j.jocn.2012.12.028.
16. Nottmeier EW, Pirris SM, Balseiro S, Fenton D. Three-dimensional image-guided placement of S2 alar screws to adjunct or salvage lumbosacral fixation. *Spine J*. 2010;10(7):595–601. https://doi.org/10.1016/j.spinee.2010.03.023.
17. Ray WZ, Ravindra VM, Schmidt MH, Dailey AT. Stereotactic navigation with the O-arm for placement of S-2 alar iliac screws in pelvic lumbar fixation. *J Neurosurg Spine*. 2013;18(5):490–495. https://doi.org/10.3171/2013.2.SPINE12813.
18. Laratta JL, Shillingford JN, Lombardi JM, et al. Accuracy of S2 alar-iliac screw placement under robotic guidance. *Spine Deform*. 2018;6(2):130–136. https://doi.org/10.1016/j.jspd.2017.08.009.
19. Shillingford JN, Laratta JL, Park PJ, et al. Human versus robot: a propensity-matched analysis of the accuracy of free hand versus robotic guidance for placement of S2 alar-Iliac (S2AI) screws. *Spine*. 2018;43(21):E1297–E1304. https://doi.org/10.1097/BRS.0000000000002694.
20. Shin JH, Hoh DJ, Kalfas IH. Iliac screw fixation using computer-assisted computer tomographic image guidance: technical note. *Oper Neurosurg*. 2012;70(suppl 1):16–20, discussion 20. https://doi.org/10.1227/NEU.0b013e318230517a.
21. Rajasekaran S, Vidyadhara S, Ramesh P, Shetty AP. Randomized clinical study to compare the accuracy of navigated and non-navigated thoracic pedicle screws in deformity correction surgeries. *Spine*. 2007;32(2):E56–E64. https://doi.org/10.1097/01.brs.0000252094.64857.ab.
22. Nagashima H, Nishi T, Yamane K, Tanida A. Case report: osteoid osteoma of the C2 pedicle: surgical technique using a navigation system. *Clin Orthop Relat Res*. 2010;468(1):283–288. https://doi.org/10.1007/s11999-009-0958-8.
23. Van Royen BJ, Baayen JC, Pijpers R, Noske DP, Schakenraad D, Wuisman PIJM. Osteoid osteoma of the spine: a novel technique using combined computer-assisted and gamma probe-guided high-speed intralesional drill excision. *Spine*. 2005;30(3):369–373. https://doi.org/10.1097/01.brs.0000152531.49095.34.
24. Moore T, McLain RF. Image-guided surgery in resection of benign cervicothoracic spinal tumors: a report of two cases. *Spine J*. 2005;5(1):109–114. https://doi.org/10.1016/j.spinee.2004.06.020.
25. Fujibayashi S, Neo M, Takemoto M, et al. Computer-assisted spinal osteotomy: a technical note and report of four cases. *Spine*. 2010;35(18):E895–E903. https://doi.org/10.1097/brs.0b013e3181dc5ed1.
26. Costa F, Porazzi E, Restelli U, et al. Economic study: a cost-effectiveness analysis of an intraoperative compared with a preoperative image-guided system in lumbar pedicle screw fixation in patients with degenerative spondylolisthesis. *Spine J*. 2014;14(8):1790–1796. https://doi.org/10.1016/j.spinee.2013.10.019.
27. Hodges SD, Eck JC, Newton D. Analysis of CT-based navigation system for pedicle screw placement. *Orthopedics*. 2012;35(8):e1221–e1224. https://doi.org/10.3928/01477447-20120725-23.
28. Watkins RG, Gupta A, Watkins RG. Cost-effectiveness of image-guided spine surgery. *Open Orthop J*. 2010;4:228–233. https://doi.org/10.2174/1874325001004010228.
29. Hecht AC, Koehler SM, Laudone JC, Jenkins A, Qureshi S. Is intraoperative CT of posterior cervical spine instrumentation cost-effective and does it reduce complications? *Clin Orthop Relat Res*. 2011;469(4):1035–1041. https://doi.org/10.1007/s11999-010-1603-2.
30. Hu JC, Gandaglia G, Karakiewicz PI, et al. Comparative effectiveness of robot-assisted versus open radical prostatectomy cancer control. *Eur Urol*. 2014;66(4):666–672. https://doi.org/10.1016/j.eururo.2014.02.015.
31. Barbash GI, Glied SA. New technology and health care costs—the case of robot-assisted surgery. *N Engl J Med*. 2010;363(8):701–704. https://doi.org/10.1056/NEJMp1006602.
32. Budäus L, Abdollah F, Sun M, et al. The impact of surgical experience on total hospital charges for minimally invasive prostatectomy: a population-based study. *BJU Int*. 2011;108(6):888–893. https://doi.org/10.1111/j.1464-410X.2010.09906.x.
33. Pearson SD, Bach PB. How Medicare could use comparative effectiveness research in deciding on new coverage and reimbursement. *Health Aff*. 2010;29(10):1796–1804. https://doi.org/10.1377/hlthaff.2010.0623.
34. Childers CP, Maggard-Gibbons M. Estimation of the acquisition and operating costs for robotic surgery. *JAMA*. 2018;320(8):835–836. https://doi.org/10.1001/jama.2018.9219.
35. Menger RP, Savardekar AR, Farokhi F, Sin A. A cost-effectiveness analysis of the integration of robotic spine technology in spine surgery. *Neurospine*. 2018;15(3):216–224. https://doi.org/10.14245/ns.1836082.041.
36. Fiani B, Quadri SA, Farooqui M, et al. Impact of robot-assisted spine surgery on health care quality and neurosurgical economics: a systemic review.. *Neurosurg Rev*. 2020;43(1):17–25. https://doi.org/10.1007/s10143-018-0971-z.
37. Hu X, Ohnmeiss DD, Lieberman IH. Robotic-assisted pedicle screw placement: lessons learned from the first 102 patients. *Eur Spine J*. 2013;22(3):661–666. https://doi.org/10.1007/s00586-012-2499-1.
38. Zahrawi F. Comparative analysis of robotic-guided pedicle screw placement accuracy and freehand controls in percutaneous adult degenerative spinal instrumentation.

Spine J. 2014;14(11): (suppl 63). https://doi.org/10.1016/j.spinee.2014.08.164.
39. Joseph JR, Smith BW, Liu X, Park P. Current applications of robotics in spine surgery: a systematic review of the literature. *Neurosurg Focus*. 2017;42(5):E2. https://doi.org/10.3171/2017.2.FOCUS16544.
40. Keric N, Doenitz C, Haj A, et al. Evaluation of robot-guided minimally invasive implantation of 2067 pedicle screws. *Neurosurg Focus*. 2017;42(5):E11. https://doi.org/10.3171/2017.2.FOCUS16552.
41. Molliqaj G, Schatlo B, Alaid A, et al. Accuracy of robot-guided versus freehand fluoroscopy-assisted pedicle screw insertion in thoracolumbar spinal surgery. *Neurosurg Focus*. 2017;42(5):E14. https://doi.org/10.3171/2017.3.FOCUS179.
42. Fan Y, Peng Du J, Liu JJ, Zhang JN, Liu SC, Hao DJ. Radiological and clinical differences among three assisted technologies in pedicle screw fixation of adult degenerative scoliosis. *Sci Rep*. 2018;8(1):890. https://doi.org/10.1038/s41598-017-19054-7.
43. Schröder ML, Staartjes VE. Revisions for screw malposition and clinical outcomes after robot-guided lumbar fusion for spondylolisthesis. *Neurosurg Focus*. 2017;42(5):E12. https://doi.org/10.3171/2017.3.FOCUS16534.
44. Hyun SJ, Kim KJ, Jahng TA, Kim HJ. Minimally invasive robotic versus open fluoroscopic-guided spinal instrumented fusions: a randomized controlled trial.. *Spine*. 2017;42(6):353–358. https://doi.org/10.1097/BRS.0000000000001778.
45. Barzilay Y, Schroeder JE, Hiller N, et al. Robot-assisted vertebral body augmentation: a radiation reduction tool. *Spine*. 2014;39(2):153–157. https://doi.org/10.1097/BRS.0000000000000100.
46. Bederman SS, Hahn P, Colin V, Kiester PD, Bhatia NN. Robotic guidance for S2-alar-iliac screws in spinal deformity correction. *Clin Spine Surg*. 2017;30(1):E49–E53. https://doi.org/10.1097/BSD.0b013e3182a3572b.
47. Hu X, Lieberman IH. Robotic-guided sacro-pelvic fixation using S2 alar-iliac screws: feasibility and accuracy. *Eur Spine J*. 2017;26(3):720–725. https://doi.org/10.1007/s00586-016-4639-5.
48. Hyun SJ, Kim KJ, Jahng TA. S2 alar iliac screw placement under robotic guidance for adult spinal deformity patients: technical note. *Eur Spine J*. 2017;26(8):2198–2203. https://doi.org/10.1007/s00586-017-5012-z.
49. Quadri SA, Capua J, Ramakrishnan V, et al. A rare case of pharyngeal perforation and expectoration of an entire anterior cervical fixation construct. *J Neurosurg Spine*. 2017;26(5):560–566. https://doi.org/10.3171/2016.10.SPINE16560.
50. Nasser R, Yadla S, Maltenfort MG, et al. Complications in spine surgery. *J Neurosurg Spine*. 2010;13(2):144–157. https://doi.org/10.3171/2010.3.SPINE09369.
51. Mortazavi MM, Quadri SA, Suriya SS, et al. Rare concurrent retroclival and pan-spinal subdural empyema: review of literature with an uncommon illustrative case. *World Neurosurg*. 2018;110:326–335. https://doi.org/10.1016/j.wneu.2017.11.082.
52. Kantelhardt SR, Martinez R, Baerwinkel S, Burger R, Giese A, Rohde V. Perioperative course and accuracy of screw positioning in conventional, open robotic-guided and percutaneous robotic-guided, pedicle screw placement. *Eur Spine J*. 2011;20(6):860–868. https://doi.org/10.1007/s00586-011-1729-2.
53. Schroerlucke SR, Wang MY, Cannestra AF, et al. Complication rate in robotic-guided vs fluoro-guided minimally invasive spinal fusion surgery: report from MIS refresh prospective comparative study. *Spine J*. 2017;17(10):S254–S255. https://doi.org/10.1016/j.spinee.2017.08.177.
54. Onen MR, Simsek M, Naderi S. Robotic spine surgery: a preliminary report. *Turk Neurosurg*. 2014;24(4):512–518. https://doi.org/10.5137/1019-5149.JTN.8951-13.1.
55. Solomiichuk V, Fleischhammer J, Molliqaj G, et al. Robotic versus fluoroscopy-guided pedicle screw insertion for metastatic spinal disease: a matched-cohort comparison. *Neurosurg Focus*. 2017;42(5):E13. https://doi.org/10.3171/2017.3.FOCUS1710.
56. Lonjon N, Chan-Seng E, Costalat V, Bonnafoux B, Vassal M, Boetto J. Robot-assisted spine surgery: feasibility study through a prospective case-matched analysis. *Eur Spine J*. 2016;25(3):947–955. https://doi.org/10.1007/s00586-015-3758-8.
57. Schroerlucke SR, Good CR, Wang MY. A Prospective, Comparative Study of Robotic-Guidance versus Freehand in Minimally Invasive Spinal Fusion Surgery: first Report from MIS ReFRESH. *Spine J*. 2016;16(10):S253. https://doi.org/10.1016/j.spinee.2016.07.166.
58. Keric N, Eum DJ, Afghanyar F, et al. Evaluation of surgical strategy of conventional vs. percutaneous robot-assisted spinal trans-pedicular instrumentation in spondylodiscitis. *J Robot Surg*. 2017;11(1):17–25. https://doi.org/10.1007/s11701-016-0597-5.
59. Devito DP, Kaplan L, Dietl R, et al. Clinical acceptance and accuracy assessment of spinal implants guided with SpineAssist surgical robot: retrospective study. *Spine*. 2010;35(24):2109–2115. https://doi.org/10.1097/BRS.0b013e3181d323ab.
60. Kim HJ, Jung WI, Chang BS, Lee CK, Kang KT, Yeom JS. A prospective, randomized, controlled trial of robot-assisted vs freehand pedicle screw fixation in spine surgery. *Int J Med Robot*. 2017;13(3):e1779. https://doi.org/10.1002/rcs.1779.
61. Mirbod SM, Yoshida H, Miyamoto K, Miyashita K, Inaba R, Iwata H. Subjective complaints in orthopedists and general surgeons. *Int Arch Occup Env Health*. 1995;67(3):179–186. https://doi.org/10.1007/BF00626350.
62. Kappert U, Tugtekin SM, Cichon R, Braun M, Matschke K. Robotic totally endoscopic coronary artery bypass: a word of caution implicated by a five-year follow-up. *J Thorac Cardiovasc Surg*. 2008;135(4):857–862. https://doi.org/10.1016/j.jtcvs.2007.11.018.
63. Hakimi AA, Feder M, Ghavamian R. Minimally invasive approaches to prostate cancer: a review of the current literature. *Urol J*. 2007;4(3):130–137.

13

Virtual and Augmented Reality in Spine Surgery

Nader Delavari, MD, and Anthony K. Frempong-Boadu, MD

INTRODUCTION OF TECHNOLOGY

The utilization of surgical intelligence technologies has evolved since the inception of medicine. Epstein et al. pioneered the use of intraoperative ultrasound for the resection of intramedullary tumors.[1] Ultrasound remains an invaluable aid during the resection of spinal cord tumors. By visualizing the echogenic signal of intramedullary tumors, the surgeon can evaluate the cranial and caudal extension of the tumor and assess the completeness of the resection. Advances in magnetic resonance imaging, such as diffusion tensor imaging, permit the surgeon to appreciate the relationship of the corticospinal tracts to intramedullary tumors.[2] When the midline is distorted by an expansile mass, an understanding of the position of the corticospinal tracts can be helpful during surgical resection and deciding placement of the initial myelotomy.[2]

While adoption of image-guided surgery for cranial tumors was advocated by Kelly as early as 1990,[3] image-guided surgery for spinal tumors has required further refinement and advances in technology. The application of an automated elastic registration algorithm allows for co-registration of intraoperative CT and preoperative MRI[4] (Fig. 13.1). This technology has been crucial in overcoming differences in spine curvature between pre- and intraoperative imaging, permitting the use of MRI to guide tumor resection. Integration of the MRI-based navigation into the operative microscope represents an application of augmented reality in spinal oncologic surgery. The tumor's borders are outlined and superimposed on the surgeon's view of the spinal cord. This technology aids the surgeon when the tumor's borders are indistinct, helps assess completeness of resection, and, when integrated with diffusion tensor imaging, can help preserve corticospinal tracts.

While (3D) tumor overlays integrated into the operative microscope view of the patient represent an application of augmented reality, 3D multimodal images viewed on a workstation or using a headset (Hololens, Microsoft) represent an application of virtual reality (Figs. 13.2 and 13.3). Multiple layers, including spinal cord, bone, and soft tissue, are constructed using CT and MRI images and subsequently fused using a virtual reality workstation (Surgical Theater, Mayfield, OH).

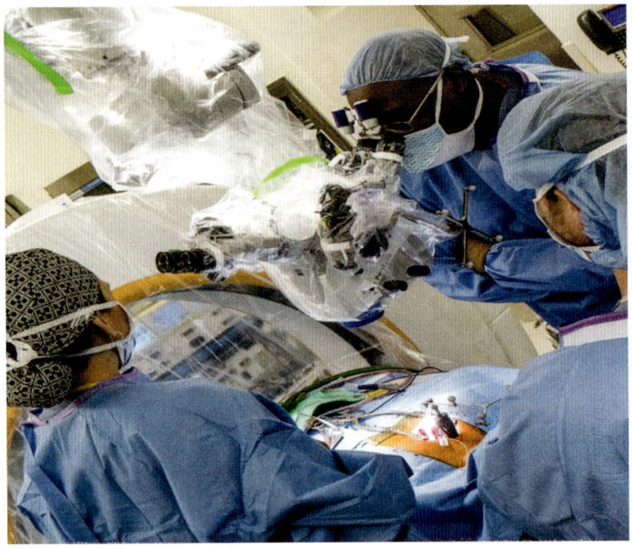

FIG. 13.1 Demonstration of operative setup including intraoperative CT scanner, neuronavigation reference array, and operating microscope with neuronavigation integration.

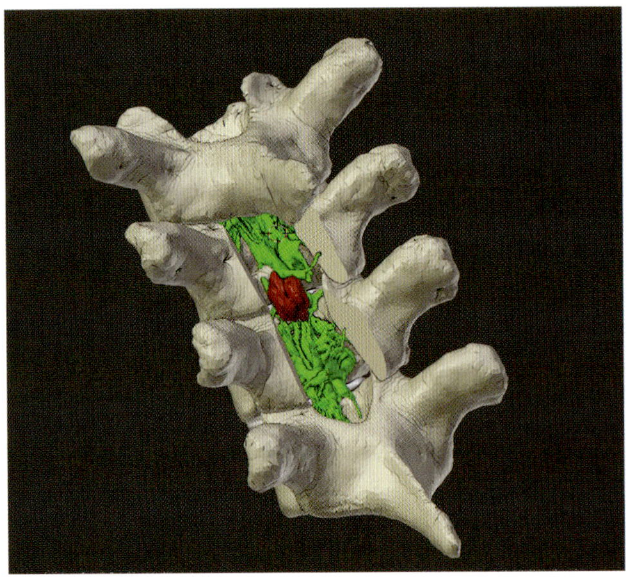

FIG. 13.2 Multimodal 3D model of an intramedullary spinal cord tumor.

Surgical Treatment for Spinal Pathology

Clinical Studies

Clinical Presentation

A 31-year-old gentleman presented with an 8-month history of declining bowel, bladder, and sexual function. He more recently developed low back pain, a right foot drop, and

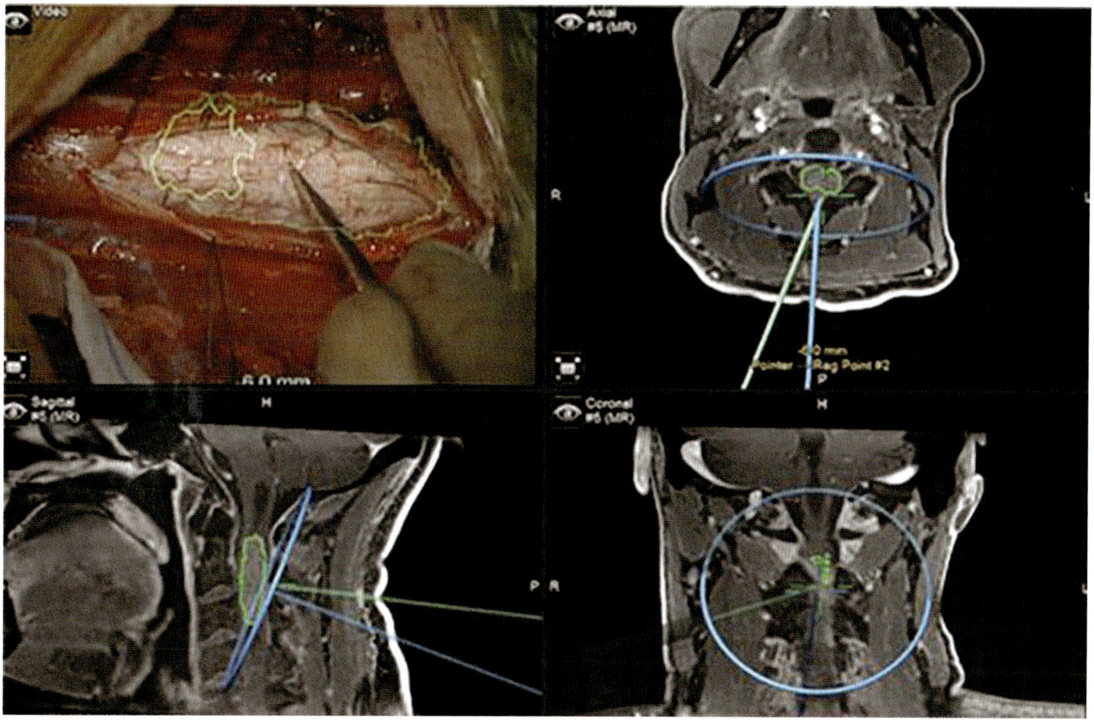

FIG. 13.3 Demonstration of tumor outlines during operative microscope integration with neuronavigation.

numbness of the right buttocks, shin, and foot. He was unable to bear weight on the right leg, resulting in an antalgic gait. The pain was worse when lying down and with Valsalva. On examination he had no movement on right dorsiflexion and plantarflexion, brisk right patellar and Achilles reflexes, and decreased sensation on the dorsum of the right foot.

Preoperative Imaging

An MRI of the lumbar spine was obtained, which demonstrated an intradural intramedullary enhancing expansile mass within the conus and proximal cauda equina. The mass did not have a cystic component and MRI of the rest of the neural axis did not reveal any further lesions (Fig. 13.4).

Surgical Plan and Intraoperative Imaging

A T11–L1 laminoplasty and microsurgical resection of the intradural intramedullary spinal mass was planned. The patient was positioned prone on a Jackson table. Using two Steinmann pins percutaneously placed into the right iliac crest, a stereotactic navigation reference array was affixed to the patient. An intraoperative CT scan (Airo, BrainLab, Munich) was obtained for computer assisted intraoperative navigation. The (prone) intraoperative CT scan was fused with the (supine) preoperative MRI using an elastic registration algorithm to account for differences in the curvature of the spine[4] (Fig. 13.5). An intraoperative 3D visualization system (Surgical Theater, Mayfield, OH) was integrated with the neuronavigation (Figs. 13.6 and 13.7). The T11–L1 levels were localized and a 3-inch incision was made. A decompressive osteoplastic laminectomy of T11–L1 was performed.

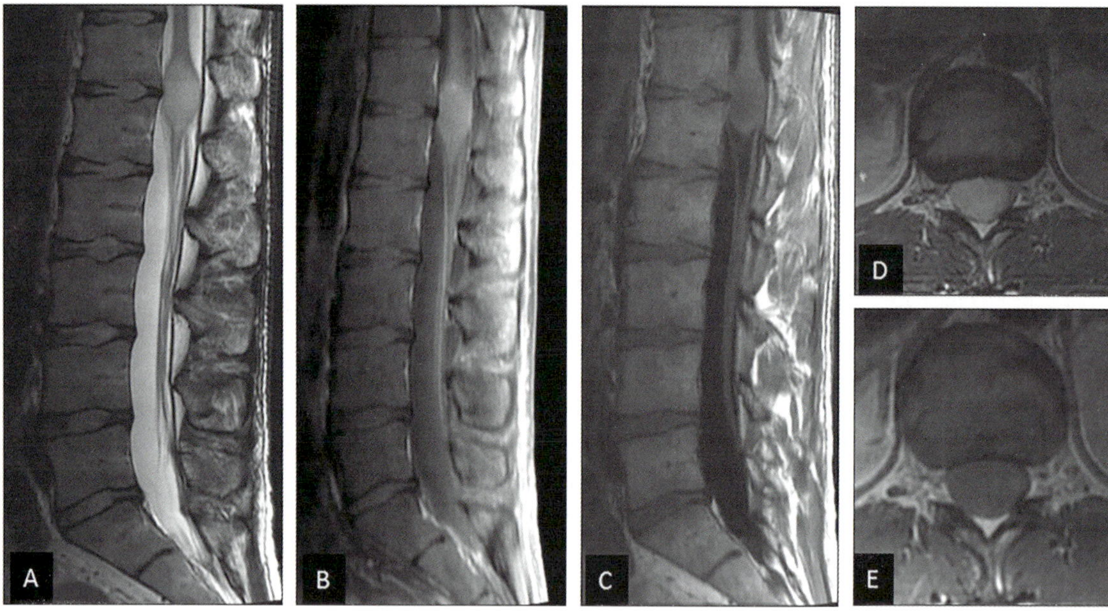

FIG. 13.4 (A) T2 sagittal MRI demonstrates an intramedullary mass within the conus medullaris. (B, D) T1 postcontrast. (C and E) T1 precontrast.

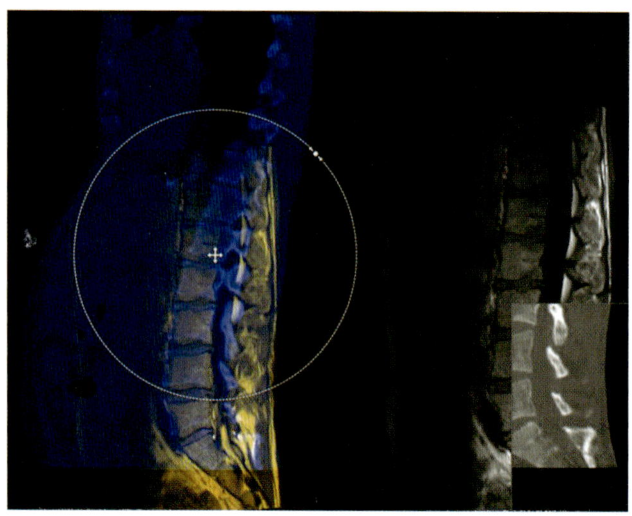

FIG. 13.5 Algorithm-based elastic fusion co-registers the preoperative MRI with intraoperative CT.

After the thecal sac was exposed, ultrasound was used to define the cranial and caudal extent of the tumor and the dura was subsequently opened. The cephalad and caudal ends of the intramedullary mass were fully exposed. Stereotactic neuronavigation with microscope integration confirmed the cranial and caudal extent of the tumor and accurately correlated with intraoperative ultrasound. A myelotomy was performed, and the mass was

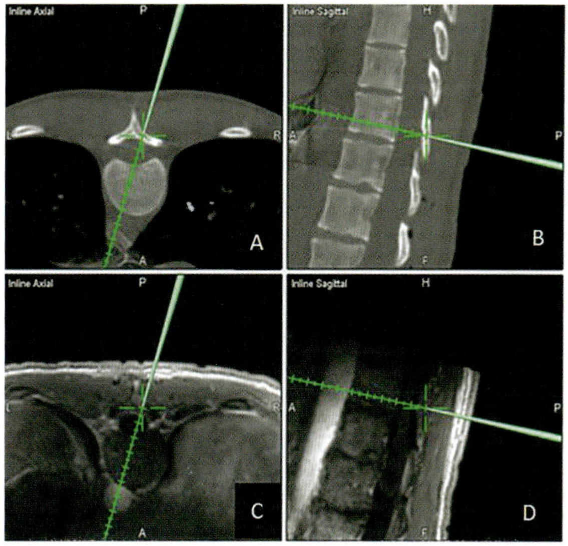

FIG. 13.6 (A, B) Intraoperative CT scan and stereotactic registration. (C, D) Co-registration with preoperative MRI.

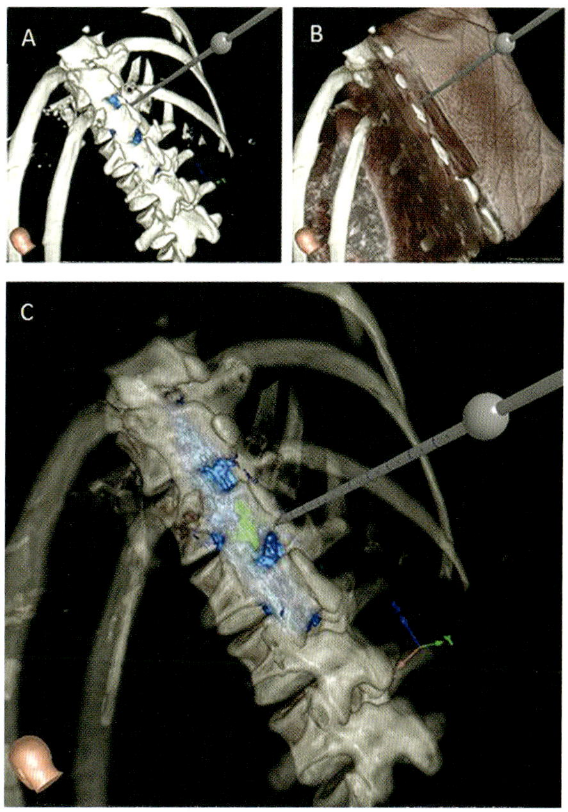

FIG. 13.7 Screenshots of multimodal 3D intraoperative visualization demonstrates the multilayered visualization of osseous anatomy (A), soft tissues (B), and tumor (C)

entered. The mass was densely adherent to the underlying neural tissue and the tumor was cyto-reduced using ultrasonic aspiration. Gross total resection was achieved. The dura was closed and reconstruction of the T11–L1 osteoplastic laminectomy was performed.

Postoperative Imaging

Fig. 13.8 shows postoperative sagittal T2-weighted MRI demonstrating no gross residual of the prior intramedullary lesion.

Postoperative Recovery and Follow-Up

The pathology was consistent with a K27 mutant midline glioma, WHO grade IV. The patient developed mild paresis of left paresis of left plantarflexion and dorsiflexion which improved after a course of steroids and rehabilitation. His preoperative bowel and bladder dysfunction, as well as right lower extremity motor and sensory deficits, persisted. He received adjuvant radiation and chemotherapy. At the 1-year follow-up, he continued on chemotherapy and was ambulating with a walker.

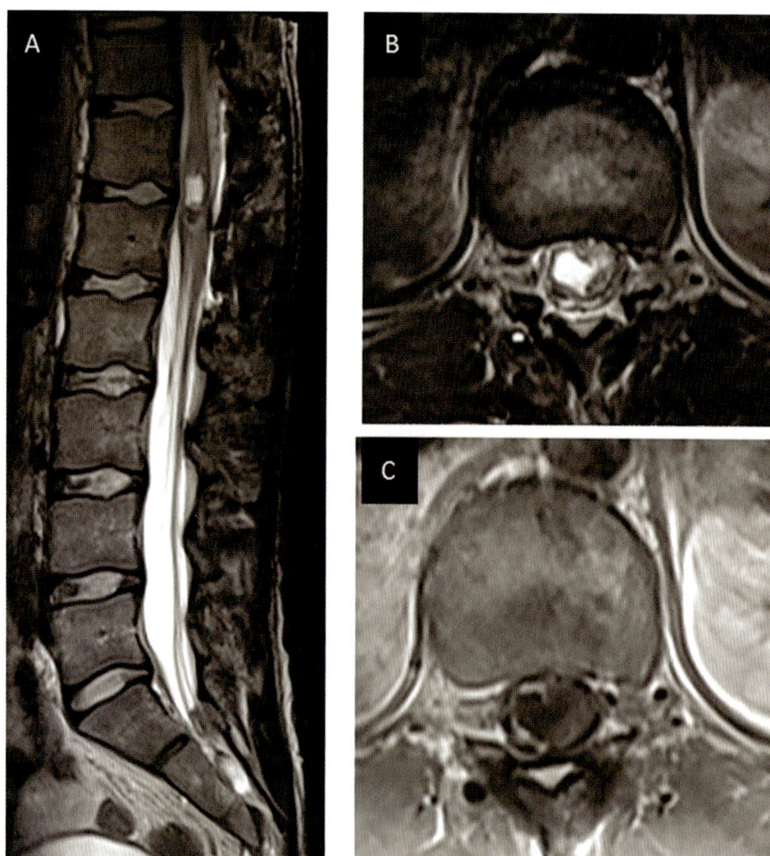

FIG. 13.8 (A) Postoperative sagittal T2-weighted MRI demonstrating no gross residual of the prior intramedullary lesion. (B, C) Axial T2-weighted and postcontrast MRI.

Clinical Studies

Clinical Presentation

A 39-year-old woman with a history of neurofibromatosis type I who had been followed for multiple intradural tumors was noted to have an intramedullary lesion at C4–C5 that had become rapidly expansile. She also had an intradural extramedullary mass at C5–C6. She was noted to have had marked changes in her neurologic function secondary to the mass, including severe distal paresis of her right upper extremity and mild proximal paresis of her right lower extremity.

Preoperative Imaging

Fig. 13.9 shows preoperative MRI demonstrating an intramedullary lesion at C4–C5 and an intradural extramedullary mass at C5–C6.

Surgical Plan and Intraoperative Imaging

After obtaining informed consent, the patient underwent general endotracheal anesthesia. Invasive arterial pressure was monitored to maintain a mean arterial pressure greater than 70 mm Hg. Neuromonitoring leads were placed for somatosensory evoked potentials and transcranial motor-evoked potentials. A Mayfield head holder was applied, and the patient was positioned prone on a Jackson table. A stereotactic reference array was attached to the Mayfield head holder and an intraoperative CT scan (Airo, BrainLab, Munich) was obtained for computer assisted navigation. The (prone) intraoperative CT scan was fused with the (supine) preoperative MRI using an elastic registration algorithm to account for differences in the curvature of the spine.[4] An intraoperative 3D visualization system (Surgical Theater, Mayfield, OH) was integrated with the neuronavigation. Prior to performing laminectomies at C3 to C6, the navigation system was used to drill lateral mass trajectories at these levels. Ultrasound and stereotactic navigation were used to identify

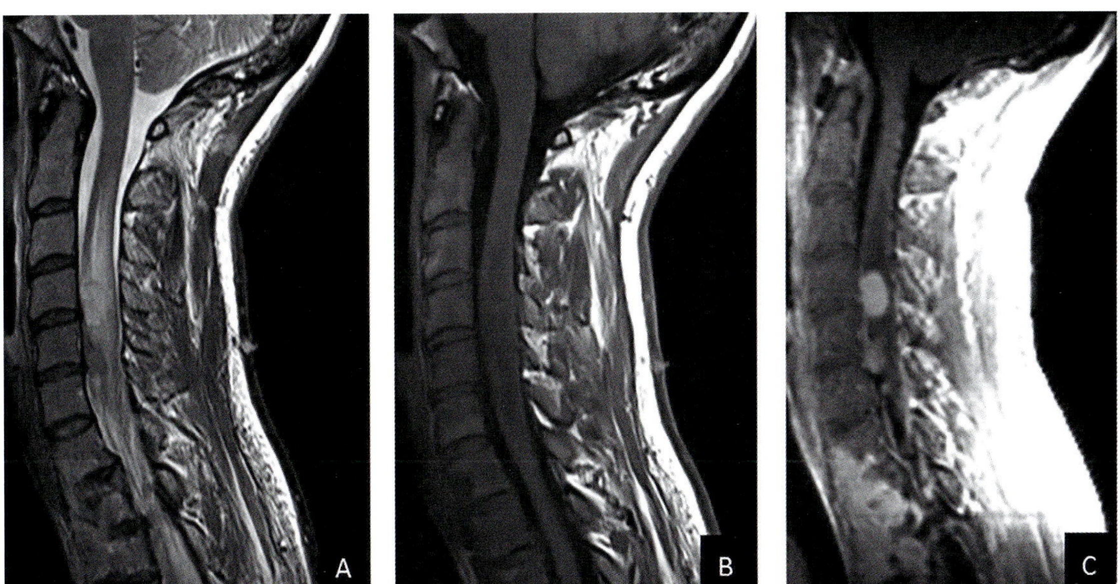

FIG. 13.9 (A) Sagittal T2-weighted preoperative MRI. (B, C) Sagittal T1-weighted pre- and postcontrast MRI.

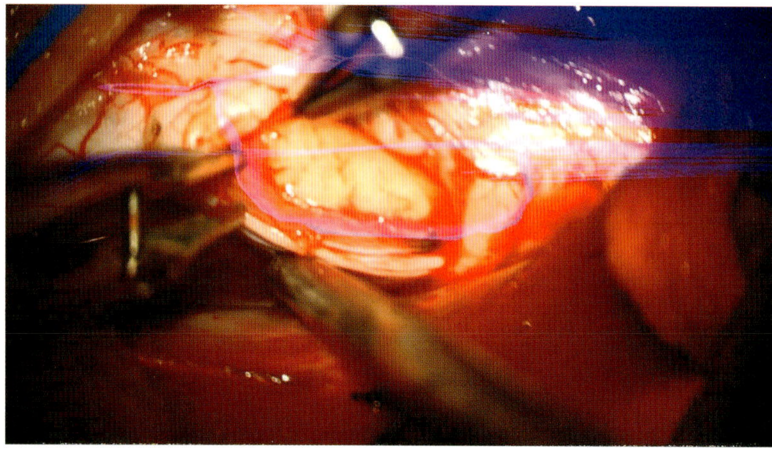

FIG. 13.10 3D tumor overlay integrated into the operative microscope view of the surgical field.

the cranial and caudal extents of the tumor, and accuracy of stereotactic navigation was confirmed. The operative microscope was brought into the field. 3D tumor overlays and diffusion tensor imaging overlays as well as stereotactic navigation were integrated with the operative microscope (Fig. 13.10). The dura was opened, and the dentate ligaments were cut. The intradural extramedullary tumor was identified with the navigation system and excised. The frozen pathology was consistent with a neurofibroma. The navigation system was used to identify the intramedullary tumor and its relation to the corticospinal tracts using overlayed diffusion tensor imaging. A myelotomy was performed and the tumor was debulked using an ultrasonic aspirator. The frozen pathology was consistent with an astrocytoma. Neuromonitoring indicated decreased amplitude of right lower extremity motor-evoked potentials and gross total resection was not pursued. After achieving hemostasis, the dura was closed with a running 6-0 prolene. Lateral mass screws were placed in the previously drilled trajectories. After securing the instrumentation, subfascial and suprafascial drains were placed and the fascia was closed with a running 0 PDS suture. After the skin was closed, the patient was positioned supine again and awoken from anesthesia.

Postoperative Imaging

Fig. 13.11 shows postoperative MRI demonstrating decompression of the cervical spinal cord.

Postoperative Recovery and Follow-Up

The pathology of the intramedullary lesion was consistent with an astrocytoma with an elevated Ki-67 proliferation index of 15%. Postoperatively the patient was noted to have increased proximal paresis of the right lower extremity (antigravity strength) but was able to ambulate with minimal assistance. Her right upper extremity weakness had mild improvement.

Procedural Concerns and Treatment Side Effects

The resection of intramedullary spinal cord lesions carries a significant risk of neurologic deterioration, and neuromonitoring can be used to guide the extent of resection.[5]

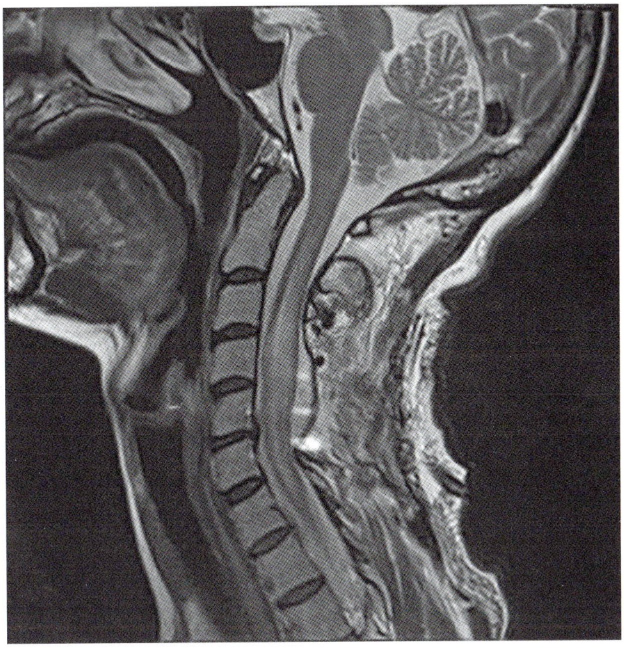

FIG. 13.11 Postoperative sagittal T2-weighted MRI.

The maximum safe resection should be pursued for malignant spinal cord astrocytomas when feasible and has been associated with improved survival in a retrospective review of 35 patients.[6]

Potential Pitfalls

Augmented reality and stereotactic navigation can be a powerful tool in the surgical resection of spinal cord tumors; however, over-reliance on these tools should be avoided. The accuracy of stereotactic navigation should be confirmed with anatomic landmarks and the use of intraoperative ultrasound. A solid anatomical understanding can aid the surgeon in early detection of inaccurate stereotaxic navigation.

Management of Complications

McGirt et al. reported neurologic decline in 40% of patients who underwent resection of malignant spinal cord astrocytomas.[6] Neurologic deficit and impaired mobility are associated with thrombo-embolic complications, and early mobilization, compressive stockings, and prophylactic anticoagulation should be implemented. Physical and occupational therapy should be pursued to maximize recovery.

SUMMARY AND FUTURE DIRECTIONS

Augmented reality with 3D tumor overlays integrated into the operative microscope represents an important advancement in image-guided surgery. The ability to integrate diffusion tensor imaging into the surgeon's view of the spinal cord can significantly aid in safe surgical resection of intramedullary spinal cord tumors. Virtual reality multimodal

3D models can aid in surgical planning. Improvements in radiologic images as well as the automation of data acquisition and registration will facilitate the broader application of these technologies.

REFERENCES

1. Epstein FJ, Farmer JP, Freed D. Adult intramedullary spinal cord ependymomas: the result of surgery in 38 patients. *J Neurol Surg*. 1993;79(2):204–209. https://doi.org/10.3171/jns.1993.79.2.0204.
2. Benjamin CG, Frempong-Boadu A, Hoch M, Bruno M, Shepherd T, Pacione D. Combined use of diffusion tractography and advanced intraoperative imaging for resection of cervical intramedullary spinal cord neoplasms: a case series and technical note. *Oper Neurosurg (Hagerstown)*. 2019;17(5):525–530. https://doi.org/10.1093/ons/opz039.
3. Kelly PJ. Image-directed tumor resection. *Neurosurg Clin N Am*. 1990;1(1):81–95. https://doi.org/10.1016/S1042-3680(18)30825-8.
4. Rashad A, Heiland M, Hiepe P, et al. Evaluation of a novel elastic registration algorithm for spinal imaging data: A pilot clinical study. *Int J Med Robot*. 2019;15(3):e1991. https://doi.org/10.1002/rcs.1991.
5. Matsuyama Y, Sakai Y, Katayama Y, et al. Surgical results of intramedullary spinal cord tumor with spinal cord monitoring to guide extent of resection. *J Neurosurg Spine*. 2009;10(5):404–413. https://doi.org/10.3171/2009.2.SPINE08698.
6. McGirt MJ, Goldstein IM, Chaichana KL, Tobias ME, Kothbauer KF, Jallo GI. Extent of surgical resection of malignant astrocytomas of the spinal cord: outcome analysis of 35 patients. *Neurosurgery*. 2008;63(1):55–60, discussion 60–61. https://doi.org/10.1227/01.NEU.0000335070.37943.09.

14

Use of Activity Monitors in Enhancing Spine Surgery

Martin Nikolaus Stienen, MD, FEBNS, and Nicolai Maldaner, MD

INTRODUCTION OF TECHNOLOGY

Outcome Measurement: Present Practice and Standard of Care

How outcomes are determined after spine surgery has shifted from subjective and solely physician-based to patient-centered and patient-reported.[1] The last few decades have seen the development and systematic validation of a wide variety of generic and disease-specific patient-reported outcome measures (PROMs).[2] Those are usually administered to patients in the form of conventional pen-and-pencil or electronic questionnaires that produce a score or value to estimate the severity of a patient's pain, disability, or restriction in health-related quality of life (HRQOL).

The benefits of these scales are evident. Firstly, they measure the patient's own (subjective) perception of symptom severity and wellbeing—a key outcome any surgical treatment aims to address.[3] Secondly, there are several specific PROMs available that measure different aspects of outcome and that can be chosen according to the leading complaints or pathology (e.g., back pain vs. radicular leg pain vs. painless weakness vs. myelopathy). Thirdly, for the more frequently used PROMs such as the Oswestry Disability Index (ODI), the Roland-Morris Disease Index (RMDI), the Core Outcome Measures Index (COMI) Back, the Zurich Claudication Questionnaire (ZCQ), or the Short-Forms 12/36 (SF-12/SF-36), there are large bodies of literature with disease-specific data, allowing the comparison and interpretation of individual patient scores.[4–6]

However, there are certain downsides to subjective outcome measures. Those include restricted comparability, as every patient rates his/her subjective pain perception differently. Subjective outcome measures are influenced by educational, cultural, and motivational inter-individual differences.[3,7,8] The questions included in PROM questionnaires can be misunderstood (especially in foreign-language patients/illiterate people) or misinterpreted, leading to reliability issues. Some questions contained in PROMs (e.g., questions about traveling or sex life) may not necessarily apply to the individual patient's situation, which lowers validity on the patient level. Most PROMs focus on pain as major complaint and are insensitive to less painful conditions where, for example, hindering motor deficits or dexterity issues dominate the clinical picture.[9] Lastly, patients do not like filling out questionnaires and typically remain unaware of the constructed score. Especially for detailed (multiple questionnaires) or repeated assessments over time, there are important compliance issues, which lead to low data quality resulting from missing data and very limited granularity.[10,11]

The use of objective outcome measures has significantly increased, especially over the past two decades. This increase was caused by both technological advances and the recognition that objective tests can easily, accurately, and repetitively measure functions that are performed by virtually all ambulant humans daily. Additionally, these measured functions are essential for patients after spine surgery to maintain activities of daily living and quality of life.[12,13] Those activities (e.g., standing up, walking, changing direction, and sitting down) can be measured by (wearable) accelerometers, global positioning systems (GPS), or simply modern smartphone devices.[12,14–18] Some of the smartphones store activity data unobtrusively, rendering a possible retrospective analysis of longitudinal "big data" with high granularity and completeness.[19] The options for physical performance tests range from brief evaluations at predefined time points,[20–23] which can be performed by the physician or physician assistants during outpatient evaluation, to extensive and longitudinal patient self-measurements generating "big data".[14,16,18,24,25] The results from objective tests of function allow the estimation of frailty and prediction of perioperative complications of patients scheduled for spine surgery, which can be helpful for risk stratification and complication avoidance.[26] Digital objective outcome measures can be self-measured and display an easily interpretable result. In doing this, patients are empowered to take a greater degree of interest and responsibility as an equal partner in their healthcare.[27] Reported objective outcome measures for degenerative lumbar spine diseases were summarized in recent reviews.[2,12,28] The available and validated options for activity monitoring are listed in Table 14.1 of this chapter.

The downsides to some objective outcome measures are their lack of thorough validation and the lack of normative data availability,[29] although the test qualities of many including the Timed-Up-and-Go (TUG) test, the app-based 6-minute walking test (6WT), the 5-Repetitions-Sit-To-Stand (5R-STS), and Motorized Treadmill Tests (MTTs) have been studied extensively and are favorable.[12,20,22,23] Moreover, there is little standardization in the test choice, conduction, and result interpretation, especially in view of the comorbidities that naturally impact mobility and can introduce significant bias (e.g., prior stroke, congestive heart failure, Parkinson disease, or hip/knee osteoarthritis). This underlines a need for agreement in order to facilitate future comparison of outcome results across cohorts, studies, and countries.[12]

Two of the key advantages of objective activity monitoring are patient convenience and preference. Many spine surgeons are aware of the difficulties associated with questionnaire-based outcome evaluations, which are regarded as tedious and patients tend to avoid filling them out. Objective outcome measures are less prone to missing data, which is a huge problem for PROM-based database studies and is known to influence results.[30] Compared to PROMs, objective tests of function were rated as superior by patients with lumbar degenerative spinal disorders to assess severity and change in spine-related symptoms, as well as significantly more convenient to perform.[11] For repeated assessments, the shift in patient preference from PROM questionnaires to objective functional assessments is more pronounced.[10] The authors of this chapter have encountered several patients who were fascinated by the fact that they were able to observe and measure themselves their positive change in functional impairment over time, for instance after epidural injections

TABLE 14.1 **Review of currently available and validated options for activity monitoring in patients with diseases of the spine**

Name	Description	Disease type	Reliability	Validity	Standardization	Responsiveness
TUG test	The participants begin with sitting on a chair. On the word "Go," they get up and walk as fast as possible to a marked line on the floor at 3 m distance. At this line, the patients turn around, return to the chair and sit down again as quickly as possible. The test result is the time between getting up and sitting down again (s).	LSS, LDH, LBP, listhesis, deformity, VCF, others	Excellent intrarater (ICC = 0.97) and interrater reliability (ICC = 0.99) with a SEM of 0.21–0.23 s	Adequate convergent validity with PROMs, including VAS back ($r = 0.25$) and VAS leg pain ($r = 0.29$), RMDI ($r = 0.38$), and ODI ($r = 0.34$) as well as the SF-12 physical component summary ($r = -0.32$) and EQ-5D ($r = -0.28$)	Transformation of raw test values into age- and sex-standardized T-scores to determine OFI is recommended. The TUG smartphone app[a] contains normative population data and facilitates the transformation of raw into standardized outcomes.	Change in raw TUG test time of 2.1–3.4 s per change in TUG test z-score of 1.5
6WT	Participants walk as fast as possible for 6 min. The main result of the test is the 6WD (m), but time (s) and distance (m) to first symptoms (TTFS/DTFS) are additional helpful outcomes.	LSS, LDH, LBP, listhesis, deformity	App-based measurements are highly reliable outdoors with unobstructed GPS signal (ICC = 0.97). Good intrarater reliability (ICC = 0.82) with a SEM of 58.3 m	Adequate convergent validity with PROMs, including COMI Back ($r = -0.31$), ZCQ symptom severity ($r = -0.32$), ZCQ physical function ($r = -0.33$), VAS back pain ($r = -0.42$), VAS leg pain ($r = -0.32$)	Transformation of raw test values into age- and sex-standardized z-scores to determine OFI is recommended. The 6WT smartphone app[b] contains normative population data and facilitates the transformation of raw into standardized outcomes.	Change in raw 6WD of 92 m per change in 6WT z-score of 1.0
MTT	Patients walk on a treadmill, usually at a predefined protocol. Test results include the time of onset or significant increase in symptoms (s), the total ambulation time (s), the total distance walked (m).	LSS, LDH, LBP, listhesis, others	Reported ICCs for different MTT protocols ranged from 0.83 to 0.98	Studies indicated moderate to high convergent validity of the MTT and self-paced walking test ($r = 0.88$), self-reported walking distance ($r = 0.62$), and the ODI ($r = -0.51$).	Various MTT protocols have been applied, but no gold standard is available. The authors are not aware of normative population data for standardized expression of test results.	No MCID has yet been reported for patients with diseases of the spine.

(Continued)

TABLE 14.1 Review of currently available and validated options for activity monitoring in patients with diseases of the spine—cont'd

Name	Description	Disease type	Reliability	Validity	Standardization	Responsiveness
5R-STS	Participants sit on a chair, firmly placed against the wall. With arms folded across the chest and feet kept flat on the ground participants then stand up fully and sit back down again five times. The test result is the time needed (s).	LSS, LDH, LBP, listhesis	Excellent intrarater (ICC = 0.98) reliability	Adequate convergent validity with PROMs, including RMDI (r = 0.49), ODI (r = 0.44), VAS back pain (r = 0.31) and EQ-5D index (r = −0.41) were observed (P < .001).	Available normative population data allow for severity stratification of raw test results into OFI categories (no, mild, moderate, or severe OFI).	No MCID has yet been reported for patients with diseases of the spine.
Accelerometers	Various (wearable) devices have been applied that measure acceleration. Depending on the device, the number of steps taken, distance walked (m), or calories expended can be calculated. Some allow for calculation of index values that combine several qualities of ambulation.[41]	LSS, LDH, LBP, CDH, CSM	There is a body of literature supporting that accelerometers are usually reliable, while detailed, device-specific data is often not reported.	Study findings generally support accelerometers as valid indicators of overall physical activity and functional disability in adult patients, while not all studies find correlations with PROMs.[14]	Although average steps per day data become increasingly available for the spine-healthy population, so far, no studies reporting standardized outcome data are available.	No MCIDs have been reported for functional impairment, defined by accelerometers.

[a]The "TUG app" is available for smartphones and can be downloaded free of charge from the Apple (https://itunes.apple.com/de/app/tug-app/id1119087707?mt=8) or Google app stores (https://play.google.com/store/apps/details?id=ch.webgearing.tugapp) in multiple languages.

[b]The "6WT app" is available for smartphones and can be downloaded free of charge from the Apple (https://apps.apple.com/ch/app/6wt-app/id1454002232) or Google app stores (https://play.google.com/store/apps/details?id=ch.webgearing.walkingapp&hl=en&gl=US) in multiple languages.

6WD, 6-Minute walking distance; *6WT*, 6-minute walking test; *CDH*, cervical disk herniation; *CSM*, cervical spondylotic myelopathy; *DTFS*, distance to first symptoms; *EQ-5D*, Euro-Qol Five-Dimension Questionnaire; *GPS*, global positioning systems; *ICC*, intraclass correlation coefficient; *LBP*, low back pain; *LDH*, lumbar disk herniation; *LSS*, lumbar spinal stenosis; *MCID*, minimum clinically important difference; *MTT*, Motorized Treadmill test; *ODI*, Oswestry Disability Index; *OFI*, Objective Functional Impairment; *PROM*, patient-reported outcome measure; *RMDI*, Roland-Morris Disability Index; *SEM*, standardized error of mean; *SF*, short form; *TTFS*, time to first symptoms; *TUG*, Timed-Up-and-Go; *VAS*, visual analog scale; *VCF*, vertebral compression fracture; *ZCQ*, Zurich Claudication Questionnaire.

Adapted from Maldaner N, Stienen MN Subjective and objective measures of symptoms, function, and outcome in patients with degenerative spine disease. Arthritis Care Res (Hoboken). 2020;72(suppl 10):183–199. https://doi.org/10.1002/acr.24210 and Stienen MN, Ho AL, Staartjes VE, et al. Objective measures of functional impairment for degenerative diseases of the lumbar spine: a systematic review of the literature. Spine J. 2019;19(7):1276–1293. https://doi.org/10.1016/j.spinee.2019.02.014.

or surgical treatment.[15,25] Many patients conducted notably more measurements than they were asked to provide; some patients even measured their objective functional conditions voluntarily on a daily basis.[25] With PROMs (at least in the authors' experience) this has never happened.

There are clinical scenarios where patient-specific features render a subjective, PROM-based evaluation less precise. For example, patients with depressive comorbidities are known to over-rate pain or disability on subjective scales,[31] whereas in patients with radiculopathy and associated motor deficits, disability may be under-appreciated by PROMs.[9] It has been shown that in cases where pain is subordinate to neurological deficits, PROMs are suboptimal to determine disability. Case 2 (see below) illustrates the benefit of activity monitoring in patient with motor deficits; hence, this topic is not expanded upon in this section.

Case Discussion: Benefits of Objective Outcome Measures

Regarding the benefits of objective outcome measures in patients with mental health issues, we would like to describe the case of a 27-year-old female who developed sciatica secondary to a relatively minor posterolateral LDH with preserved motor function and a history of depression. Her initial TUG test was 25.3 s (age- and sex-adjusted T-score 218.4), indicative of severe objective functional impairment (TUG T-scores of >123 indicate disability). After oral pain medication and epidural steroid injections were administered, she showed significant progressive improvement in the TUG test from 22.0 s (T-score 198.2) to 18.8 s (T-score 178.5), and down to 12.8 s (T-score 141.7). At the same time, she rated her subjective back and leg pain as unchanged, always ranging from 8 to 10 on the visual analog scale (VAS), and was requesting surgical treatment. When realizing the marked improvement in her TUG test T-score over time, however, she became motivated to pursue nonoperative treatment, which lead to complete alleviation within 4 weeks. We have the impression that patients, specifically those with depressive comorbidities, experience difficulties in realizing their rehabilitation progress. In these situations, objective activity monitoring, for example, by serial TUG tests, is useful to objectify improvement and reinforce motivation at the same time.[31]

GUIDING DECISION-MAKING BY ACTIVITY MONITORS WHEN PROM RESULTS ARE CONFLICTING—CASE 1

Case Description

History/Clinical Presentation

A 56-year-old male (BMI 25.4 kg/m^2) presented to our outpatient department with a 2-week history of sudden onset and progressive radiating pain into his right lateral thigh and malleolus lateralis without paresis. His PROMs indicated considerable pain and disability (Numeric Rating Scale [NRS] 6/10, ODI 12/100, COMI Back 5.7/10, Fig. 14.1C–E). He had undergone right-sided L4/5 sequestrectomy due to a lumbar disk herniation 13 months prior but has been pain-free until now.

Preoperative Assessment

Lumbar MRI revealed a recurrent disk herniation at the level L4/5 compromising the right-sided L5 nerve in the intervertebral recess (see Fig. 14.1A and B). His baseline 6-minute walking distance (6WD) was below the age- and sex-adjusted healthy population reference (487 m; z-score −1.00), indicative of mild disability (see Fig. 14.1C). For a screenshot of the "6WT app" depicting his baseline 6WT result, see Fig. 14.2.

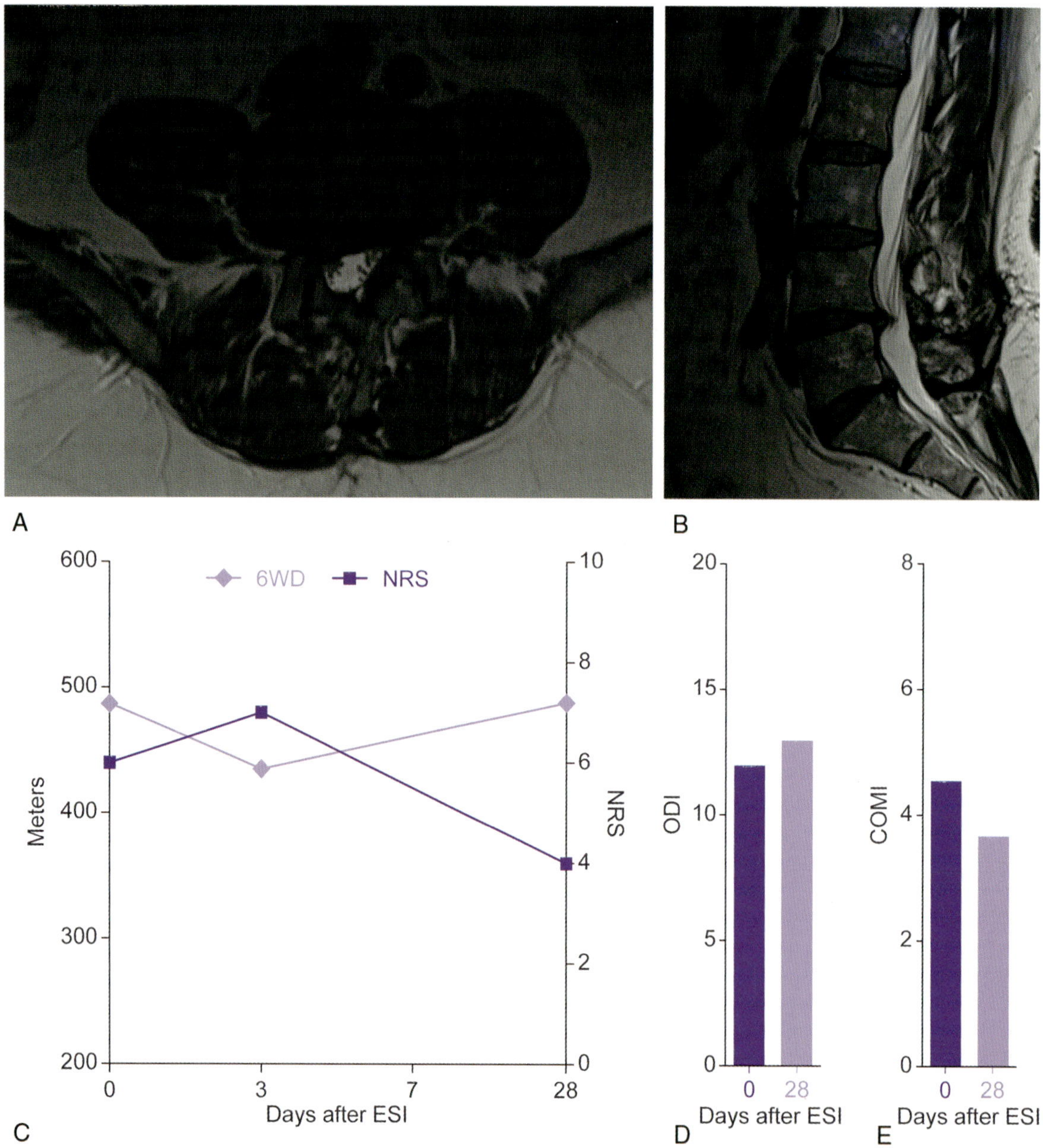

FIG. 14.1 Case vignette 1. The case vignette was published before,[15] but permission for re-use was obtained from the journal. (A) axial T2-weighted MRI; (B) sagittal T2-weighted MRI; (C) On the left x-axis the 6-minute walking distance (*6WD*) in meters before and after lumbar epidural steroid injection (*ESI*) is displayed while the change in numeric rating scale (*NRS*) is depicted on the right x-axis; (D and E) Displays the Core Outcome Measures Index (*COMI*) Back and the Oswestry Disability Index (*ODI*) before and 4 weeks after the ESI.

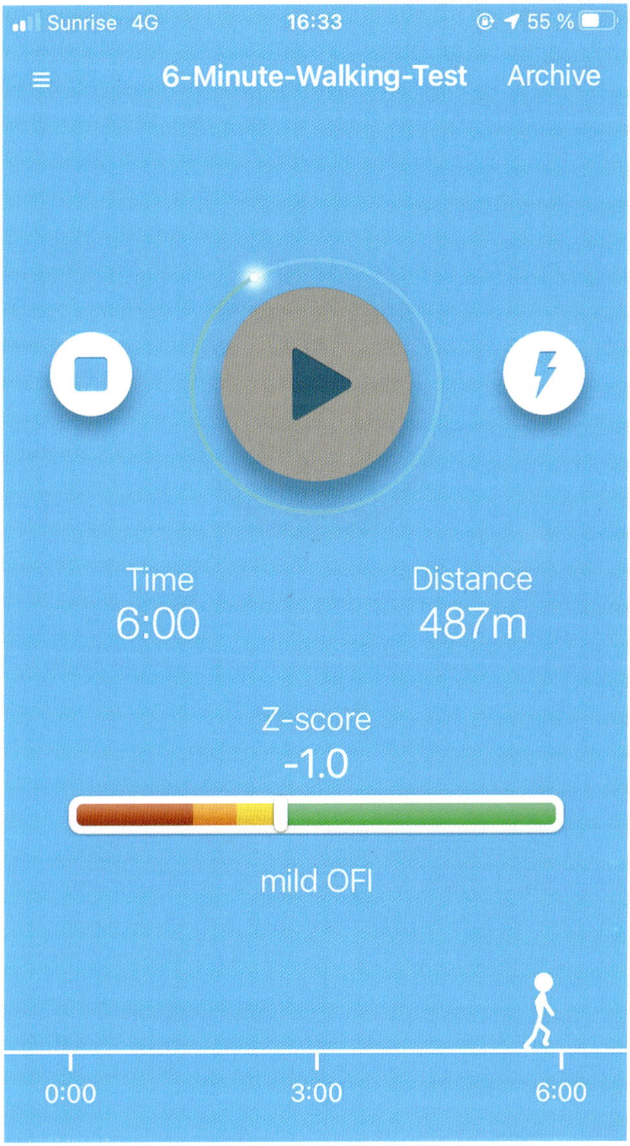

FIG. 14.2 Screenshot of the 6-minute walking test smartphone application (6WT app). To start the test, the patient pushes the "Play" button and the application then begins to measure the distance walked within 6 minutes as the main outcome. The distance, time, and a standardized disability z-score are displayed continuously while walking. In our example, the patient achieved a 6-minute walking distance (6WD) of 487 m, resulting in an age- and sex-adjusted disability z-score of −1.00 (indicating a test result one standard deviation below the normative value). The free 6WT app can be downloaded from the Android Google Play Store (https://play.google.com/store/apps/details?id=ch.webgearing.walkingapp&hl=en) or the Apple App Store (https://apps.apple.com/us/app/6wt/id1454002232). *OFI*, Objective functional impairment.

Surgical Plan

As his pain worsened despite oral pain medication and physiotherapy treatment, we performed a left-sided transforaminal epidural steroid injection. The procedure was successfully conducted without difficulties or complications during, or immediately after, the intervention.

Postoperative Assessment

The patient reported moderate pain relief to NRS at 4 weeks after the injection, with conflicting results in the PROMs. The ODI increased during follow-up (13/100) while the COMI Back Score showed minor improvements (4.6/10; see Fig. 14.1C–E). Serial objective assessments by the 6WT showed temporary, minor improvements in walking ability after the intervention; however, there was no substantial improvement over the 4 weeks' follow-up.

Long-Term Recovery and Follow-Up

Despite moderate pain relief on the NRS, the PROM results were conflicting and the patient did not show clinically meaningful improvement in objective functional impairment. The results were interpreted as persisting symptoms and gait disturbance secondary to lumboradicular pain from the known lumbar disk herniation, without neurological deficits. The patient was not satisfied with his clinical condition and the final outcome after the injection. He signed up for, and subsequently underwent, microsurgical L4/5 sequestrectomy shortly after, which resulted in a clinically meaningful improvement in his 6WD to 650 m (z-score 0.63). Management of complications was not applicable to this case.

Discussion

This case highlights the ability of activity monitoring to differentiate between treatment responders and non-responders, even in the case of conflicting PROM results. Because of the monoradicular pain pattern without associated neurological deficits, we initially opted for transforaminal epidural steroid injection. Despite a moderate pain relief, the patient's 6WD did not improve. Persisting walking difficulties resulting from worsening pain when ambulating prevented the patient from improving on the objective functional impairment metric. In the case of conflicting PROM results, the objective evaluation of walking capacity using the 6WT provides meaningful and quantifiable additional information for the surgeon, which aids in the decision-making process.

In most setups where activity is monitored, including the Self-Paced-Walking-Test (SPWT) or the 6WT,[12,24,32–34] patients are instructed to use their self-selected speed to walk as long and far as possible. For the 6WT, a specifically designed smartphone application is employed for distance measurement. Since patients select their own walking speed without external influence and the measurements simulate a basic activity of daily routine, there are no added risks to otherwise healthy patients. However, any physical activity may pose a risk to patients with certain comorbidities. If in doubt, patients should consult their physicians before conducting measurements.[35]

To avoid adverse events related with the assessment and biased results, we use the following criteria to exclude patients with high-risk profiles:

- Inability to walk (extreme pain or severe neurological deficits)
- Severe chronic obstructive lung disease (COPD) corresponding to ≥Gold III
- Severe heart failure corresponding to ≥NYHA III
- Lung cancer and diffuse parenchymal lung disease

- Other medical reasons interfering with the patient's ability to walk and perform activity monitoring for spinal disorders (e.g., osteoarthritis of the lower extremities, Parkinson disease, heart failure, hip or knee prosthesis, etc.)

While the potential benefits of the smartphone-based assessment of physical activity is evident, we must still overcome some obstacles that might prevent the widespread adoption of digital objective outcome assessment in spine patients. All-new outcome measures have to be rigorously examined in their psychometric properties to enter clinical routine.[2,12,28,36] Secondly, both patients and physicians need to be confident that their personal data is protected against theft and abuse. Finally, patients who do not, or cannot, use smartphone devices must be included, as failure to include these patients may discriminate against those of older age or lower socioeconomic status.[17,27]

EVALUATING DISABILITY WHEN MOTOR DEFICITS ARE THE PREDOMINATING SYMPTOM—CASE 2

Case Description

History/Clinical Presentation

A non-obese (BMI 22.0 kg/m^2), 54-year-old, female patient (smoker, no known comorbidities, light physical work 3 days/week) was admitted to our hospital for a brief period of excruciating pain (shooting down from the lower back into the right buttock and posterior thigh). Within hours, and until admission, the pain resolved to a large extent, but she developed a foot weakness in parallel, for which she consulted the emergency department.

Preoperative Assessment

In her admission examination, a right-sided Medical Research Council (MRC) grade 3 plantar flexion weakness, a loss of tactile sensitivity at the sole of the foot including the last two toes, and a positive straight-leg sign were remarkable. Her admission pain level was 2/10 on the VAS for the back and 1/10 on the VAS for the leg. In terms of subjective disability, she scored 12/100 on the ODI and 4/24 on the RMDI. Her HRQOL was reasonably high, with a Short-Form 12 physical component summary (SF-12 PCS) of 41.5, Short-Form 12 mental component summary (SF-12 MCS) of 44.5, and Euro-Qol Five-Dimension Questionnaire (EQ-5D) index of 0.846.

Her objective functional assessment with the Timed-Up-and-Go (TUG) test was 17.2 s, indicative of moderate objective functional impairment (age- and sex-adjusted T-score 168.5).

MRI studies of the lumbar spine revealed a relatively large, right-sided paramedian disk herniation at the L5/S1 level, caudally sequestered, with recessal compression of the right S1 nerve root (Fig. 14.3A and B).

Surgical Plan

Considering the acute and higher-grade neurological deficits in conjunction with the conclusive pathological finding on MRI, we recommended, and subsequently performed, an uneventful microsurgical L5/S1 discectomy/sequestrectomy.

Postoperative Assessment

The patient was mobilized early and intensive physiotherapy was initiated. Her plantar flexion strength had improved to MRC grade 4 at this time. She was re-evaluated on postoperative day 3, when she had 0/10 VAS back and/or leg pain, her subjective disability was low (ODI 10/100; RMDI 1/24) and HRQOL-measures were similar to the preoperative values. On the TUG test, she showed residual signs of impairment (12.2 s; T-score 138.0; mild OFI).

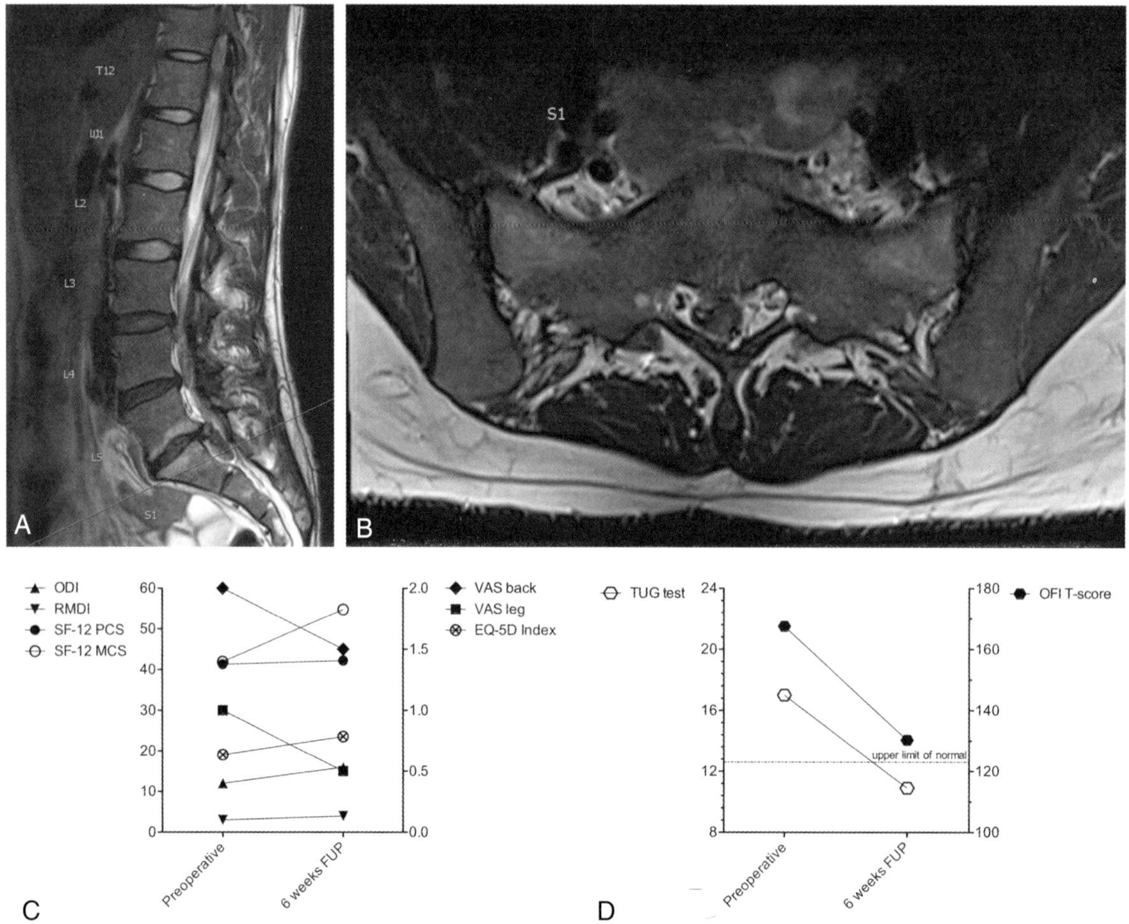

FIG. 14.3 **Case vignette 2.** The case vignette was published before,[9] but permission for re-use was obtained from the journal. (A) Sagittal T2-weighted MRI. (B) Axial T2-weighted MRI. (C) Change in subjective PROMs preoperative to 6 weeks postoperative. (D) Change in objective functional impairment, measured by the TUG test raw value in seconds and standardized OFI T-score preoperative to 6 weeks postoperative. The *dotted line* indicates the OFI T-score threshold of 123, under which a TUG test result is considered within the normal population range (upper limit of normal). *EQ-5D*, EuroQol-5D; *ODI*, Oswestry Disability Index; *OFI*, objective functional impairment; *RMDI*, Roland-Morris Disability Index; *SF-12 MCS*, Short-Form 12 mental component summary; *SF-12 PCS*, Short-Form 12 physical component summary; *TUG*, Timed-Up and Go; *VAS*, visual analog scale.

Long-Term Recovery and Follow-Up

At the 6-week follow-up, her plantar flexion weakness had improved substantially (MRC 4+). Her condition according to subjective PROMs can be summarized as: VAS back 1.5/10, VAS leg 0.5/10, ODI 15/100, RMDI 5/24, SF-12 PCS 42.4, and SF-12 MCS 55.2 (see Fig. 14.3C).

The objective TUG-based assessment revealed a clinically meaningful improvement in function, compared to the preoperative value,[37] while still indicating minor residual impairment (10.8 s; T-score 129.2; mild OFI; see Fig. 14.3D). Management of complications was not applicable to this case.

Discussion

In the era of evidence-based medicine, the outcome after spine surgery is typically determined based on PROMs, but those usually focus on pain as predominant symptom. Disability resulting from motor deficits may be ignored by PROMs, whereas objective outcome measures may be more sensitive here.[9]

This example demonstrates that the degree and severity of OFI paralleled the rehabilitation process. The better the regained plantar flexion strength, the better also was the ambulation, which translated into faster TUG test times. In patients with motor deficits, PROM outcomes should ideally be accompanied by either a neurological examination (focusing on the affected function loss) or by an objective test that evaluates the affected function.

To the best of the authors' knowledge, there have not been reports of adverse events associated with the listed, recommended, objective tests of function (see Table 14.1). However, patients should be reminded that while ideally performing (timed) tests at a high pace, falls/accidents or medical complications (resulting from known comorbidities) must be avoided, even if that lowers the test result. Depending on the test, the examiner may accompany frail patients to make sure that they do not tremble and fall (Video 14.1).

An appropriate objective test must be chosen for each patient according to the prevailing symptom. PROMs will fail to measure patient outcome if the set of symptoms present in the individual patient are not contained in the items of the questionnaire. A patient with lumbar spinal stenosis, for example, who feels mild paresthesia or leg heaviness without painful sensations during ambulation, will not score significantly worse than a healthy individual on the VAS pain scale, the ODI, or the COMI questionnaire. This is also true for activity monitoring. The same patient may not be limited in his walking ability as measured by the TUG or 6WT; hence, those tests would be inappropriate to measure disability. Here, a carefully selected PROM questionnaire, accounting for this particular symptom, for example, the ZCQ, may be superior.

VIDEO OF ACTIVITY MONITORING

The video demonstrates the objective functional assessment of a 55-year-old patient with lumbar spinal stenosis, scheduled for elective microsurgical decompression at the L4/5 level for failed conservative treatment. Her subjective disease severity can be described as relatively mild with PROM scores as follows: VAS back pain 3/10, VAS leg pain 2/10, ODI 30/100, RMDI 12/24, SF-12 PCS 45.6, and SF-12 MCS 52.4. Accordingly, the TUG test result is within the range of the spine-healthy normal population (7.9 s; age- and sex-adjusted T-score 111.7; no OFI). The video serves to demonstrate how the TUG test is conducted in a patient without obvious disability.

SUMMARY

Current Added Value of Activity Monitors

Currently, activity monitors add another dimension of outcome by determining objective functional impairment in spine patients undergoing conservative or operative treatment. As more and more objective outcome measures are being validated in the context of spine diseases, they may overcome certain disadvantages that are inherent to the subjective nature of PROM questionnaires. Unlike PROMs, activity monitors that are worn like smartwatches, or carried like smartphones, allow patients to determine their disability in an environment that matters most to them (e.g., home or work).[17] This is especially helpful in a time where the experience from the COVID pandemic has resulted in increased patient demand for remote (tele-)medicine. Several standardized measures, like the TUG test, the 5R-STS, or the 6WT, are easily administered, supported with dedicated smartphone applications, and based on thoroughly examined psychometric properties.[2,12,15,22,24,38] By applying activity monitors in patient care, physicians are able to collect longitudinal outcome date with high granularity to detect and objectify change in a patient's functional status over time. Patients, on the other hand, are able to use these outcome measures repeatedly, at their own discretion, to appreciate their change in function; change of function is usually shown on simple and relatable metrices (e.g., speed of standing/sitting, distance walked, or steps taken).[14, 27, 39] The ability to objectify a patient's disability is therefore of benefit to both the patient and the treating physician as the digital technology may help optimize processes, stratify risks, and lower overall costs in healthcare.[10,11,40]

Future Directions

There exist ample, unexploited opportunities for remote and real-time objective outcome analyses that may not only serve to document treatment efficacy but could even be used to detect adverse events or complications at early stages.[14,18] There is room to develop activity measurement devices that determine several different qualities in parallel, including step count, velocity, step length, and posture, which can be used together in order to calculate index scores that more accurately represent the patient's physical condition.[41] It is only a question of time until start-ups or established medical device companies will provide spine surgeons with implantable solutions for objective activity monitoring. Small implantable devices could be fit into both pedicle screws and cages. This transition may additionally be promoted by the recently introduced CPT code or reimbursement for remote patient monitoring by the US Centers for Medicare and Medicaid Services (CPT code 99091).

Objective activity monitoring for patient-centered spine care has a potentially bright digital future. This relies on physicians, scientists, and industry all collaborating to set the grounds for meaningful and responsible ways to collect, analyze, and protect this highly sensitive personal data against theft and abuse.[17,27]

REFERENCES

1. Stienen MN, Bellut D, Regli L, Hausmann ON, Gautschi OP. Praxis. (Bern 1994). *Praxis*. 2017;106(19):1041–1052. https://doi.org/10.1024/1661-8157/a002779.
2. Maldaner N, Stienen MN. Subjective and objective measures of symptoms, function, and outcome in patients with degenerative spine disease. *Arthritis Care Res (Hoboken)*. 2020; 72(suppl 10):183–199. https://doi.org/10.1002/acr.24210.
3. Gautschi OP, Corniola MV, Schaller K, Smoll NR, Stienen MN. The need for an objective outcome measurement in spine surgery—the timed-up-and-go test. *Spine J*. 2014;14(10):2521–2522. https://doi.org/10.1016/j.spinee.2014.05.004.
4. Deyo RA, Battie M, Beurskens AJ, et al. Outcome measures for low back pain research. A proposal for standardized

use. *Spine*. 1998;23(18):2003–2013. https://doi.org/10.1097/00007632-199809150-00018.
5. Harrop J. The Bull or the Horn—What Are Outcomes Data? *Neurospine*. 2020;17:281–282.
6. Mannion AF, Elfering A, Staerkle R, et al. Outcome assessment in low back pain: how low can you go? *Eur Spine J*. 2005;14(10):1014–1026. https://doi.org/10.1007/s00586-005-0911-9.
7. Gautschi OP, Corniola MV, Smoll NR, et al. Sex differences in subjective and objective measures of pain, functional impairment, and health-related quality of life in patients with lumbar degenerative disc disease. *Pain*. 2016;157(5):1065–1071. https://doi.org/10.1097/j.pain.0000000000000480.
8. Gautschi OP, Smoll NR, Joswig H, et al. Influence of age on pain intensity, functional impairment and health-related quality of life before and after surgery for lumbar degenerative disc disease. *Clin Neurol Neurosurg*. 2016;150:33–39. https://doi.org/10.1016/j.clineuro.2016.08.024.
9. Stienen MN, Maldaner N, Sosnova M, et al. Lower extremity motor deficits are underappreciated in patient-reported outcome measures: added value of objective outcome measures. *Neurospine*. 2020;17(1):270–280. https://doi.org/10.14245/ns.1938368.184.
10. Joswig H, Stienen MN, Smoll NR, et al. Patients' preference of the timed up and go test or patient-reported outcome measures before and after surgery for lumbar degenerative disk disease. *World Neurosurg*. 2017;99:26–30. https://doi.org/10.1016/j.wneu.2016.11.039.
11. Sosnova M, Zeitlberger AM, Ziga M, et al. Patients undergoing surgery for lumbar degenerative spinal disorders favor smartphone-based objective self-assessment over paper-based patient-reported outcome measures. *Spine J*. 2021;21(4):610–617. https://doi.org/10.1016/j.spinee.2020.11.013.
12. Stienen MN, Ho AL, Staartjes VE, et al. Objective measures of functional impairment for degenerative diseases of the lumbar spine: a systematic review of the literature. *Spine J*. 2019;19(7):1276–1293. https://doi.org/10.1016/j.spinee.2019.02.014.
13. Yamaguchi S. Does the rise of objective measure of functional impairment mean the fall of PROMs? *Neurospine*. 2020;17(1):283–284. https://doi.org/10.14245/ns.2040112.056.
14. Stienen MN, Rezaii PG, Ho AL, et al. Objective activity tracking in spine surgery: a prospective feasibility study with a low-cost consumer grade wearable accelerometer. *Sci Rep*. 2020;10(1):4939. https://doi.org/10.1038/s41598-020-61893-4.
15. Zeitlberger AM, Sosnova M, Ziga M, et al. Smartphone-based self-assessment of objective functional impairment (6-minute walking test) in patients undergoing epidural steroid injection. *Neurospine*. 2020;17(1):136–142. https://doi.org/10.14245/ns.2040022.011.
16. Bostelmann R, Schneller S, Cornelius JF, Steiger HJ, Fischer I. A new possibility to assess the perioperative walking capacity using a global positioning system in neurosurgical spine patients: a feasibility study. *Eur Spine J*. 2016;25(3):963–968. https://doi.org/10.1007/s00586-015-3922-1.
17. Maldaner N, Tomkins-Lane C, Desai A, et al. Digital transformation in spine research and outcome assessment. *Spine J*. 2020;20(2):310–311. https://doi.org/10.1016/j.spinee.2019.06.027.
18. Akeret K, Vasella F, Geisseler O, et al. Time to be "smart"-Opportunities arising from smartphone-based behavioral analysis in daily patient care. *Front Behav Neurosci*. 2018;12:303. https://doi.org/10.3389/fnbeh.2018.00303.
19. Basil GW, Sprau AC, Eliahu K, Borowsky PA, Wang MY, Yoon JW. Using smartphone-based accelerometer data to objectively assess outcomes in spine surgery. *Neurosurgery*. 2021;88(4):763–772. https://doi.org/10.1093/neuros/nyaa505.
20. Gautschi OP, Smoll NR, Corniola MV, et al. Validity and reliability of a measurement of objective functional impairment in lumbar degenerative disc disease: the timed up and go (TUG) test. *Neurosurgery*. 2016;79(2):270–278. https://doi.org/10.1227/NEU.0000000000001195.
21. Hartmann S, Hegewald AA, Tschugg A, Neururer S, Abenhardt M, Thomé C. Analysis of a performance-based functional test in comparison with the visual analog scale for postoperative outcome assessment after lumbar spondylodesis. *Eur Spine J*. 2016;25(5):1620–1626. https://doi.org/10.1007/s00586-015-4350-y.
22. Staartjes VE, Schröder ML. The five-repetition sit-to-stand test: evaluation of a simple and objective tool for the assessment of degenerative pathologies of the lumbar spine. *J Neurosurg Spine*. 2018;29(4):380–387. https://doi.org/10.3171/2018.2.SPINE171416.
23. Stienen MN, Smoll NR, Joswig H, et al. Validation of the baseline severity stratification of objective functional impairment in lumbar degenerative disc disease. *J Neurosurg Spine*. 2017;26(5):598–604. https://doi.org/10.3171/2016.11.SPINE16683.
24. Maldaner N, Sosnova M, Zeitlberger AM, et al. Evaluation of the 6-minute walking test as a smartphone app-based self-measurement of objective functional impairment in patients with lumbar degenerative disc disease. *J Neurosurg Spine*. 2020:1–10.
25. Sosnova M, Zeitlberger AM, Ziga M, et al. Longitudinal smartphone-based self-assessment of objective functional impairment in patients undergoing surgery for lumbar degenerative disc disease: initial experience. *Acta neurochir*. 2020;162(9):2061–2068. https://doi.org/10.1007/s00701-020-04377-8.
26. Komodikis G, Gannamani V, Neppala S, Li M, Merli GJ, Harrop JS. Usefulness of timed up and go (TUG) test for prediction of adverse outcomes in patients undergoing thoracolumbar spine surgery. *Neurosurgery*. 2020;86(3):E273–E280. https://doi.org/10.1093/neuros/nyz480.
27. Maldaner N, Desai A, Gautschi OP, et al. Improving the patient-physician relationship in the digital era—transformation from subjective questionnaires into

objective real-time and patient-specific data reporting tools. *Neurospine*. 2019;16(4):712–714. https://doi.org/10.14245/ns.1938400.200.

28. Anderson DB, Mathieson S, Eyles J, et al. Measurement properties of walking outcome measures for neurogenic claudication: a systematic review and meta analysis. *Spine J*. 2019;19(8):1378–1396. https://doi.org/10.1016/j.spinee.2019.04.004.
29. Brodie MA, Pliner EM, Ho A, et al. Big data vs accurate data in health research: large-scale physical activity monitoring, smartphones, wearable devices and risk of unconscious bias. *Med Hypo*. 2018;119:32–36. https://doi.org/10.1016/j.mehy.2018.07.015.
30. Basques BA, McLynn RP, Fice MP, et al. Results of database studies in spine surgery can be influenced by missing data. *Clin Orthop Relat Res*. 2017;475(12):2893–2904. https://doi.org/10.1007/s11999-016-5175-7.
31. Stienen MN, Smoll NR, Joswig H, et al. Influence of the mental health status on a new measure of objective functional impairment in lumbar degenerative disc disease. *Spine J*. 2017;17(6):807–813. https://doi.org/10.1016/j.spinee.2016.12.004.
32. Conway J, Tomkins CC, Haig AJ. Walking assessment in people with lumbar spinal stenosis: capacity, performance, and self-report measures. *Spine J*. 2011;11(9):816–823. https://doi.org/10.1016/j.spinee.2010.10.019.
33. Smuck M, Muaremi A, Zheng P, et al. Objective measurement of function following lumbar spinal stenosis decompression reveals improved functional capacity with stagnant real-life physical activity. *Spine J*. 2018;18(1):15–21. https://doi.org/10.1016/j.spinee.2017.08.262.
34. Tomkins-Lane CC, Battié MC. Predictors of objectively measured walking capacity in people with degenerative lumbar spinal stenosis. *J Back Musculoskelet Rehabil*. 2013;26(4):345–352. https://doi.org/10.3233/BMR-130390.
35. Fletcher GF, Balady GJ, Amsterdam EA, et al. Exercise standards for testing and training: a statement for healthcare professionals from the American Heart Association. *Circulation*. 2001;104(14):1694–1740. https://doi.org/10.1161/hc3901.095960.
36. Smeets RJ, Hijdra HJ, Kester AD, Hitters MW, Knottnerus JA. The usability of six physical performance tasks in a rehabilitation population with chronic low back pain. *Clin Rehabil*. 2006;20(11):989–997. https://doi.org/10.1177/0269215506070698.
37. Gautschi OP, Stienen MN, Corniola MV, et al. Assessment of the minimum clinically important difference in the timed up and go test after surgery for lumbar degenerative disc disease. *Neurosurgery*. 2017;80(3):380–385. https://doi.org/10.1227/NEU.0000000000001320.
38. Tosic L, Goldberger E, Maldaner N, et al. Normative data of a smartphone app-based 6-minute walking test, test-retest reliability, and content validity with patient-reported outcome measures. *J Neurosurg Spine*. 2020:1–10. https://doi.org/10.3171/2020.3.SPINE2084.
39. Staartjes VE, Beusekamp F, Schröder ML. Can objective functional impairment in lumbar degenerative disease be reliably assessed at home using the five-repetition sit-to-stand test? A prospective study. *Eur Spine J*. 2019;28(4):665–673. https://doi.org/10.1007/s00586-019-05897-3.
40. Pendharkar AV, Shahin MN, Ho AL, et al. Outpatient spine surgery: defining the outcomes, value, and barriers to implementation. *Neurosurg Focus*. 2018;44(5):E11. https://doi.org/10.3171/2018.2.FOCUS17790.
41. Ghent F, Mobbs RJ, Mobbs RR, Sy L, Betteridge C, Choy WJ. Assessment and post-intervention recovery after surgery for lumbar disk herniation based on objective gait metrics from wearable devices using the gait posture index. *World Neurosurg*. 2020;142:e111–e116. https://doi.org/10.1016/j.wneu.2020.06.104.

15

Artificial Intelligence and Machine Learning in Spine Surgery

Michael Jin, BS, Marc Schröder, MD, PhD, and Victor E. Staartjes, MD

INTRODUCTION OF TECHNOLOGY

While investigations into incorporating machine learning (ML) and artificial intelligence (AI) into medicine have been numerous and diverse, their aggregate contributions have altered and revolutionized clinical practice. Fundamentally, ML and AI approaches seek to leverage automata for pattern recognition and extrapolation. Generally, approaches are classified as one of two predominant forms: supervised and unsupervised learning. *Supervised learning* describes those approaches that use a prelabeled "training" dataset to discover relationships between model features and the outcome-of-interest that can subsequently be applied to generate risk or likelihood predictions in unlabeled "test" datasets. Such methods are commonly used for modeling peri- and postoperative outcomes and for automated interpretation of written clinical reports through natural language processing (NLP). *Unsupervised learning* refers to the *de novo* identification of patterns and relationships in unlabeled datasets through discovery and reconstruction of often complex and non-linear relationships within data. Examples of unsupervised learning applications within medicine include the contouring of radiology and pathology studies. Within spine surgery specifically, we will review common approaches to three clinical themes: *outcome prediction*, *image analysis*, and *NLP*. We will further describe the notable current applications of ML and AI within these themes and discuss, in depth, an example of how automata may shape patient care within spine surgery.

Outcome Prediction

Perhaps the theme most frequently associated with ML in medicine has been the prediction of clinical outcomes. The early efforts to design intelligent clinical prediction systems generally revolved around semi-automated rule-based systems, such as MYCIN and PLEXXUS.[1–3] However, while such models augmented real-time decision-making using stored knowledge compiled by subfield experts, rule-based approaches were limited by low flexibility and adaptability. Since the 1970s, continued advancements in computer architecture and hardware have facilitated growth, diversity, and complexity of predictive modeling approaches. Clinical predictive modeling now offers innumerable options for algorithm design and opportunities to anticipate short- and long-term patient outcomes accurately.

With external validation and implementation, these approaches may help shape the care delivery framework toward a more personalized archetype enabling improvements in both healthcare efficiency and patients' care experiences.

The practice of clinical predictive modeling can be generalized into two broad categories: shallow learning and deep learning. *Shallow learning* describes the approaches designed to identify relationships among pre-defined features of a dataset and an outcome-of-interest. Examples of shallow learning frameworks frequently applied to clinical medicine include regression and classification approaches such as generalized linear models (GLMs), decision trees, and support vector machines. In contrast, *deep learning* requires no pre-defined feature set, instead allowing the computer system to identify, arrange, and weight important contributors within the data during the process of model development and tuning. Approaches such as convolutional neural networks (CNNs) can recognize and decompose complex signals for the identification of underlying patterns and relationships.[4] Deep learning offers numerous advantages, particularly in the setting of feature-rich datasets or intricate pattern recognition tasks; however, its disadvantages must also be highlighted, foremost among them being the reduced interpretability of model parameters and component contribution. Deep neural networks, especially, are frequently referred to as "black boxes," a metaphor that highlights the difficulty of deconvoluting and explaining the transformation of input components into an output decision.[5] Ongoing research aims to develop "explainers" to ameliorate this concern[6]; nevertheless, the practical utility of deep learning approaches will largely depend on clinicians weighing the marginal importance of incremental performance boosts (and downstream implications for clinical care) against the heightened difficulty in model interpretation and increased computational resources required by such architectures.

Within the realm of spine surgery, clinical predictive modeling has been applied to outcomes ranging from postoperative complications and readmissions to long-term postoperative recovery and opioid dependence. Goyal et al. sought to develop an approach to predict non-home discharge and early readmission following cervical or lumbar vertebral fusion.[7] The performance across modeling approaches (GLM, gradient boosting machines, Elastic Net GLM, and artificial neural networks [ANN], among others) was comparable, reaching Area Under the Receiver Operating Characteristic curve (AUROCs) of 0.87 and 0.66 for prediction of non-home discharge and early unplanned readmission, respectively. Similar methods have also been applied to predict postsurgical outcome[8–11] and complications,[12,13] long-term narcotic use,[14,15] healthcare costs,[16] and mortality.[17] It remains important to note that, while increasing interest in ML models for clinical outcome prediction has yielded numerous promising candidates for introduction into clinical practice, there remains a paucity of studies demonstrating objective utility in secondary prospective investigations. Clinical trials applying validated predictors and appropriate care interventions (such as personalized pain management regimens, increased postoperative vigilance, or re-evaluation of post-discharge care) remain important "next-steps" in the translation of ML models from theory into practice.

ANNs and CNNs, outside of image interpretation and NLP (topics that will be addressed in the following sections), have also been explored in the context of clinical predictive modeling. Studies have compared the performance of neural networks to that of alternative approaches such as logistic regression,[18] proposing these more complex model designs as feasible alternatives and potential improvements to the more frequently applied regression- and tree-based methods. In support of this, a prior study by Dreiseitl and Ohno-Machado demonstrated that, in a subset of applications and settings, ANNs may offer better class discrimination than does logistic regression. These investigations, while reflective of the broadening interest within the medical community in harnessing increasingly complex models, emphasize the recognition of important considerations. As described by Dreiseitl and Ohno-Machado, logistic regression performed comparably to ANNs in the majority of examined cases.[19] It certainly is possible that, under many practical circumstances, ANNs offer indistinguishable performance compared to simpler approaches; as previously discussed, a cost-benefit assessment should be conducted by the prospective user to determine whether the increased resource utilization and development complexity is justified by the expected marginal improvements in performance. Lastly, in contexts where developers hope to use model development and validation to identify modifiable factors informative for subsequent prospective studies, the loss of interpretability associated with higher complexity models may hinder informed research design.

Image Classification

The manual interpretation of imaging incurs several downsides that may be ameliorated by automata. First, the low throughput nature of manual radiology review can result in reduced workflow speed and efficiency.[20] Automated and semi-automated MRI interpretation can leverage the multithreaded and superior computational capabilities of modern-day computers to streamline radiology review. Second, heterogeneity in image interpretation across reviewers may compromise confidence in evaluation results. In prior evaluations of interrater concordance, reliability of findings generally ranged broadly from moderate to good.[21,22] Improved reliability may be achieved by integrating deep learning approaches as either an independent or adjunctive process for establishing diagnoses.[23] Third, detection of surreptitious pathologies may be difficult even for experienced radiologists. Studies evaluating application of deep sCNNs for sensitive diagnosis of these lesions have yielded promising results.[24] Taken together, these potential drawbacks suggest that the integration of AI into spine surgery diagnostics and practice may streamline radiologic evaluation while potentially improving interpretation accuracy and consistency.

While the interpretation of spinal imaging by automated systems has historically relied on shallow learning architectures such as support vector machine[25] and random forest,[26] the recent literature has shown an ever-increasing presence of deep learning in image classification. By the early 2010s, the potential of deep learning in imaging classification had been spotlighted by the development of graphics processing unit (GPU)-implemented CNNs capable of attaining previously unachievable levels of prediction accuracy with accelerated computational speed.[27,28] Among the most recognizable was AlexNet, an eight-layer CNN that reduced misclassification error on the ImageNet Large Scale Visual Recognition Challenge 2012 dataset by more than 40%.[29] During the development of early CNN-based computer vision approaches such as AlexNet, model performance was significantly limited by the heavy computational and memory resources required by deep learning frameworks. However, the growing understanding of neural network architecture and construction has yielded algorithms with increased resource and computational efficiency[30,31]; further augmenting research in deep learning has been the industry-wide progression of computing power and data availability facilitating high dimensional analyses. Broadly, the impact of deep learning constructs on image recognition tasks may be best summarized by the sophistication of recent algorithms harnessing hundreds of millions of parameters that have now achieved classification errors orders of magnitude lower than that of AlexNet.[32,33]

Specifically pertaining to spinal pathologies and spine surgery, the application of machine-assisted image recognition approaches may impact both presurgical diagnostics and perioperative management. Automating segmentation and annotation of vertebrae using CNNs may facilitate opportunities for sensitive detection and characterization of degenerative disk disease and acute spinal cord injury.[34,35] Both Huang et al.[34] and McCoy et al.[35] modeled their approaches on the often-employed U-net architecture[36] purposed for segmentation of T2-weighted MRI. The former introduced *Spine Explorer*, an algorithm for the automated detection and quantification of vertebral body and vertebral disk measurements (metrics including diameter, height, area, and signal intensity). Compared to gold standard manual expert segmentation, *Spine Explorer* achieved high contour accuracy (97.4% as evaluated by the Jaccard index, which measures the regional intersection of automated and gold standard countours over their union). Disk measurables obtained by *Spine Explorer* were compared to previously developed indices grading disk degeneration,[37] demonstrating strong inverse correlation between CSF-adjusted disk intensity and disk degeneration severity. The latter study developed *BASICseg* for auto-segmentation of the spinal cord and spinal cord lesions. Compared to gold standard expert manual segmentation, *BASICseg* achieved a high Dice coefficient (a measure reflecting degree of regional overlap[38]) of 0.93 during spinal cord segmentation. Notably, segmenting acute spinal cord injury lesions proved more difficult and, despite *BASICseg* achieving higher test set accuracy than prior algorithms, further research is necessary to improve contour fidelity. Taken together, these studies introduce approaches to the automated quantification of spinal anatomy and pathology that may supplement surgeon clinical experience when localizing and explaining symptomatology.

Deep learning may guide not only the diagnosis of spinal pathologies but also the practice of spine surgery itself. In a study aimed at automating surgical planning for pedicle screw insertion, Cai et al. constructed a deep CNN for digital three-dimensional segmentation and pedicle screw path simulation in spinal CT imaging.[39] On withheld imaging series, segmentation achieved a Dice coefficient of nearly 97% and a Jaccard coefficient of over 93%. The pedicle screw localization was also accurate, with a mean squared error of 1.34 voxels during five-fold cross validation. Despite promising results, the notable limitations of the study include input imaging requirements and missing physiological qualities, such as biomechanical characterization of the planned surgical path. Regarding the former, limited computational resources necessitated scaling down input bulk and restricting CNN size. The latter concerns the importance of biophysical factors beyond anatomical setting and location. The biomechanical properties and composition of individual vertebral bodies, particularly in the setting of degenerative pathologies, may significantly alter surgical planning and should be considered in fully automated surgical planning workflows.[40] Although such an approach has yet to be developed and validated, the implementation of current methods in a semi-automated manner and future elucidation of improved fully automated algorithms may improve surgical planning efficiency while reducing variance. Lastly, deep learning-enhanced planning and reduction of radiation in instrumented spine surgery through generation of synthetic CT images, as will be discussed later in this chapter, are promising developments.[41]

Natural Language Processing

Beyond the enhanced interpretation of radiologic imaging using computer vision, automated dissection and interpretation of unstructured clinical reports offers tantalizing opportunities for optimizing spine surgery workflows. From origins reaching back to the 1960s, free-text parsing has remained a significant challenge. One of the earliest efforts to transform human-interpretable language into machine-understandable features was the Linguistic String Project whose development, led by Dr. Naomi Sager, served for decades as the archetype of NLP.[42] The application of NLP frameworks to clinical, radiology, and pathology reports have yielded promising results, often outperforming manual alternatives in terms of reliability and accuracy.[43,44] At a high level, NLP algorithms in medicine generally comprise two phases: the conversion of unstructured or semi-structured reports into a constellation of machine-interpretable information, ranging from semantics to syntactical context, and feature engineering for development of discriminative models for classification tasks. The expanded prevalence of electronic health records in the 21st century to near-ubiquitous presence[45] has concocted significant opportunity for incorporation of NLP into medical practice. Increasing access to large, shared healthcare datasets, such as the MIMIC databases curated by the Beth Israel Deaconess Medical Center in Boston, Massachusetts,[46] has also aided efforts to optimize NLP algorithms for the clinical setting. Together with increasing physician eagerness to improve care efficiency and effectiveness, the past two decades have seen rapid acceleration of NLP-related medical research and publications.[47]

The formalization of an NLP system capable of processing free-text clinical records is a multistep process, requiring fragmentation of the document into text subunits called *tokens* that can subsequently be interpreted as discrete concepts using appropriate lexicons and the syntactical context it was identified in. Language databanks, such as the Unified Medical Language system and the frequently used SPECIALIST medical lexicon it encapsulates, are necessary to define and standardize identified tokens. Those systems geared toward extraction of data from clinical reports, such as MEDLEE,[48] cTAKES,[49] and MetaMap,[50] consolidate these steps within an encompassing wrapper. The encoded language can then be contextualized using databases such as SNOMED-CT[51–53] and can also serve as feature sets for additional classification algorithms. In an early example of NLP implementation in medicine, Murff et al. surveyed surgical inpatient admission records using the Multi-Threaded Clinical Vocabulary Server to identify postoperative complications and compare performance against manually coded complications.[54] While both manual review and NLP-based queries offered high specificity, the latter achieved significantly higher sensitivity particularly for identification of postoperative acute renal failure, sepsis, and pneumonia.

While still fledgling, NLP has been assessed for application in spine surgery primarily as a means of automated detection and surveillance of complications. Karhade et al. developed an NLP pipeline for the identification of incidental durotomy during spine surgery using free-text operative notes and benchmarked predictions against ground truth established by multiple independent expert review.[55] Post-tokenization feature importance was established based on term frequency-inverse document frequency, which seeks to quantify differential prevalence of candidate tokens between the documents of differing strata in the training set (in this case, classified by the presence of incidental durotomy). Downstream classification was performed using gradient-boosted decision trees and performance significantly higher than durotomy identification using CPT and ICD codes (AUROC of 0.99 vs. 0.64 in the test set); subsequent external validation confirmed robust model performance.[56] Similar approaches have been applied for the identification of other spinal pathologies, including low back pain,[57] surgical site infections,[58] and Modic type 1 endplate change.[59]

While few modern NLP approaches used for interpretation of clinical reports leverage deep learning models, studies in informatics and AI have suggested that deep CNNs may significantly improve model accuracy.[60] Machine automation of complex tasks, such as language translation and natural language interpretation (NLI), could spearhead significant shifts in applied clinical medicine.[61,62] For example, accurate translators may facilitate collaborative efforts to query aggregated clinical records from diverse geographic regions by facilitating information transfer and standardization. NLI, which includes subtasks such as sentiment analysis and question answering, may also increase care efficiency and effectiveness through task multithreading and intelligent understanding of written and spoken language (both in the physician-physician and physician-patient settings). However, estimations of current resource requirements for state-of-the-art NLP models such as BERT[63] and XLNet[64] suggest improved algorithm efficiency may be required for increased scalability.[60] Current industry efforts include those directed at increasing algorithm efficiency, such as the advent of the SustaiNLP 2020 workshop to emphasize sustainable NLP practices and exploration of more minimalistic model designs, such as qQRNN, which can approximate the performance of state-of-the-art approaches while reducing resource use by more than 300-fold.[65]

MACHINE LEARNING IN CLINICAL PRACTICE: SYNTHETIC CT AND PREDICTIVE ANALYTICS

In complex lumbar spine surgery, the combination of MRI and CT has long proven complementary.[41] While the strength of CT imaging lies in visualizing osseous structures and allows assessment of spinal integrity and stability, MRI excels at soft tissue imaging, including nervous tissue. Still, CT images are often required for neuronavigation and treatment planning, such as for image-guided navigated biopsies or pedicle screw placement.[66] CT inherently leads to radiation exposure, with an average lumbar spinal CT equaling an effective dose of around 3.5 mSv up to 19.5 mSv.[67–71] In addition, multiple imaging sessions increase the logistic burden for patients and healthcare providers alike, and also drive overall costs. The independent acquisition of both imaging modalities can also introduce complex workflows, with the potential for inter-modality registration errors.

For these reasons, MRI-only workflows, especially in radiotherapy, have increased markedly in recent years.[72,73] The ability to derive synthetic CT images from routinely collected MR sequences, which are usually mandated anyway in spine surgery due to the necessity of delineating the neural structures, without radiation and a second imaging session would thus prove beneficial. As detailed before, deep learning can at times enable tackling such complex tasks that may have appeared impossible beforehand.

Similarly, predictive analytics can guide decision-making by producing accurate and, most importantly, individualized risk profiles, also enabling more confident patient counseling preoperatively.

In the following two case presentations, we aim to demonstrate the clinical use of synthetic CT along with predictive analytics in instrumented lumbar spine surgery.

Please note that while pedicle screw trajectory planning was successfully performed using synthetic CTs and the robot workstation, pedicle screw insertion was effectively carried out based on spiral CT, as there is not yet an ethical and scientific basis to operate patients based on synthetic CT alone. The two cases are, however, real cases treated at our center using robotic guidance, and both pertain to lumbar spinal fusion augmented by the two aforementioned ML applications.

History and Clinical Presentation

Patient A

Patient A (female, 62 years) presented to us with predominant chronic low back pain (CLBP; Numeric Rating Scale [NRS] 7) as well as right-sided radiating pain in the L4 dermatome (NRS 5), and had previously undergone three decompression procedures at L3–L4 at another center, leading to a clinical conclusion of a failed back surgery syndrome (FBSS). Walking down stairs had become more difficult with the right leg. The patient had no left-sided complaints. Conservative therapy and analgesic interventions had no lasting effect; the patient was largely unable to work and indicated being unable to go on further with her CLBP. The adipose and hypertensive smoker was otherwise healthy and worked as a civil servant. The SCOAP-CERTAIN model predicted a high likelihood of clinically significant improvement in all of subjective functional impairment, back pain, and leg pain.[9] Prior to considering surgery, the patient was required by us to cease smoking and lose weight.

Patient B

Patient B (male, 53 years) presented to us with progressive mechanical low back pain upon standing up and walking that had been existing for over 17 years, without radiating leg pain, but with constant hypesthesia in the right thigh. Upon flexion, the pain increased in intensity. A pantaloon cast test (PCT)[74] was carried out to simulate a fusion procedure, which led to a 90% reduction in back pain and the disappearance of the hypesthesia. After the removal of the pantaloon cast (re-challenge), the patient again developed low back pain and hypesthesia in the right thigh. The patient had never undergone spine surgery before, but had undergone multiple analgesic interventions (facet blocks and thermolesional facet interventions at L5–S1). These interventions and other conservative therapies had no lasting effects. The patient was adipose but otherwise healthy, and the SCOAP-CERTAIN model predicted high chances of success after lumbar spinal fusion. We required the patient to lose weight to at least 100 kg before offering surgery.

Preoperative Imaging

Patient A

The preoperative imaging is demonstrated in Fig. 15.1, including MRI, spiral CT, and synthetic CT. The preoperative MRI demonstrated a status post-three-fold exploration at L3–L4 on the right side, severe discopathy at L3–L4, as well as facet joint degeneration at L3–L4 on the right side.

Patient B

The preoperative imaging is demonstrated in Fig. 15.1, including MRI, spiral CT, and synthetic CT, as well as a 3D-volume render and x-ray imaging. The preoperative MRI and CT demonstrate a bilateral spondylolysis of L5 with consequent Meyerding Grade 1 spondylolisthesis and the obliteration of both neuroforamina at L5–S1.

Surgical Plan

Patient A

Due to the unilateral radiculopathy and CLBP, we opted for a single-level, minimally invasive, robotic-guided, transforaminal lumbar interbody fusion (MI-TLIF) at L3–L4, as described before.[75] The pedicle screw trajectories were planned on a Mazor SpineAssist

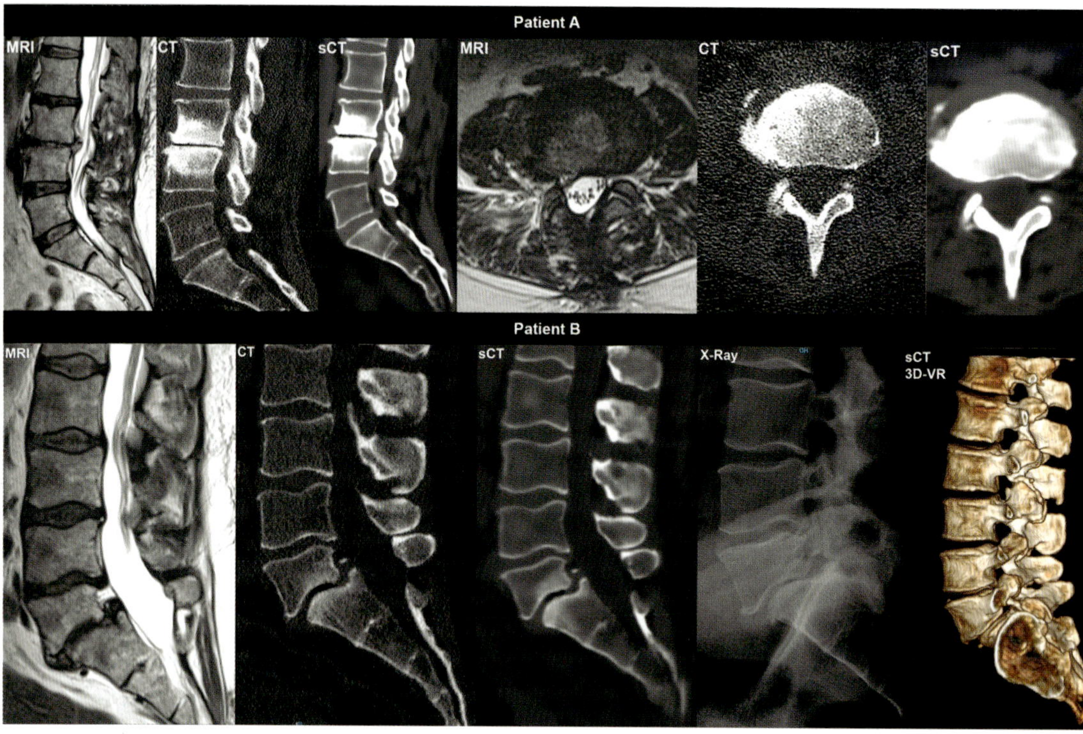

FIG. 15.1 *Patient A* is depicted in the top panel. It demonstrates preoperative imaging in sagittal and axial multiplanar reconstructions. T2-weighted MRI, conventional spiral CT, and synthetic CT (sCT) based on the BoneMRI technique are shown. *Patient B* is depicted in the bottom panel. It demonstrates preoperative imaging in a sagittal reconstruction. T2-weighted MRI, conventional spiral CT, and sCT based on the BoneMRI technique. In addition, the preoperative lumbosacral x-ray and a 3D-volume render based on the synthetic CT demonstrates spondylolisthesis due to the bilateral L5 spondylolysis.

workstation based on the synthetic CT derived using the BoneMRI technique (Fig. 15.2). The patient was included in our Enhanced Recovery After Surgery (ERAS) program.[76,77]

Patient B

Because of the bilateral neuroforaminal stenosis, we opted for a single-level, mini-open, robot-guided, posterior lumbar interbody fusion (PLIF) at L5–S1 as described before.[75] The pedicle screw trajectories were planned on a Mazor SpineAssist workstation based on the synthetic CT derived using the BoneMRI technique (see Fig. 15.2). The patient was included in our ERAS program.[76]

Intraoperative Imaging

In both cases, fluoroscopy was the only imaging technique applied intraoperatively. First, the correct spinal level was localized, and anteroposterior and oblique shots were taken to register the robot in relation to the patient. Fluoroscopy was also used to control the positioning of K-wires, cages, pedicle screws, and rods.

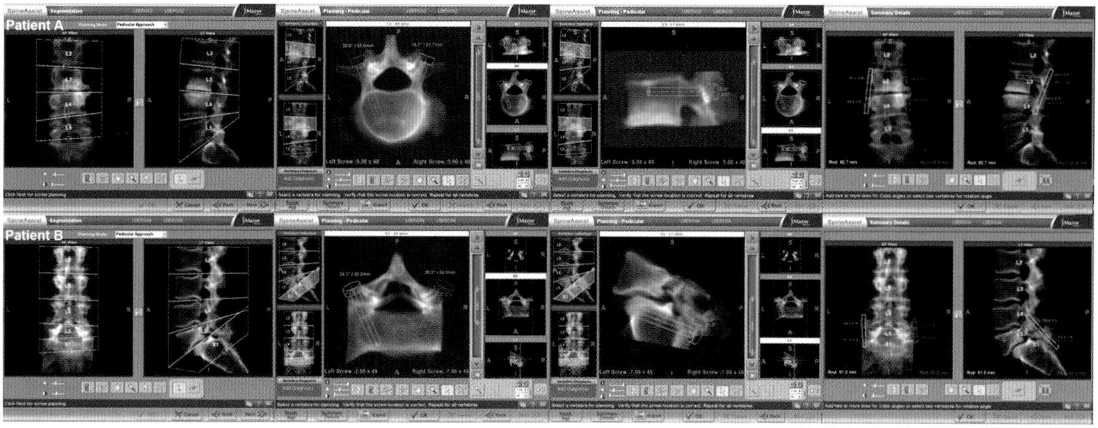

FIG. 15.2 The top panel (*Patient A*) demonstrates the planning process for an L3–L4 pedicle screw instrumentation on the Mazor Robotics SpineAssist workstation. The bottom panel (*Patient B*) demonstrates the planning process for an L5–S1 pedicle screw instrumentation on the Mazor Robotics SpineAssist workstation.

Postoperative Imaging

Both patients underwent radiological follow-up with lateral and anteroposterior lumbosacral x-ray imaging at 6 weeks and 12 months postoperatively. As demonstrated in Fig. 15.3, the position of the interbody cages and the pedicle screws was adequate at 12 months postoperatively, with beginning bony fusion in both cases. *Patient B's* spondylolisthesis was reduced by 6 mm.

Postoperative Recovery and Follow-Up

Patient A

The patient was mobilized on the morning of the first postoperative day and reported that, immediately after surgery, back and leg pain had somewhat improved. The patient was followed up clinically and radiographically at 6 weeks and 12 months postoperatively, where the patient indicated that the chief complaint of low back pain had regressed almost completely, and that the right-sided radiating leg pain was also significantly less but still present when lying down. The patient was discharged from follow-up after 12 months.

Patient B

The patient was swiftly mobilized on the same day after surgery and was discharged home the following morning. After surgery, the hypesthesia in the thigh was no longer present. Clinical and radiographic follow-ups at 6 weeks and 12 months postoperatively were carried out, where the patient reported the disappearance of the hypesthesia and clinically significant improvement of the low back pain. No complications were observed. The patient was discharged from follow-up after 12 months.

Procedural Concerns in Detail

Generation of Synthetic CTs

A research prototype of the BoneMRI synthetic CT generation method (BoneMRI, MRIguidance B.V., Utrecht, The Netherlands) was used.[41,78-80] The methods are laid out in more detail in Staartjes et al.[41] and Florkow et al.[78] The CT images were acquired in the

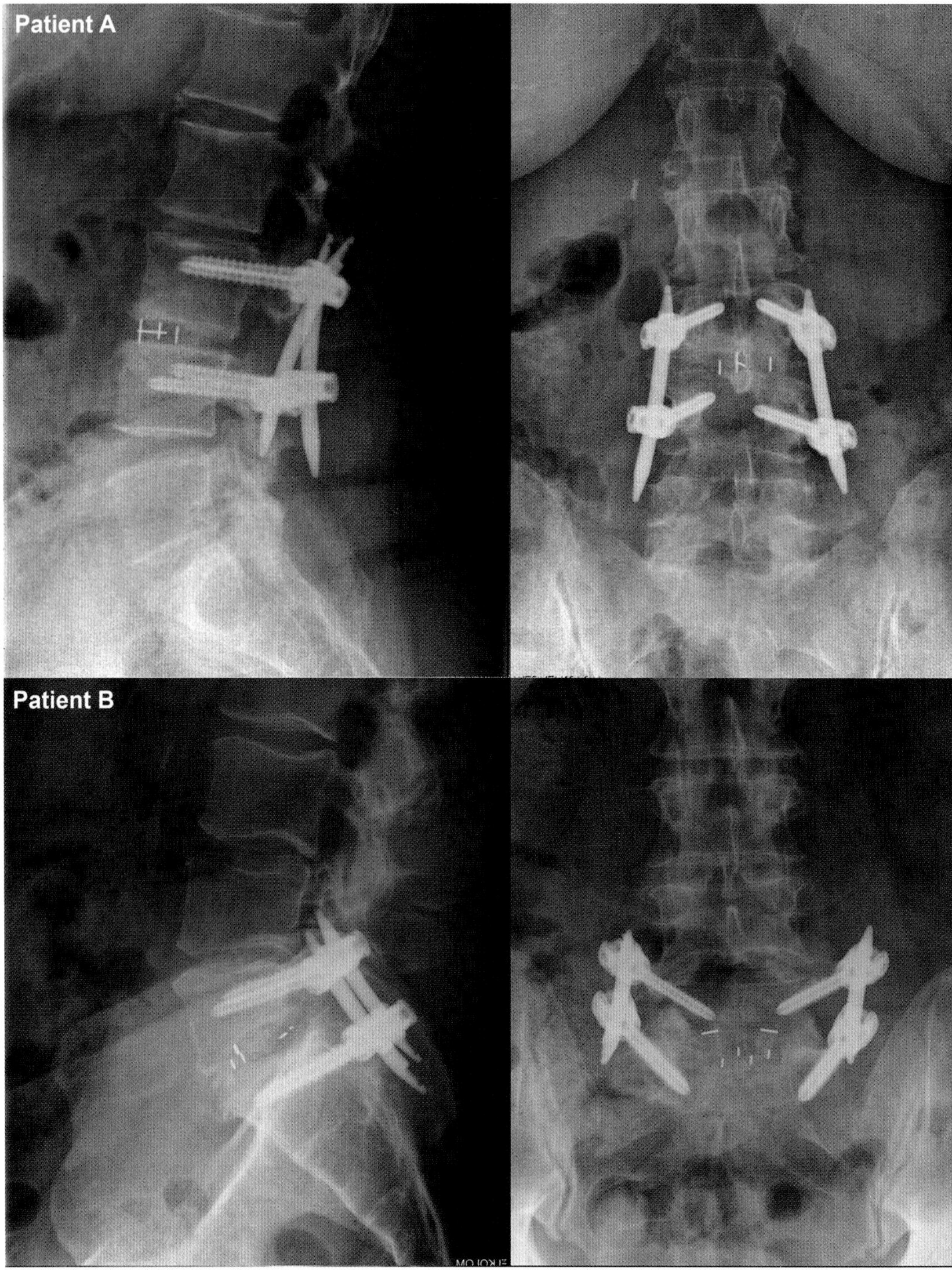

FIG. 15.3 Lateral and anterioposterior lumbosacral x-ray follow-up imaging at 12 months postoperatively, demonstrating the proper positioning of the cage and pedicle screws.

supine position using a Philips ICT 256 scanner (318 slices/1-mm thickness), while the MRI images were acquired in a fixed supine position using a Siemens Magnetom Essenza (1.5 T). A standard lumbar spine protocol including conventional T_1W and T_2W sequences (acquisition time = 15 min and 4 s), was complemented with a sagittal 3D rf-spoiled T_1-weighted multiple gradient echo (T_1W-MGE) sequence for BoneMRI reconstruction. The deep learning model was trained using paired MRI and CT data of eight patients scheduled for robotic lumbar spinal fusion. Synthetic CTs were generated from MRI inputs using a patch-based CNN.[41,78,81] These synthetic CTs were subsequently uploaded to a Mazor Robotics SpineAssist workstation.

Predictive Analytics of Outcome After Lumbar Spinal Fusion Surgery

To predict the likelihood of a clinically relevant improvement in subjective functional impairment (Oswestry Disability Index) and pain scores (back and leg pain) at 12 months after surgery, the spine surgical care and outcomes assessment program/comparative effectiveness translational network (SCOAP-CERTAIN) model described by Khor et al.[9] and externally validated by Quddusi et al.[10] was implemented. The model is based on logistic regression; includes several clinical input variables such as preoperative questionnaires, indications for surgery, and patient demographics; and has achieved AUROCs of 0.71 to 0.83 at external validation.[9,10] The SCOAP-CERTAIN model has been integrated as a freely accessible web app, making its clinical use feasible.

Treatment Side Effects

Elective lumbar spinal fusion for degenerative disease has a well-described complication profile.[75,82] Neither the generation of synthetic CTs nor predictive analytics are expected to lead to any additional side effects, although some potential downfalls and limitations have to be delineated.

Potential Downfalls

Synthetic CT is not yet established in spine surgery and is poorly validated. In patients with implants from prior surgeries or other artefactants such as aortic stents, neurostimulators, analgesic pumps, etc., the validity of a synthetic CT is currently unknown. Similarly, the method has not yet been validated in patients with for example, highly dysplastic or scoliotic pedicles, bone metastases, Modic type endplate changes, etc. In addition, although preliminary measurements have demonstrated that synthetic lumbar spinal CT is isometric to spiral CT to an extent that would allow navigated or robotic-guided surgery,[41] MRI is sometimes said to be inaccurate for distance measurements due to geometric distortions.[83] Further development and validation on larger cohorts are needed before clinically applying the method, which may also further improve the quality of the images produced. A case series is currently underway for clinical validation of the use of synthetic CT for near radiationless, accurate, robotic-guided surgery. As with any surgical adjunct, the technique may also fail outright and require conversion. In the early stages of adoption of the technique, it may be wise to have either an intraoperative CT or a preoperative spiral CT at hand as a backup, should registration fail to produce the necessary accuracy.

Concerning predictive analytics in medicine, the potential downfalls have been described in detail.[84] Apart from more mundane problems such as overfitting and poor external validation/generalization, the issue of extrapolation is critical. Predicting the future remains a virtually impossible task, not only due to the balance that has to be struck between creating parsimonious (i.e., simple enough to be used in clinical practice, e.g., regarding their inputs) models and providing extremely granular information about a patient to the model. Outcomes after spinal fusion are governed by thousands of influencing factors, of which the SCOAP-CERTAIN model, for example, takes only 22. Lastly, extrapolating not only into the future but also to even slightly different patient populations (i.e., deformity, pediatric patients, underrepresented demographics, patients with psychosomatic syndromes, and so forth) will almost certainly lead to erroneous results.

Management of Complications

For these reasons, techniques such as ML-based predictive analytics and synthetic imaging should only be used as ancillary tools in a large toolbox. Patient counseling should not rely too heavily on the predictions made by an algorithm, and diagnostic imaging as well as construct planning should not solely be carried out based upon the synthetic voxels generated by a deep neural network.

SUMMARY AND FUTURE DIRECTIONS

Continued advances in computing capability and data sharing will enable the advent of increasingly intricate ML approaches in spine surgery. As noted in the previous sections, the resource and computational costs associated with model training and parameter tuning present logistical barriers in the development of highly complex automated solutions to sophisticated medical tasks. The increased quantity and granularity of publicly available data may unveil opportunities to devise approaches of higher intricacy and to investigate events of extreme rarity. More broadly, increased inter-institutional collaboration may facilitate model benchmarking and validation in efforts to further optimize performance and generalizability. This section will review future directions for increasing AI integrations into clinical workflows to further guide spine surgery practice and outcomes.

Regarding outcome prediction, the focus of investigations should center around the development of models that provide insight into actionable aspects of the care process. Improvements in model design and performance are clinically significant only insofar as their ability to improve healthcare delivery, patient recovery, and long-term outcomes. For example, significant effort has been placed into defining risk classifiers able to predict pharmacological dependence and, more indirectly, durable pain management. The secondary investigations stemming from these models may therefore explore alternative pain management protocols earlier during the postsurgical (or even peri- and pre-surgical) periods in situations where long-term narcotic reliance is likely. Given this need to understand, to a certain extent, decision-making by predictive models, future efforts should emphasize interpretability and modularity. Furthermore, additional efforts to externally validate models using independently sourced data, preferably from diverse clinical settings, are necessary prior to incorporation in standard clinical practice.[85]

Given the increased difficulty of image and free-text interpretation, technical improvements on those frontiers will likely be more challenging. Apart from poor or missing external validation, there are other aspects that render scaling complex deep learning approaches to widespread clinical adoption relatively difficult. Often, the resulting models, particularly in imaging and NLP, are rather large and computationally expensive to run, which does not necessarily lend well to mobile- or tablet-based clinical applications. Naturally, mobile applications would constitute the most beneficial clinical use case for scaling deep learning models into daily practice. A potential solution to this issue is the implementation of algorithms into mobile web apps running the algorithm server-side. This however produces further issues regarding data security and privacy, as medical data are becoming increasingly traceable. For example, the upload of cranial imaging has recently been heavily discussed due to the fact that facial reconstructions can relatively easily be made from these images, rendering true anonymization difficult. The final issue in scaling these models to clinical practice is of a regulatory nature. Apart from approval processes, whenever algorithms would need to be updated with more training data to improve performance further, they essentially constitute a new medical device and require a new external validation study. The desired and frequently discussed "living algorithm" that improves over time through further input data could thus run aground not only due to issues with data privacy, but also regulatory challenges.

Image translation algorithms, while having previously gained interested in radiotherapy for MRI-only workflows,[86,87] has not yet reached its potential and is currently poorly adopted in spine surgery. The BoneMRI technique[41] demonstrated in our clinical vignettes is a deep learning-based method based on a specific, 4-minute MRI sequence, that, due to its dual-echo approach, can extract more information about proton density, water and fat fractions, relaxation constants, and susceptibility.[78] As demonstrated before,[41,79] the results of the BoneMRI technique appear promising in providing high-fidelity synthetic CT images from MRI, with reliable error margins for instrumented spine surgery.[41] The implementation of image translation algorithms in clinical spine surgery could lead to relevant improvements in overall logistic efficacy, and a reduction in total examination time, as well as the elimination of radiation exposure. In combination with neuronavigation or robotics, this could enable the concept of "radiationless navigated surgery" (RANAS), with the the use of computer assistance based on preoperative MRI imaging only and without the need for additional radiation, apart from intraoperative fluoroscopy for registration and control. Even when the benefits of intraoperative CT imaging in spine surgery are considered, one could imagine that, using image translation techniques, fast intraoperative MRI sequences could be used to reproduce radiationless bone imaging, especially considering that intraoperative MRI scanners are increasingly implemented in neurosurgical departments around the world, and that the BoneMRI sequence only runs for a total of 4 minutes. In the near future, however, we expect that the clinical applications of image translation will revolve around preoperative surgical planning for complex cases, implant sizing, and RANAS.

This research has not been previously submitted for review or presented at any conferences.

DISCLOSURES

Conflict of Interest: The authors declare that the article and its content were composed in the absence of any commercial or financial relationships that could be construed as a potential conflict of interest.

Grants and Support: This research did not receive any specific grant from funding agencies in the public, commercial, or not-for-profit sectors.

Ethical Considerations: The development and proof-of-concept testing of the model, and the associated use of patient data, was approved by the local ethical review board (Medical Ethics Committees United [MEC-U], Registration Number: W18.157). All patients signed informed consent forms that allow for the use of their data for research and publication purposes.

ACKNOWLEDGMENT

We thank Marijn van Stralen, PhD and Peter Seevinck, PhD of the Image Science Institute, University Medical Center Utrecht and MRIguidance B.V. for supplying the BoneMRI sequences.

REFERENCES

1. Shortliffe EH, Davis R, Axline SG, Buchanan BG, Green CC, Cohen SN. Computer-based consultations in clinical therapeutics: explanation and rule acquisition capabilities of the MYCIN system. *Comput Biomed Res.* 1975;8(4):303–320. https://doi.org/10.1016/0010-4809(75)90009-9.
2. Shortliffe EH, Axline SG, Buchanan BG, Merigan TC, Cohen SN. An artificial intelligence program to advise physicians regarding antimicrobial therapy. *Comput Biomed Res.* 1973;6(6):544–560. https://doi.org/10.1016/0010-4809(73)90029-3.
3. Fisher WS. Computer-aided intelligence: application of an expert system to brachial plexus injuries. *Neurosurgery.* 1990;27(5):837–843, discussion 843. https://doi.org/10.1227/00006123-199011000-00029.
4. Aloysius N, Geetha M. A review on deep convolutional neural networks. *Int Conf Commun Signal Process (ICCSP):2017 IEEE.* 2017:0588–0592. https://doi.org/10.1109/ICCSP.2017.8286426.
5. Castelvecchi D. Can we open the black box of AI? *Nature.* 2016;538(7623):20–23. https://doi.org/10.1038/538020a.
6. Buhrmester V, Münch D, Arens M. Analysis of explainers of black box deep neural networks for computer vision: a survey. *arXiv Prepr ArXiv.* 2019 1911.12116. Published online.
7. Goyal A, Ngufor C, Kerezoudis P, McCutcheon B, Storlie C, Bydon M. Can machine learning algorithms accurately predict discharge to nonhome facility and early unplanned readmissions following spinal fusion? Analysis of a national surgical registry: presented at the 2019 AANS/CNS Section on Disorders of the Spine and Peripheral Nerves. *J Neurosurg Spine.* 2019;31(4):1–11. https://doi.org/10.3171/2019.3.SPINE181367.
8. Siccoli A, de Wispelaere MP, Schröder ML, Staartjes VE. Machine learning–based preoperative predictive analytics for lumbar spinal stenosis. *Neurosurg Focus.* 2019;46(5):E5. https://doi.org/10.3171/2019.2.FOCUS18723.
9. Khor S, Lavallee D, Cizik AM, et al. Development and validation of a prediction model for pain and functional outcomes after lumbar spine surgery. *JAMA Surg.* 2018;153(7):634–642. https://doi.org/10.1001/jamasurg.2018.0072.
10. Quddusi A, Eversdijk HAJ, Klukowska AM, et al. External validation of a prediction model for pain and functional outcome after elective lumbar spinal fusion. *Eur Spine J.* 2020;29(2):374–383. https://doi.org/10.1007/s00586-019-06189-6.
11. Staartjes VE, de Wispelaere MP, Vandertop WP, Schröder ML. Deep learning-based preoperative predictive analytics for patient-reported outcomes following lumbar discectomy: feasibility of center-specific modeling. *Spine J.* 2019;19(5):853–861. https://doi.org/10.1016/j.spinee.2018.11.009.
12. Han SS, Azad TD, Suarez PA, Ratliff JK. A machine learning approach for predictive models of adverse events following spine surgery. *Spine J.* 2019;19(11):1772–1781. https://doi.org/10.1016/j.spinee.2019.06.018.
13. Arvind V, Kim JS, Oermann EK, Kaji D, Cho SK. Predicting surgical complications in adult patients undergoing anterior cervical discectomy and fusion using machine learning. *Neurospine.* 2018;15(4):329–337. https://doi.org/10.14245/ns.1836248.124.
14. Jin MC, Ho AL, Feng AY, et al. Predictive modeling of long-term opioid and benzodiazepine use after intradural tumor resection. *Spine J.* 2021;21(10):1687–1699. https://doi.org/10.1016/j.spinee.2020.10.010.
15. Karhade AV, Cha TD, Fogel HA, et al. Predicting prolonged opioid prescriptions in opioid-naive lumbar spine surgery patients. *Spine J.* 2020;20(6):888–895. https://doi.org/10.1016/j.spinee.2019.12.019.
16. Kuo CY, Yu LC, Chen HC, Chan CL. Comparison of models for the prediction of medical costs of spinal fusion in Taiwan diagnosis-related groups by machine learning algorithms. *Healthc Inf Res.* 2018;24(1):29–37. https://doi.org/10.4258/hir.2018.24.1.29.
17. DiSilvestro KJ, Veeramani A, McDonald CL, et al. Predicting postoperative mortality after metastatic intraspinal neoplasm excision: development of a machine-learning approach. *World Neurosurg.* 2021;146:e917–e924. https://doi.org/10.1016/j.wneu.2020.11.037.
18. Kim JS, Merrill RK, Arvind V, et al. Examining the ability of artificial neural networks machine learning models to accurately predict complications following posterior lumbar spine

fusion. *Spine*. 2018;43(12):853–860. https://doi.org/10.1097/BRS.0000000000002442.

19. Dreiseitl S, Ohno-Machado L. Logistic regression and artificial neural network classification models: a methodology review. *J Biomed Inf*. 2002;35(5–6):352–359. https://doi.org/10.1016/S1532-0464(03)00034-0.
20. McGrath H, Li P, Dorent R, et al. Manual segmentation versus semi-automated segmentation for quantifying vestibular schwannoma volume on MRI. *Int J Comput Assist Radiol Surg*. 2020;15(9):1445–1455. https://doi.org/10.1007/s11548-020-02222-y.
21. Doktor K, Jensen TS, Christensen HW, et al. Degenerative findings in lumbar spine MRI: an inter-rater reliability study involving three raters. *Chiropr Man Ther*. 2020;28(1):8. https://doi.org/10.1186/s12998-020-0297-0.
22. Carrino JA, Lurie JD, Tosteson ANA, et al. Lumbar spine: reliability of MR imaging findings. *Radiology*. 2009;250(1):161–170. https://doi.org/10.1148/radiol.2493071999.
23. Lewandrowski KU, Muraleedharan N, Eddy SA, et al. Reliability analysis of deep learning algorithms for reporting of routine lumbar MRI scans. *Int J Spine Surg*. 2020;14(s3):7132 https://doi.org/10.14444/7132. Published online on October 29, 2020.
24. Roth HR, Wang Y, Yao J, Lu L, Burns JE, Summers RM. Deep convolutional networks for automated detection of posterior-element fractures on spine CT. *Int Soc Opt Photonics*. 2016:97850P.
25. Duong L, Cheriet F, Labelle H. Automatic detection of scoliotic curves in posteroanterior radiographs. *IEEE Trans Bio Med Eng*. 2010;57(5):1143–1151. https://doi.org/10.1109/TBME.2009.2037214.
26. Baka N, Leenstra S, van Walsum T. Random forest-based bone segmentation in ultrasound. *Ultrasound Med Biol*. 2017;43(10):2426–2437. https://doi.org/10.1016/j.ultrasmedbio.2017.04.022.
27. Ciregan D, Meier U, Schmidhuber J. Multi-column deep neural networks for image classification. *IEEE*. 2012:3642–3649.
28. Ciresan D.C., Meier U., Masci J., Gambardella L.M., Schmidhuber J. Flexible, high performance convolutional neural networks for image classification. In: 2011.
29. Krizhevsky A, Sutskever I, Hinton GE. Imagenet classification with deep convolutional neural networks. *Adv Neural Inf Process Syst*. 2012;25:1097–1105. https://proceedings.neurips.cc/paper/2012/file/c399862d3b9d6b76c8436e924a68c45b-Paper.pdf.
30. Cong J, Xiao B. Minimizing computation in convolutional neural networks. In: Wermter S, Weber C, Duch W, eds. *Artificial Neural Networks and Machine Learning–ICANN 2014*. Springer International Publishing; 2014:281–290.
31. Li C, Yang Y, Feng M, Chakradhar S, Zhou H. Optimizing memory efficiency for deep convolutional neural networks on GPUs. *Interface Sci16: Int Conf High Perform Computing, Networking, Storage Anal IEEE*. 2016:633–644. https://doi.org/10.1109/SC.2016.53.
32. Dosovitskiy A, Beyer L, Kolesnikov A, et al. An image is worth 16 × 16 words: transformers for image recognition at scale. *arXiv Prepr ArXiv*. 2020. 2010.11929. Published online.
33. Pham H, Xie Q, Dai Z, Le QV. Meta pseudo labels. *arXiv Prepr ArXiv*. 2020:2003.10580. Published online.
34. Huang J, Shen H, Wu J, et al. Spine explorer: a deep learning based fully automated program for efficient and reliable quantifications of the vertebrae and discs on sagittal lumbar spine MR images. *Spine J*. 2020;20(4):590–599. https://doi.org/10.1016/j.spinee.2019.11.010.
35. McCoy DB, Dupont SM, Gros C, et al. Convolutional Neural Network. Convolutional Neural Network-Based automated segmentation of the spinal cord and contusion injury: deep learning biomarker correlates of motor impairment in acute spinal cord injury. *AJNR Am J Neuroradiol*. 2019;40(4):737–744. https://doi.org/10.3174/ajnr.A6020.
36. Ronneberger O, Fischer P, Brox T. *U-net: Convolutional networks for biomedical image segmentation. Lecture Notes in Computer Science*: Springer; 2015:234–241. https://doi.org/10.1007/978-3-319-24574-4-28.
37. Pfirrmann CW, Metzdorf A, Zanetti M, Hodler J, Boos N. Magnetic resonance classification of lumbar intervertebral disc degeneration. *Spine (Phila Pa 1976)*. 2001;26(17):1873–1878. https://doi.org/10.1097/00007632-200109010-00011.
38. Dice LR. Measures of the amount of ecologic association between species. *Ecology*. 1945;26(3):297–302. https://doi.org/10.2307/1932409.
39. Cai D, Wang Z, Liu Y, Zhang Q, Han X, Liu W. Automatic path planning for navigated pedicle screw surgery based on Deep. *Neural Network. IEEE*. 2019:62–67.
40. Cho W, Cho SK, Wu C. The biomechanics of pedicle screw-based instrumentation. *J Bone Jt Surg Br*. 2010;92(8):1061–1065. https://doi.org/10.1302/0301-620X.92B8.24237.
41. Staartjes VE, Seevinck PR, Vandertop WP, van Stralen M, Schröder ML. Magnetic resonance imaging-based synthetic computed tomography of the lumbar spine for surgical planning: a clinical proof-of-concept. *Neurosurg Focus*. 2021;50(1):E13. https://doi.org/10.3171/2020.10.FOCUS20801.
42. Sager N, Friedman C, Lyman M. Medical language processing: computer management of narrative data. 1987.
43. Wadia R, Akgun K, Brandt C, et al. Comparison of natural language processing and manual coding for the identification of cross-sectional imaging reports suspicious for lung cancer. *JCO Clin Cancer Inf*. 2018;2(2):1–7. https://doi.org/10.1200/CCI.17.00069.
44. Glaser AP, Jordan BJ, Cohen J, Desai A, Silberman P, Meeks JJ. Automated extraction of grade, stage, and quality information from transurethral resection of bladder tumor pathology reports using natural language processing. *JCO Clin Cancer Inf*. 2018;2:1–8. https://doi.org/10.1200/CCI.17.00128.
45. Henry J. Adoption of Electronic Health Record Systems among U.S. Non-Federal Acute Care Hospitals: 2008–2015: Office of the National Coordinator for Health Information Technology; 2008:15 Data Brief ONC:35.

46. Johnson AEW, Pollard TJ, Shen L, et al. MIMIC-III, a freely accessible critical care database. *Sci Data*. 2016;3(1):160035. https://doi.org/10.1038/sdata.2016.35.
47. Wang J, Deng H, Liu B, et al. Systematic evaluation of research progress on natural language processing in medicine over the past 20 years: bibliometric study on PubMed. *J Med Internet Res*. 2020;22(1):e16816. https://doi.org/10.2196/16816.
48. Friedman C. A broad-coverage natural language processing system. *Proc AMIA Symp*. 2000:270–274. Published online.
49. Savova GK, Masanz JJ, Ogren PV, et al. Mayo clinical Text Analysis and Knowledge Extraction System (cTAKES): architecture, component evaluation and applications. *J Am Med Inf Assoc*. 2010;17(5):507–513. https://doi.org/10.1136/jamia.2009.001560.
50. Aronson AR, Lang FM. An overview of MetaMap: historical perspective and recent advances. *J Am Med Inf Assoc*. 2010;17(3):229–236. https://doi.org/10.1136/jamia.2009.002733.
51. Stearns MQ, Price C, Spackman KA, Wang AY. SNOMED Clinical Terms: overview of the development process and project status. Proceedings: AMIA Symposium; 2001:662–666.
52. Donnelly K. SNOMED-CT: the advanced terminology and coding system for eHealth. *Stud Health Technol Inf*. 2006;121:279.
53. Elkin PL, Brown SH, Husser CS, et al. Evaluation of the content coverage of SNOMED CT: ability of SNOMED clinical terms to represent clinical problem lists. *Mayo Clin Proc*. 2006;81(6):741–748. https://doi.org/10.4065/81.6.741.
54. Murff HJ, FitzHenry F, Matheny ME, et al. Automated identification of postoperative complications within an electronic medical record using natural language processing. *JAMA*. 2011;306(8):848–855. https://doi.org/10.1001/jama.2011.1204.
55. Karhade AV, Bongers MER, Groot OQ, et al. Natural language processing for automated detection of incidental durotomy. *Spine J*. 2020;20(5):695–700. https://doi.org/10.1016/j.spinee.2019.12.006.
56. Ehresman J, Pennington Z, Karhade AV, et al. Incidental durotomy: predictive risk model and external validation of natural language process identification algorithm. *J Neurosurg Spine*. 2020;33(3):1–7. https://doi.org/10.3171/2020.2.SPINE20127.
57. Tan WK, Hassanpour S, Heagerty PJ, et al. Comparison of natural language processing rules-based and machine-learning systems to identify lumbar spine imaging findings related to low back pain. *Acad Rad*. 2018;25(11):1422–1432. https://doi.org/10.1016/j.acra.2018.03.008.
58. Thirukumaran CP, Zaman A, Rubery PT, et al. Natural language processing for the identification of surgical site infections in orthopaedics. *J Bone Jt Surg*. 2019;101(24):2167–2174. https://doi.org/10.2106/JBJS.19.00661.
59. Huhdanpaa HT, Tan WK, Rundell SD, et al. Using natural language processing of free-text radiology reports to identify Type 1 Modic endplate changes. *J Digit Imaging*. 2018;31(1):84–90. https://doi.org/10.1007/s10278-017-0013-3.
60. Strubell E, Ganesh A, McCallum A. *Energy and Policy Considerations for Deep Learning in NLP. Proceedings of the 57th Annual Meeting of the Association for Computational Linguistics*. Association for Computational Linguistics; 2019:3645–3650. https://doi.org/10.18653/v1/P19-1355.
61. Peters ME, Neumann M, Iyyer M, et al. Deep contextualized word representations. *arXiv Prepr ArXiv*. 2018:180205365. Published online.
62. So D, Le Q, Liang C. *The evolved transformer. PMLR*. 2019:5877–5886.
63. Devlin J, Chang M-W, Lee K, Toutanova K. BERT: pre-training of deep bidirectional transformers for language understanding. *arXiv Prepr ArXiv*. 2018:181004805. Published online.
64. Yang Z, Dai Z, Yang Y, Carbonell J, Salakhutdinov R, Le QV. Xlnet: generalized autoregressive pretraining for language understanding. *arXiv Prepr ArXiv*. 2019:190608237. Published online.
65. Kaliamoorthi P, Siddhant A, Li E, Johnson M. Distilling large language models into tiny and effective students using pQRNN. *arXiv Prepr ArXiv*. 2021:210108890. Published online.
66. Härtl R, Lam KS, Wang J, Korge A, Kandziora F, Audigé L. Worldwide survey on the use of navigation in spine surgery. *World Neurosurg*. 2013;79(1):162–172. https://doi.org/10.1016/j.wneu.2012.03.011.
67. Bohl DD, Hijji FY, Massel DH, et al. Patient knowledge regarding radiation exposure from spinal imaging. *Spine J*. 2017;17(3):305–312. https://doi.org/10.1016/j.spinee.2016.09.017.
68. Biswas D, Bible JE, Bohan M, Simpson AK, Whang PG, Grauer JN. Radiation exposure from musculoskeletal computerized tomographic scans. *J Bone Jt Surg Am*. 2009;91(8):1882–1889. https://doi.org/10.2106/JBJS.H.01199.
69. Lin EC. Radiation risk from medical imaging. *Mayo Clin Proc*. 2010;85(12):1142–1146, quiz 1146. https://doi.org/10.4065/mcp.2010.0260.
70. Papachristodoulou A, Pliamis N, Volford G, et al. Radiation Dose of Lumbar Spine CT: Analysis and Comparison Between Different Modes of Acquisition in Two European Imaging Centers. ECR 2016 Epos. https://epos.myesr.org/poster/esr/ecr2016/C-2386. Accessed August 22, 2020.
71. Richards PJ, George J, Metelko M, Brown M. Spine computed tomography doses and cancer induction. *Spine*. 2010;35(4):430–433. https://doi.org/10.1097/BRS.0b013e3181cdde47.
72. De Silva T, Uneri A, Ketcha MD, et al. Registration of MRI to intraoperative radiographs for target localization in spinal interventions. *Phys Med Biol*. 2017;62(2):684–701. https://doi.org/10.1088/1361-6560/62/2/684.
73. Owrangi AM, Greer PB, Glide-Hurst CK. MRI-only treatment planning: benefits and challenges. *Phys Med Biol*. 2018;63(5):05TR01. https://doi.org/10.1088/1361-6560/aaaca4.

74. Staartjes VE, Vergroesen P-PA, Zeilstra DJ, Schröder ML. Identifying subsets of patients with single-level degenerative disc disease for lumbar fusion: the value of prognostic tests in surgical decision making. *Spine J*. 2018;18(4):558–566. https://doi.org/10.1016/j.spinee.2017.08.242.
75. Schröder ML, Staartjes VE. Revisions for screw malposition and clinical outcomes after robot-guided lumbar fusion for spondylolisthesis. *Neurosurg Focus*. 2017;42(5):E12. https://doi.org/10.3171/2017.3.FOCUS16534.
76. Staartjes VE, de Wispelaere MP, Schröder ML. Improving recovery after elective degenerative spine surgery: 5-year experience with an enhanced recovery after surgery (ERAS) protocol. *Neurosurg Focus*. 2019;46(4):E7. https://doi.org/10.3171/2019.1.FOCUS18646.
77. Wang MY, Chang P-Y, Grossman J. Development of an Enhanced Recovery After Surgery (ERAS) approach for lumbar spinal fusion. *J Neurosurg Spine*. 2017;26(4):411–418. https://doi.org/10.3171/2016.9.SPINE16375.
78. Florkow MC, Zijlstra F, Willemsen K, et al. Deep learning-based MR-to-CT synthesis: the influence of varying gradient echo-based MR images as input channels. *Magn Reson Med*. 2020;83(4):1429–1441. https://doi.org/10.1002/mrm.28008.
79. van der Kolk BYM, van Stralen M, Podlogar M, et al. Reconstruction of Osseous Structures in MRI Scans of the Cervical Spine With BoneMRI: A Quantitative Analysis. ASNR Meeting. 2018.
80. van Stralen M, Podlogar M, Hendrikse J, et al. Bone MRI of the Cervical Spine: Deep Learning-Based Radiodensity Contrast Generation for Selective Visualization of Osseous Structures. *ISMRM Meeting*. 2019.
81. Cui Z, Yang J, Qiao Y. Brain MRI segmentation with patch-based CNN approach. In *CCC 35th Chinese Control Conference* 2016:7026–7031. https://doi.org/10.1109/ChiCC.2016.7554465.
82. Wong AP, Smith ZA, Stadler JA, et al. Minimally invasive transforaminal lumbar interbody fusion (MI-TLIF): Surgical technique, long-term 4-year prospective outcomes, and complications compared with an open TLIF cohort. *Neurosurg Clin N Am*. 2014;25(2):279–304. https://doi.org/10.1016/j.nec.2013.12.007.
83. Rogers JJ. NEMA Standards Publication MS. 1991. Published online; 2008;14:6.
84. Kernbach JM, Staartjes .VE. Machine learning-based clinical prediction modeling—a practical guide for clinicians. arXiv:200615069 [cs, stat]. 2020. http://arxiv.org/abs/2006.15069. Accessed March 13, 2021.
85. König IR, Malley JD, Weimar C, Diener HC, Ziegler A. German Stroke Study Collaboration. Practical experiences on the necessity of external validation. *Stat Med*. 2007;26(30):5499–5511. https://doi.org/10.1002/sim.3069.
86. Pollard JM, Wen Z, Sadagopan R, Wang J, Ibbott GS. The future of image-guided radiotherapy will be MR guided. *Br J Radiol*. 2017;90(1073):20160667. https://doi.org/10.1259/bjr.20160667.
87. Dirix P, Haustermans K, Vandecaveye V. The value of magnetic resonance imaging for radiotherapy planning. *Semin Radiat Oncol*. 2014;24(3):151–159. https://doi.org/10.1016/j.semradonc.2014.02.003.

16

Databases, Study Groups, and Evidence in Robotic Spine Surgery

Jason I. Liounakos, MD, Anand Veeravagu, MD, FAANS, and Michael Y. Wang, MD, FAANS

INTRODUCTION

A large amount of literature related to spine surgery is plagued by retrospective design and small sample sizes resulting in a lack of statistical power. This is particularly true for literature regarding the validation of cutting-edge technologies, including robotic guidance systems.[1–4] The methods by which researchers have attempted to provide studies of a higher yield than small institutional case series and cohort studies include the utilization of large administrative databases and forming multicenter study groups. This chapter will discuss the current evidence for robotic-assisted spine surgery and the importance of database utilization in research, particularly in the context of multicenter spinal robotics study groups.

CURRENT EVIDENCE FOR ROBOTIC-ASSISTED SPINE SURGERY

The majority of literature available for robotic-assisted spine surgery centers on the accuracy of pedicle screw placement and is often compared to other techniques including freehand and CT navigation. The Gertzbein and Robbins (GR) classification[5] is typically used to grade the accuracy of screw placement, with accurate screws defined as those meeting either GR A (no breach) or B (breach <2 mm) criteria. The Ravi classification is also used.[6] Numerous studies have reaffirmed the high accuracy of robotic-assisted pedicle screw placement since the FDA approval of the first robotic system in 2004. Multiple studies have verified the high accuracy of SpineAssist® (Mazor Robotics Ltd., Caesarea, Israel), with screws graded GR A or B ranging from 93.4% to 98.3%.[7,8] A 2017 randomized controlled trial compared minimally invasive robotic-assisted and fluoroscopic-guided spinal fusions, utilizing the Renaissance® (Mazor Robotics Ltd., Caesarea, Israel) robotic guidance system.[9] The study graded 97.7% of pedicle screws placed as GR A and 2.3% as GR B.[9] Four studies have directly evaluated the accuracy of the Mazor X™ robotic guidance system (Medtronic, Dublin, Ireland) with clinical accuracy ranging from 97.5% to 100%.[2,10–12] Further studies of recent generation robotic guidance systems have reaffirmed these high accuracy rates. At present, only seven studies have evaluated the accuracy of thoracolumbar pedicle screw placement with the current generation of navigated robotic guidance systems including the

TABLE 16.1 Summary of Accuracy Data Related to Current Generation Navigated Robotic Guidance Systems

Reference	Study Type	Device	Technique	Number of Patients	Number of Robotically Placed Screws	Screw Accuracy	Screw Grading
O'Connor et al.[17]	Technical note	Mazor XSE	Not Specified	Not specified	90	100% (A)	GR
Godzik et al.[18]	Retrospective case series	ExcelsiusGPS	Percutaneous	31	116	96.6% (1) / 2.59% (2)	Ravi
Jiang et al.[3]	Retrospective cohort study	ExcelsiusGPS	Both - open and percutaneous	24	113	86.7% (A) / 10.6% (B)	GR
Vardiman et al.[16]	Retrospective case series	ExcelsiusGPS	Percutaneous	56	348	97.7% (A or B)	GR
Jain et al.[15]	Retrospective case series	ExcelsiusGPS	Both - open and percutaneous	101	636	99% (A or B)	GR
Benech et al.[19]	Retrospective case series	ExcelsiusGPS	Percutaneous	53	292	98.3% (A or B)	GR
Fayed et al.[14]	Retrospective cohort study	ExcelsiusGPS	Percutaneous	20	100	94.2% (A) / 3.88% (B)	GR

GR, Gertzbein and Robbins Classification.

Mazor X Stealth Edition™ (XSE) (Medtronic, Dublin, Ireland) and ExcelsiusGPS™ (Globus Medical Inc, Audubon, Pennsylvania) (Table 16.1). These studies report accuracy ranging from 97.3% to 100%.[13–19]

Multiple studies exist comparing robotic-assisted surgery with CT navigation and fluoroscopic-guided techniques.[1,13,20–23] These individual studies suggest equal to superior accuracy with robotic assistance, while minimizing radiation burden and complications. However, these studies are limited primarily by their retrospective nature and small sample sizes. This is confirmed by four systematic reviews with the consensus being that while robotic-assisted spine surgery may have potential benefits, the available literature contains significant limitations and heterogeneity that precludes a complete comparison with conventional techniques (Table 16.2).[24–27] Moreover, compared to determinations of accuracy, few studies have explored the postoperative complication rates and associated readmissions and surgical revisions. In fact, a recent meta-analysis comparing robotic assistance with CT navigation and fluoroscopic guidance for thoracolumbar instrumented fusion surgeries was unable to make any conclusions about differences in complication rates due to the lack of robotic data.[26] Likely owing to a lack of single institutional data, some have turned to large administrative databases to explore this subject. The turn to database research has not been without challenges, however. For example, studies attempting to identify robotic-assisted procedures using billing codes will not be able to differentiate between robotic guidance and other forms of navigation, as a specific CPT code for robotic guidance does not currently exist. For this reason, and to be discussed in further detail later, an answer may lie in large multicenter institutional databases built with a focus on robotic surgery. Through our own inter-institution collaboration, we recently published the results of a retrospective analysis of a prospective database comparing free-hand with robotic-assisted thoracolumbar fusion

TABLE 16.2 Summary of Systematic Reviews Evaluating Robotic Guidance Systems

Reference	Comparison Groups	Number of Studies	Findings	Conclusions
Yu et al.[24]	RA, Free-hand	9	No differences in accuracy, complication rate, radiation exposure	Future well-designed studies are necessary to adequately compare techniques
Staartjes et al.[25]	RA, Navigation, Free-hand	37	Decreased rate of postoperative screw revisions in navigation and RA compared to free-hand	RA has potential to reduce incidence of revisions related to screw malposition
Siccoli et al.[26]	RA, Navigation, Free-hand	32	No differences in radiation, length of surgery, EBL, LOS, or complication rate for RA compared to free-hand	Findings attributable to a lack of statistical power; future high-quality studies required
Joseph et al.[27]	RA	25	RA accuracy 85%–100%	RA associated with high degree of implant placement accuracy

EBL, Estimated blood loss; *LOS*, length of stay; *RA*, robotic-assisted.

surgery. We found an 83.20% reduction in the overall 90-day complication rate associated with robotic guidance ($P < .001$).[23] While these results show promise, further research into the overall postoperative complication, revision, and readmission rates, as well as long-term patient outcomes for robotic-assisted spine surgery will be necessary and likely take center stage in the near future.

DATABASE UTILIZATION

Database research in spine surgery has increased significantly over the past 20 years. Government-maintained administrative databases, as well as national organization-affiliated databases tracking the quality and outcomes of healthcare delivery, contain enormous amounts of data for analysis. The large heterogenous sample sizes and resulting high statistical power constitute a primary benefit of database research. Heterogeneity among both institutions and locales also decreases the risk of institutional/regional biases and helps standardize the available data. In addition, database research largely circumvents the need for costly and time-consuming institutional review board applications. On the other hand, database research is not without limitations. Large administrative databases can be difficult to process and statistical analysis can be challenging. The data may contain inconsistencies, coding errors, or be incomplete and it may be impossible to determine the degree to which any of these potential issues are present. Finally, the researcher is dependent on the available data to formulate clinical questions, limiting the analyses that may be performed.

Several large national databases currently exist and have been featured in spine research, including but not limited to the National Inpatient Sample (NIS), Medicare claims databases, private insurance databases, and the American College of Surgeons—National Surgical Quality Improvement Project (ACS-NSQIP).[28] The NIS is the largest public inpatient healthcare database and contains information regarding the inpatient utilization of resources, access, charges, quality, and outcomes.[29] Medicare and other private insurance claims databases also collect data related to charges and, importantly, contain data beyond that of just the inpatient admission. The ACS-NSQIP also has distinct advantages in that its data is derived from clinical charts and is not based on insurance claims or billing data.

In addition, the data is both risk-adjusted and case-mix-adjusted and contains data through 30 days postoperatively, avoiding inpatient bias.[30] Completely understanding the advantages and disadvantages of each major database, as well as the scope of the included data, is critical for study formulation and execution.

STUDY GROUPS IN SPINE SURGERY

In much the same fashion as a think tank, multicenter study groups bring like-minded individuals with a passion for research and innovation together in order to produce high-quality research and advance the field of spine surgery. Several major study groups today include the International Spine Study Group (ISSG), Harms Study Group (HSG), and the European Spine Study Group (ESSG). Central to these organizations is the development of their own respective databases to evaluate clinical outcomes in spine surgery. These databases possess many of the advantages of the aforementioned large administrative databases but are clinically generated and constructed by individuals with a high-level understanding of the degree of granularity needed to address many of the current questions in this field adequately. This granularity, combined with large sample sizes and minimized practitioner and institutional bias, provides the basis for the publication of high-quality studies. Just as large administrative databases, like the NIS, are well powered to analyze rare conditions and special patient populations, focused study groups with a special interest in cutting-edge technologies, such as spinal robotics, are well suited to evaluate these less widely utilized surgical tools.

COMBINING METHODOLOGIES: SPINAL ROBOTICS STUDY GROUPS AND DATABASES

In order to increase the power of research studies (a main criticism of robotics research) and gather a large amount of granular data, the formation of study groups with a special interest in spinal robotics with the goal of producing large clinical databases is necessary. By bringing together leaders in the field of robotics and combining clinical data from multiple institutions we may produce large datasets of sufficient granularity and sample size to draw more meaningful conclusions about the true impact of robotics on spine surgery. Most recently, our center, along with eight others, came together to form the first spinal robotics study group. While still in its infancy, the retrospective database produced by the joint efforts of the members led to the construction of a database of over 1000 robotic-assisted operations with well over 5000 thoracolumbar pedicle screws placed.

There are several salient aspects of database construction that need to be emphasized in order to improve the ease at which data is collected and to avoid missed fields that may result in unnecessary and time-consuming revisions. Databases should first and foremost capture all the possible fields which may foreseeably be used for data analysis. This includes all the data related to patient demographics and comorbidities, which could potentially be used for propensity-matching. Specific data related to robotic utilization are important and the majority of this data can be pulled directly from the robotic system. This includes information related to specific utilization times and time-per-screw placement, as well as changes to trajectories and screw revisions. Perhaps the most important information moving forward however is that related to patient-reported outcome measures (PROMs), such as Visual Analog Scale (VAS) and Oswestry Disability Index (ODI) scores, collected both preoperatively and postoperatively with long-term follow-up. Given the recent emphasis on value-based care and outcomes, this information will be critical in establishing whether robotic-assisted spine surgery provides true value over the conventional approaches. While the initial databases will be retrospective, the shift to prospectively collected data will be critical in order to increase the research quality and impact of our conclusions.

SUMMARY

Large, ideally prospective, multi-institution databases built specifically to study robotic-assisted spine surgery are necessary to fully understand its true value over conventional approaches. Such databases will improve upon the limitations of current single-institution (limited sample sizes with underpowered studies, institutional biases, inadequate comparator groups) and large administrative databases (inconsistent data, inpatient bias, coding errors, lack of granularity, inability to differentiate robotic-assisted surgery from other forms of navigation). While the accuracy and safety of robotic guidance has already been established, large-volume, outcomes-based studies will be most important in the future. One of the ways to meet this need will be through the construction and expansion of multicenter spinal robotics study groups.

REFERENCES

1. Schatlo B, Molliqaj G, Cuvinciuc V, Kotowski M, Schaller K, Tessitore E. Safety and accuracy of robot-assisted versus fluoroscopy-guided pedicle screw insertion for degenerative diseases of the lumbar spine: A matched cohort comparison. *J Neurosurg Spine*. 2014;20(6):636–643. https://doi.org/10.3171/2014.3.SPINE13714.
2. Mao G, Gigliotti MJ, Myers D, Yu A, Whiting D. Single-Surgeon Direct Comparison of O-arm *Neuronavigation versus Mazor* X Robotic-Guided Posterior Spinal Instrumentation. *World Neurosurg*. 2020;137:e278–e285. https://doi.org/10.1016/j.wneu.2020.01.175.
3. Jiang B, Pennington Z, Azad T, et al. Robot-assisted versus freehand instrumentation in short-segment lumbar fusion: experience with real-time image-guided spinal robot. *World Neurosurg*. 2020;136:e635–e645. https://doi.org/10.1016/j.wneu.2020.01.119.
4. Solomiichuk V, Fleischhammer J, Molliqaj G, et al. Robotic versus fluoroscopy-guided pedicle screw insertion for metastatic spinal disease: a matched-cohort comparison. *Neurosurg Focus*. 2017;42(5):E13. https://doi.org/10.3171/2017.3.FOCUS1710.
5. Keric N, Doenitz C, Haj A, et al. Evaluation of robot-guided minimally invasive implantation of 2067 pedicle screws. *Neurosurg Focus*. 2017;42(5):E11. https://doi.org/10.3171/2017.2.FOCUS16552.
6. Gertzbein SD, Robbins SE. Accuracy of pedicular screw placement in vivo. *Spine (Phila Pa 1976)*. 1990;15(1):11–14. https://doi.org/10.1097/00007632-199001000-00004.
7. Ravi B, Zahrai A, Rampersaud R. Clinical accuracy of computer-assisted two-dimensional fluoroscopy for the percutaneous placement of lumbosacral pedicle screws. *Spine (Phila Pa 1976)*. 2011;36(1):84–91. https://doi.org/10.1097/BRS.0b013e3181cbfd09.
8. Devito DP, Kaplan L, Dietl R, et al. Clinical acceptance and accuracy assessment of spinal implants guided with SpineAssist surgical robot: retrospective study. *Spine (Phila Pa 1976)*. 2010;35(24):2109–2115. https://doi.org/10.1097/BRS.0b013e3181d323ab.
9. Molliqaj G, Schatlo B, Alaid A, et al. Accuracy of robot-guided versus freehand fluoroscopy-assisted pedicle screw insertion in thoracolumbar spinal surgery. *Neurosurg Focus*. 2017;42(5):E14. https://doi.org/10.3171/2017.3.FOCUS179.
10. Hyun SJ, Kim KJ, Jahng TA, Kim HJ. Minimally invasive robotic versus open fluoroscopic-guided spinal instrumented fusions: a randomized controlled trial. *Spine (Phila Pa 1976)*. 2017;42(6):353–358. https://doi.org/10.1097/BRS.0000000000001778.
11. Khan A, Meyers JE, Yavorek S, et al. Comparing next-generation robotic technology with 3-dimensional computed tomography navigation technology for the insertion of posterior pedicle screws. *World Neurosurg*. 2019;123:e474–e481. https://doi.org/10.1016/j.wneu.2018.11.190.
12. Khan A, Meyers JE, Siasios I, Pollina J. Next-generation robotic spine surgery: first report on feasibility, safety, and learning curve. *Oper Neurosurg (Hagerstown)*. 2019;17(1):61–69. https://doi.org/10.1093/ons/opy280.
13. Huntsman KT, Ahrendtsen LA, Riggleman JR, Ledonio CG. Robotic-assisted navigated minimally invasive pedicle screw placement in the first 100 cases at a single institution.

J Robot Surg. 2020;14(1):199–203. https://doi.org/10.1007/s11701-019-00959-6.

14. Fayed I, Tai A, Triano M, et al. Robot-assisted percutaneous pedicle screw placement: evaluation of accuracy of the first 100 screws and comparison with cohort of fluoroscopy-guided screws. *World Neurosurg.* 2020;143:e492–e502. https://doi.org/10.1016/j.wneu.2020.07.203.
15. Jain D, Manning J, Lord E, et al. Initial single-institution experience with a novel robotic-navigation system for thoracolumbar pedicle screw and pelvic screw placement with 643 screws. *Int J Spine Surg.* 2019;13(5):459–463. https://doi.org/10.14444/6060.
16. Vardiman AB, Wallace DJ, Crawford NR, Riggleman JR, Ahrendtsen LA, Ledonio CG. Pedicle screw accuracy in clinical utilization of minimally invasive navigated robot-assisted spine surgery. *J Robot Surg.* 2020;14(3):409–413. https://doi.org/10.1007/s11701-019-00994-3.
17. O'Connor TE, O'Hehir MM, Khan A, et al. Mazor X stealth robotic technology: a technical note. *World Neurosurg.* 2021;145:435–442. https://doi.org/10.1016/j.wneu.2020.10.010.
18. Godzik J, Walker CT, Hartman C, et al. A quantitative assessment of the accuracy and reliability of robotically guided percutaneous pedicle screw placement: technique and application accuracy. *Oper Neurosurg (Hagerstown).* 2019;17(4):389–395. https://doi.org/10.1093/ons/opy413.
19. Benech CA, Perez R, Benech F, Greeley SL, Crawford N, Ledonio C. Navigated robotic assistance results in improved screw accuracy and positive clinical outcomes: an evaluation of the first 54 cases. *J Robot Surg.* 2020;14(3):431–437. https://doi.org/10.1007/s11701-019-01007-z.
20. Kochanski RB, Lombardi JM, Laratta JL, Lehman RA, O'Toole JE. Image-guided navigation and robotics in spine surgery. *Neurosurgery.* 2019;84(6):1179–1189. https://doi.org/10.1093/neuros/nyy630.
21. Fichtner J, Hofmann N, Rienmüller A, et al. Revision rate of misplaced pedicle screws of the thoracolumbar spine-comparison of three-dimensional fluoroscopy navigation with freehand placement: a systematic analysis and review of the literature. *World Neurosurg.* 2018;109:e24–e32. https://doi.org/10.1016/j.wneu.2017.09.091.
22. Jamshidi AM, Massel DH, Liounakos JI, et al. Fluoroscopy time analysis of a prospective, multi-centre study comparing robotic- and fluoroscopic-guided placement of percutaneous pedicle screw instrumentation for short segment minimally invasive lumbar fusion surgery. *Int J Med Robot.* 2021;17(2):e2188. https://doi.org/10.1002/rcs.2188.
23. Liounakos JI, Kumar V, Jamshidi A, et al. Reduction in complication and revision rates for robotic-guided short-segment lumbar fusion surgery: results of a prospective, multi-center study. *J Robot Surg.* 2021;15(5):793–802. https://doi.org/10.1007/s11701-020-01165-5.
24. Yu L, Chen X, Margalit A, Peng H, Qiu G, Qian W. Robot-assisted vs. freehand pedicle screw fixation in spine surgery—a systematic review and a meta-analysis of comparative studies. *Int J Med Robot.* 2018;14(3):e1892. https://doi.org/10.1002/rcs.1892.
25. Staartjes VE, Klukowska AM, Schröder ML. Pedicle screw revision in robot-guided, navigated, and freehand thoracolumbar instrumentation: a systematic review and meta-analysis. *World Neurosurg.* 2018;116:433–443.e8. https://doi.org/10.1016/j.wneu.2018.05.159.
26. Siccoli A, Klukowska AM, Schröder ML, Staartjes VE. A systematic review and meta-analysis of perioperative parameters in robot-guided, navigated, and freehand thoracolumbar pedicle screw instrumentation. *World Neurosurg.* 2019;127:576–587.e5. https://doi.org/10.1016/j.wneu.2019.03.196.
27. Joseph JR, Smith BW, Liu X, Park P. Current applications of robotics in spine surgery: a systematic review of the literature. *Neurosurg Focus.* 2017;42(5):E2. https://doi.org/10.3171/2017.2.FOCUS16544.
28. Sebastian AS. Database research in spine surgery. *Clin Spine Surg.* 2016;29(10):427–429. https://doi.org/10.1097/BSD.0000000000000464.
29. Overview of the. National (Nationwide) Inpatient Sample (NIS). Accessed. https://www.hcup-us.ahrq.gov/nisoverview.jsp.
30. About ACS NSQIP. https://www.facs.org/Quality-Programs/ACS-NSQIP/About.

17

Combinatorial Technologies Leveraging Robotics in Spine Surgery

Ibrahim Hussain, MD, and Michael Y. Wang, MD, FAANS

INTRODUCTION

Technological innovations over the past several decades have enabled spine surgeons to steadily increase the safety and efficacy of procedures performed with a focus on improving outcomes, while minimizing the surgical footprint. Innovations in microscopic and endoscopic visualization systems, screw and rod instrumentation, expandable and 3D printed interbody cages, and three-dimensional computer assisted navigation capabilities are among these advancements. Robotic surgery has been revolutionized by the way surgeries are performed in other areas of medicine, including urology, gynecology, and cardiothoracic surgery. The adaptation of robotic technology has now provided a new and innovative avenue for safely performing spine surgery. Robotic-assisted spine surgery is the newest iteration of navigation-based, minimally invasive technology that is still relatively in its infancy, but has already yielded significant impact in multiple perioperative metrics in an era where evidence-based and cost-effective outcomes are being increasingly recognized.

As described in detail in the preceding chapters, multiple studies evaluating robotic-assisted screw placement to the traditional free-hand and fluoroscopic-guided techniques have demonstrated improved accuracy rates of 91% to 98.5%, based on the definition of pedicle breach used in each study.[1–4] Some studies have reported up to 100% accuracy when using the "clinically acceptable" threshold.[5] Apart from pedicle breaches, robotic-assisted surgery has shown reduction in proximal facet joint violation, thereby mitigating a major factor in adjacent segment disease; from an educational standpoint, this allows accuracy to be maintained when accounting for differences between an attending and a resident.[6] Furthermore, reductions in the radiation dose to the surgical team and patient (for fluoroscopy-guided procedures), complications, revision rates, blood loss, and length of stay have been reported across multiple retrospective and prospective studies.[3,4,7–11]

As spinal robotics become increasingly affordable and cost-effective, it is only natural that further innovations will drive new applications. Leveraging combinatorial technologies to augment the precision and minimal invasiveness of robotic spine surgery is an active area of evolution and presents unique opportunities for novice and experienced spine surgeons. In this chapter, we review the literature examining combinatorial technologies leveraging robotics in spine surgery and look into future possibilities (Table 17.1).

TABLE 17.1 Studies Describing Combinatorial Technologies With Robotics in Spine Surgery.

Author	Year	Technology	Summary
Liounakos et al.[12]	2020	Endoscopic TLIF	Robotic guidance allows the selection of either a safe or ideal trajectory for endoscopic transforaminal discectomy and interbody graft placement that minimizes the risk to DRG.
Burström et al.[13]	2020	Hybrid OR and augmented reality surgical navigation (ARSN) system	A robotic arm is used to place screws that have been pre-planned by an ARSN in a hybrid OR that relies on optical tracking eyes placed around the OR, and therefore controls the trajectory of the screw that is being placed through a rigid robotic arm.
Sun et al.[14]	2020	Artificial Intelligence	Force and sound sensors programmed into the robot based on artificially obtained intelligence from ex vivo dynamic experimentation allow for the robot to autonomously stop drilling if a breach in the cortex is detected within a time much faster than a human could.
Li et al.[15]	2021	Endoscopic decompression	Robotic guidance allows predetermined areas and depths of lamina to be localized and drilled from a single small incision to minimize excessive bony resection and instability, while utilizing a unique adapter for the robotic arm to aid in control and mitigate surgeon fatigue.

DRG, Dorsal root ganglia; *OR*, operating room; *TLIF*, transforaminal lumbar interbody fusion.

SPINAL ROBOTICS AND ENDOSCOPY

Spinal endoscopy has witnessed a resurgence over the past decade paralleled by advancements in lens and resolution optics and compatible instrumentation. When combined with increased awareness of healthcare economic costs, narcotic dependency, and COVID-19-era hospital restrictions, this has fueled a push for "ultra" minimally invasive approaches for decompression and fusion procedures that allow patients to mobilize, leave the hospital, and wean off pain medications faster than ever before. Endoscopic spine surgery has witnessed enormous strides over the last two decades, fueled by advancements in narrower rigid endoscopes, light-emitting diode (LED) illumination sources, ultra-high-definition optical displays, radiofrequency electrode probes for cauterization, high-speed drills, disk preparation instruments, and expandable interbody grafts. Combining robotics with endoscopy is an example of two distinct but rapidly evolving technologies that can synergize to offer advanced, minimally invasive solutions for common spinal pathologies. We herein present two unique cases leveraging these combinatorial technologies.

Case #1: Robotic-Assisted Endoscopic Transforaminal Lumbar Interbody Fusion (TLIF)

History and Clinical Presentation

A 78-year-old male with an extensive cardiac history on antiplatelet therapy and history of an L4/5 decompression over a decade prior presented with symptoms of back pain and bilateral lower extremity radiculopathy that had been progressively worsening over the past year. The patient's back pain had a mechanical component, which was worse when going from sitting to standing and also while ambulating, but relieved during rest. His lower extremity pain was constant and encompassed the L3 and L4 dermatomes. His lower extremity radiculopathy had previously been responsive to epidural steroid injections;

however, the injections became less efficacious over the course of a year, while his low back pain simultaneously worsened. The patient had also failed other conservative measures including various oral medications, physical therapy, and chiropractic manipulation. On physical examination, the patient had intact motor strength and sensation without evidence of myelopathy.

Preoperative Imaging

Magnetic resonance imaging revealed multilevel lumbar spondylosis with moderate central stenosis and moderate-to-severe bilateral foraminal stenosis at the L3/4 and L4/5 levels. There was also bilateral lateral recess stenosis at both levels, caused by a combination of disk bulge, ligamentum hypertrophy, and facet arthropathy (Fig. 17.1).

Surgical Plan

Given the patient's foraminal nerve root compression and symptoms of mechanical instability, a two-level L3–L5 transforaminal lumbar interbody fusion (TLIF) was recommended for the purposes of stabilization and indirect decompression. The patient had previously had a midline, traditional open L4–L5 laminectomy; therefore, scar tissue formation in this region was a consideration given the higher risk of potential cerebrospinal fluid leak. Considering the potential scar tissue formation combined with the patient's comorbidities, a minimally invasive, robotic-assisted endoscopic TLIF was recommended.

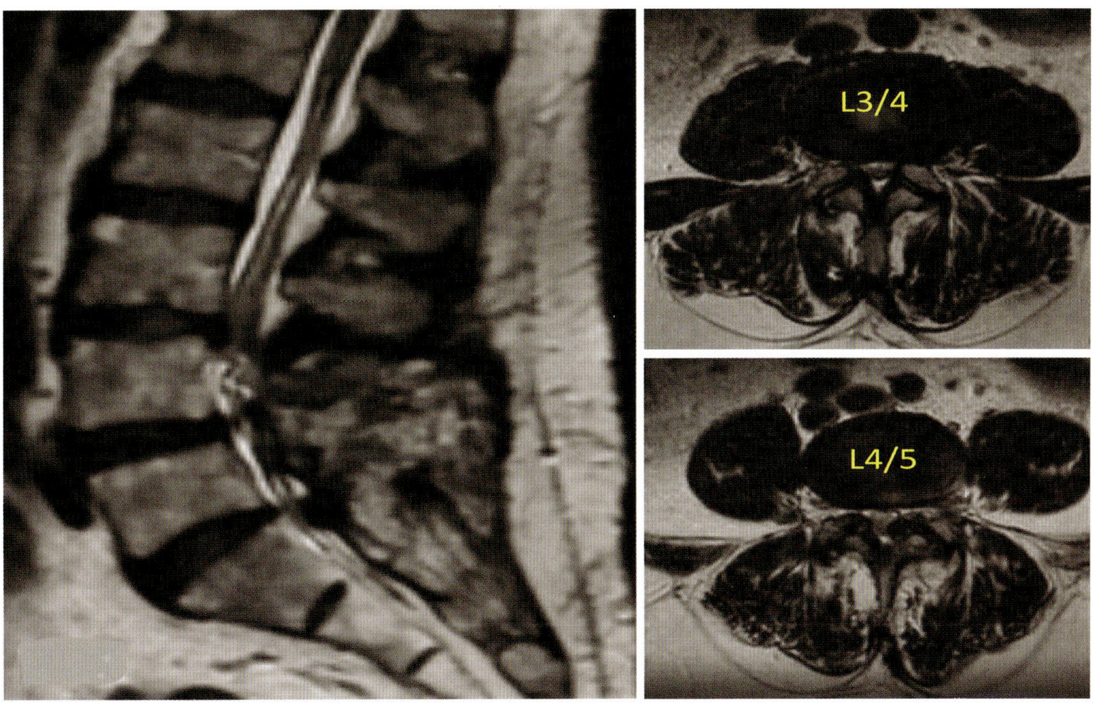

FIG. 17.1 Sagittal and axial T2-weighted MRI demonstrating central, lateral recess, and foraminal stenosis at the L3/4 and L4/5 levels. The stenosis was caused by a combination of disk bulge, ligamentum flavum hypertrophy, and facet arthropathy.

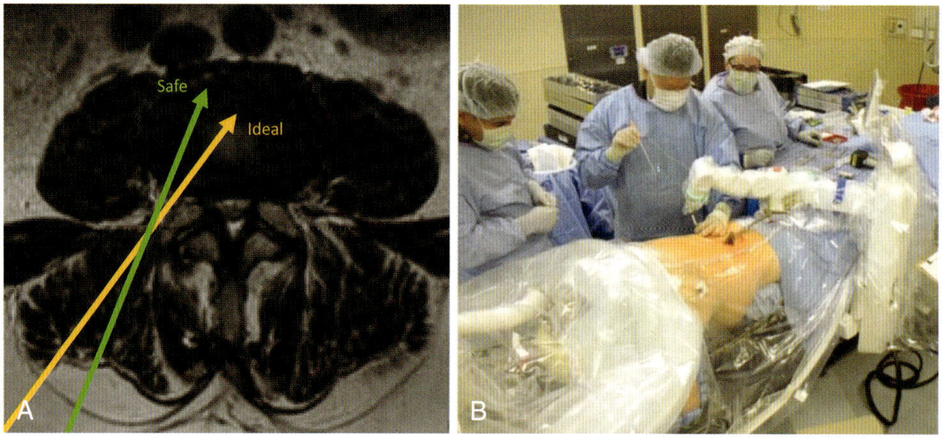

FIG. 17.2 (A) Axial T2-weight MRI of the L3/4 level demonstrating the two trajectories tested for robotic-assisted endoscopic approach for transforaminal discectomy and interbody graft insertion. The ideal (*orange*) trajectory has a more a lateral starting point and targets the center of the disk; however, it places the dorsal root ganglia at higher risk of iatrogenic injury. The safe (*green*) trajectory uses a more medial starting point that allows access to the disk space in the most medial portion of the Kambin triangle, yielding the lowest risk to the dorsal root ganglia but a slightly less optimal trajectory within the disk. Ultimately both trajectories are tested with triggered electromyography and the trajectory with the lowest feedback on stimulation is selected. (B) Intraoperative photograph demonstrating the surgical robotic arm localizing a trajectory while triggered EMG with a stimulating probe is used to assess the proximity to the exiting nerve root.

After the placement of percutaneous pedicle screws utilizing navigation-guided robotic assistance, the robot was also utilized to determine the safest and best trajectory for accessing the L3/4 and L4/5 disk spaces to performed the endoscopic discectomy. Two trajectories were tested: the ideal trajectory, which aimed toward the center of the disk with a more lateral starting point, and the safe approach, which allowed passage through the most medial portion of the Kambin triangle and therefore the largest safe zone, with a more medial starting point and anterior target within the disk space. The trajectory that was ultimately chosen was that which elicited the least feedback based on triggered EMG (Fig. 17.2). Ultimately, a safe trajectory was used for L3/4 and an ideal trajectory for L4/5. Once the trajectory for each space was selected, the endoscopic TLIF was performed as previously described.[16] Various pituitary rongeurs were used to complete the endoscopic discectomy, creating a centrum cavity across the disk. Next, C-arm fluoroscopy was brought in and further endplate preparation was completed with the use of various disk shaving instruments including a hand drill, wire brushes, and a butterfly shaver. A radiopaque dye-filled balloon was used to confirmed adequate discectomy prior to bone morphogenetic protein (BMP) sponge and collapsed mesh implantation (Fig. 17.3). Finally, the mesh implant was inserted and expanded with allograft until adequate lift was achieved. Rods were passed submuscularly into the screw heads and locking caps were placed and finally tightened to complete the construct.

Postoperative Course

The patient was discharged on postoperative day three, remaining sensorimotor intact. At the 6-week follow-up, he reported improving axial low back pain and resolution of the

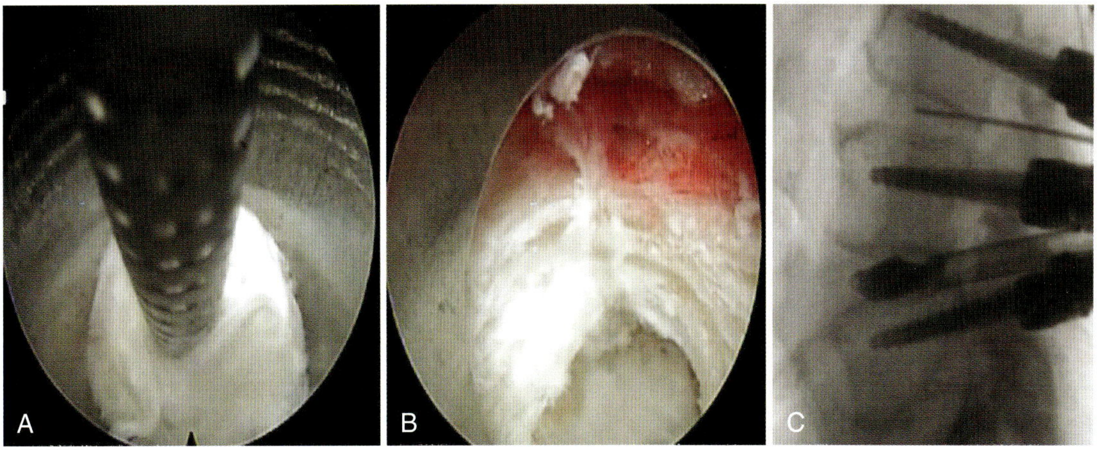

FIG. 17.3 (A) Intraoperative endoscopic view of the discectomy being performed with a pituitary rongeur. (B) The annular defect and centrum of the disk cavity are visualized during the endoscopic discectomy. (C) A radiopaque dye-filled balloon is used to determine the extent of discectomy in preparation for the final placement of the mesh interbody graft through the 8-mm working cannula.

lower extremity radiculopathy. There was no evidence of hardware abnormalities or pathologic motion on standing flexion/extension x-rays at that time (Fig. 17.4).

Procedural Advantages

The transforaminal approach in endoscopic surgery provides a versatile trajectory that can be used for discectomy, foraminoplasty, and disk preparation for interbody fusion. This approach requires accessing pathology through the Kambin triangle, entering through a window between the exiting nerve root, the superior articulating process, and the superior endplate of the inferior vertebrae. The exact site of the incision and trajectory is dependent on multiple factors, including the goal of surgery, anatomic location of pathology, habitus of the patient, and safety profile of working in the Kambin triangle to avoid exiting nerve root injury.[17]

For example, in order to access the disk space for disk preparation for a TLIF, a trajectory parallel to the disk space is required. This 1 A approach allows the safest trajectory to avoid the exiting nerve root but limits access to central disk pathology. The 1B approach is used for discectomy or transforaminal epidural injections, with a slight caudal angulation. This approach narrows the safe working corridor of the Kambin triangle and requires a medial starting point to avoid injury to the dorsal root ganglia. The 1 C approach is similar to the trajectory used in 1B in that it is aimed caudally, but is also directed more horizontally in the axial plane to optimize the trajectory for safe foraminotomy and resection of the superior articulating process.[17] In addition to the trajectory utilized, the exact entry point from the midline of the spine is also critical with the transforaminal endoscopic approach. Distances of anywhere from 8 to 12 cm from the midline have been reported, but this again depends on the exact nature of the pathology being treated as well as the habitus of the patient. Typically, a more lateral starting point allows for easier access to the disk space, but places the dorsal root ganglia at greater risk of injury.

The challenge in assessing the optimal starting point in endoscopic surgery provides an opportunity to leverage robotic assistance. Robotic surgery has already been well described

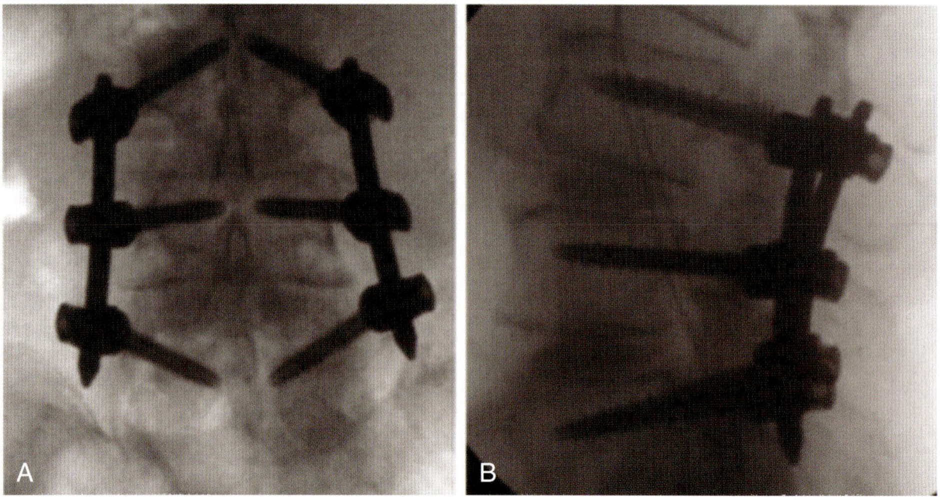

FIG. 17.4 Postoperative (A) Antero-posterior (AP) radiograph. (B) Lateral radiograph and lateral x-rays demonstrating the appropriate pedicle screw placement and interbody grafts at L3/4 and L4/5 following robotic-assisted endoscopic transforaminal lumber interbody fusion (TLIF).

in placing percutaneous pedicle screw instrumentation, which is involved in the first half of the operation described. With recent reports describing endoscopic TLIF, the utility of combining robotic and endoscopic technologies is completentary to each other and allows for a seamless operation and also for the selection of the optimal trajectory for the interbody portion of the case.[12] As described here, this single procedure combines multiple technologies as adjuncts to robotic surgery. These include triggered EMG, endoscopic visualization and discectomy, and endplate preparation under C-arm guidance.

Case #2: Robotic-Assisted Endoscopic Laminotomy

History and Clinical Presentation

A 27-year-old female with no significant past medical or surgical history presented with over 2 years of progressively worsening left lower extremity radicular pain in the L5 distribution. She endorsed paresthesias in the left lower leg and foot and had minimal back pain. Her symptoms failed to respond to multiple conservative measures including oral medications, physical therapy, and epidural steroid injections. On physical examination, she had a positive straight leg test on the left and had 4/5 strength in the left the extensor longus hallicus.

Preoperative Imaging

Magnetic resonance imaging revealed a large, caudally migrated L4/5 disk herniation with compression of the traversing L5 nerve (Fig. 17.5). There was no indication of instability with flexion/extension x-rays. Given the significant impact on her quality of life as well as refractoriness to conservative measures, surgery was indicated.

Surgical Plan

Given the patient's young age, goal of getting back to activity and work as quickly as possible, and lack of prior surgeries or other symptomatic levels or deformity, a minimally invasive endoscopic laminotomy and discectomy was recommended. In order to increase the accuracy

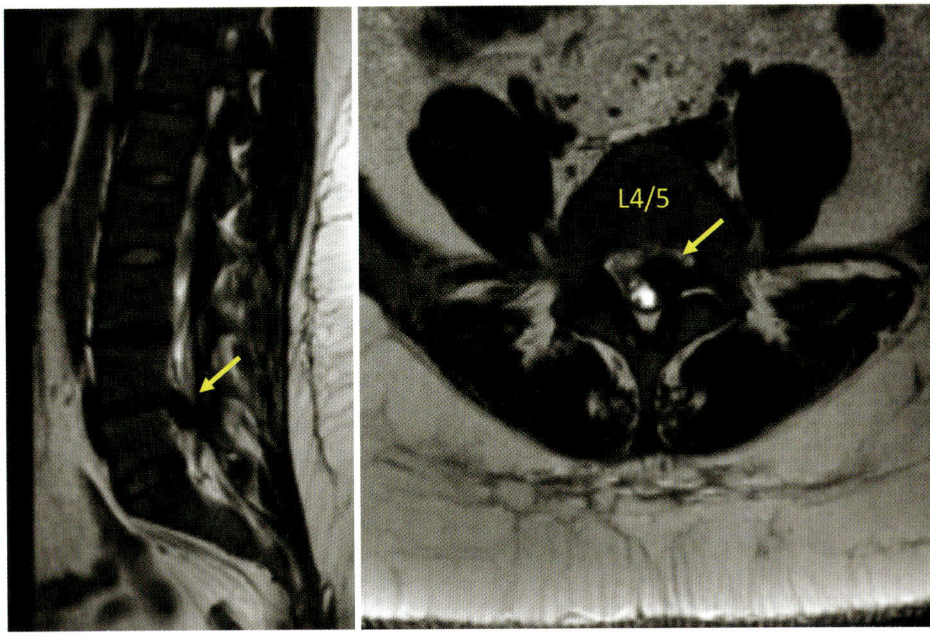

FIG. 17.5 Preoperative sagittal and axial T2-weighted MRI images demonstrating a large, caudally migrated left L4/5 disk herniation with compression of the traversing L5 nerve root.

of decompression to preserve as much healthy tissues as possible and to aid in the safety of the procedure, a robotic-assisted interlaminar endoscopic laminotomy was performed.

The procedure consisted of obtaining an intraoperative CT scan and mounting the robotic arm to the surgical table. From this CT scan, 11 different trajectories were made, which overlapped by 1 mm and had a diameter at the distal tip of 3.5 mm (equal to the drill bit) (Fig. 17.6). All the trajectories ensured that there was no greater than 10% of the medical facet resected and that the pars interarticularis was not violated, both in order to avoid iatrogenic instability. All the trajectories pivoted around a single 1-cm left paramedian incision site. The robotic arm was attached to the surgical table and used to localize the skin incision, which was then expanded subdermally with dilators followed by a docking tube on the cranial portion of the L5 lamina. The bone margins were confirmed prior to the placement of a custom-made adapter, placed in the robotic arm, through which the endoscope and endoscopic drill could pass (Fig. 17.7A). The adapter also secondarily served as a depth-stop, and the planned trajectories took into account the distance of the drill bit from the top of the adapter to prevent the inadvertent plunging of the drill.

The adapter and planned trajectories further ensured that the drill did not violate the inner cortical surface of the lamina, therefore mitigating the possibility of iatrogenic drilling of the dura or nerve root. This was especially pertinent given that the top of the L5 lamina had to be drilled, where it was partially cranial to the insertion of the ligamentum and therefore had exposed dura beneath it. The robotic arm was lowered into position and sequentially moved into each planned trajectory for drilling to be performed through the arm (Fig. 17.7B and C). Once the robotic-assisted laminotomy was completed, a Kerrison rongeur was used to bite away the egg-shelled inner cortical layer of remaining bone easily. Following this, the standard endoscopic techniques were utilized to bite away the

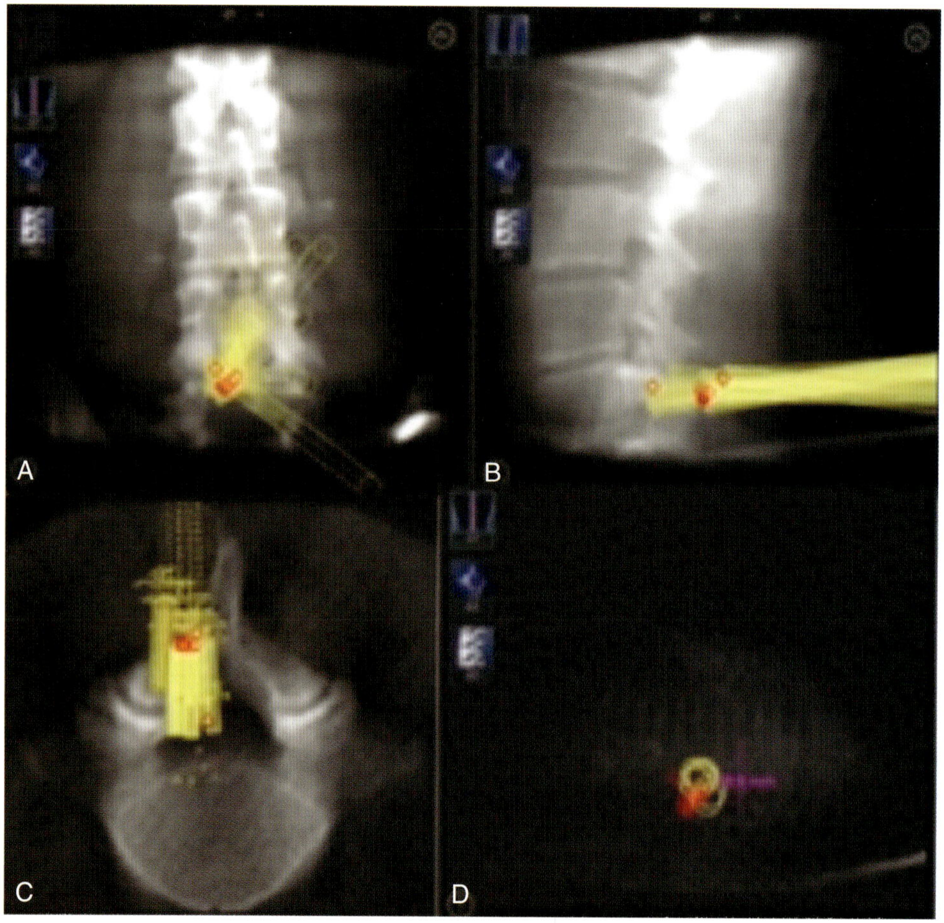

FIG. 17.6 (A) Coronal, (B) sagittal, (C) axial, and (D) probe's eye views of a 3D reconstruction of the patient's lumbar spine with robotic-assisted planning trajectories for a targeted L4/5 interlaminar endoscopic laminotomy. Note that each trajectory is 3.5 mm at the tip, which is the size of the drll bit used for the endoscopic bony decompression. All the trajectories converge on a single slightly paramedian 1-cm incision site and overlap by 1 mm to ensure that the total laminotomy area is accounted for when drilling.

ligamentum flavum, and then discectomy was performed with the assistance of endoscopic instruments. Endoscopic visualization of the pulsating L5 nerve root confirmed adequate decompression.

Postoperative Course

The patient remained in the hospital for less than 24 hours and was discharged home with full strength. Her preoperative left lower extremity radiculopathy resolved immediately and her paresthesias had resolved by the 2-week follow-up. The postoperative CT (which was obtained for the purposes of checking the intraoperative extent of bony resection and is otherwise not obtained in clinically stable patients) demonstrated precise bony resection of the pre-planned target of the lamina and medial facet joint (Fig. 17.8).

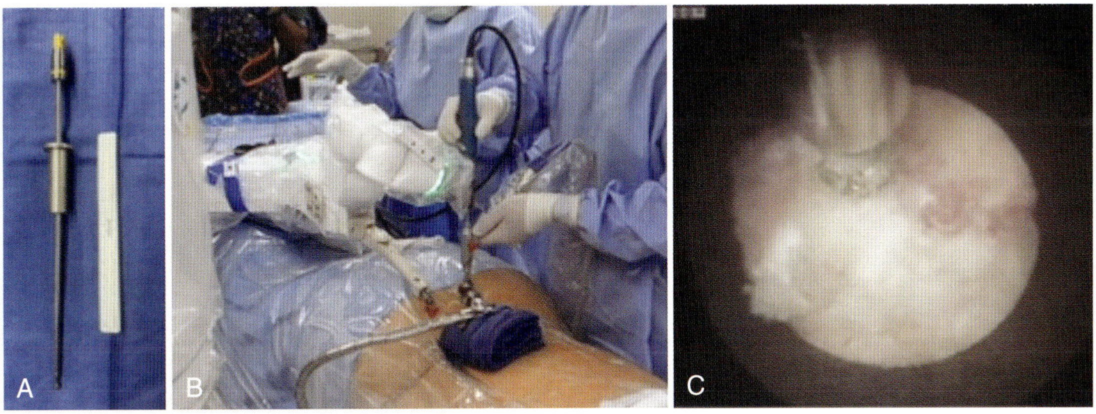

FIG. 17.7 (A) A custom-made adapter that is placed into the robotic arm through which the endoscope with working channels (including one for the hand-powered drill) are passed through. The adapter serves to stabilize the endoscope during drilling and also acts as a depth-stop to prevent inadvertent plunging through the lamina and into the dura or nerve root. (B) Intraoperative photograph demonstrating the equipment setup with the robotic arm and surgeon holding the endoscope in the non-dominant hand and the endoscopic drill in the dominant hand. (C) Intraoperative endoscopic view of the 3.5-mm diamond drill bit resecting the lamina without violating the inner cortical surface.

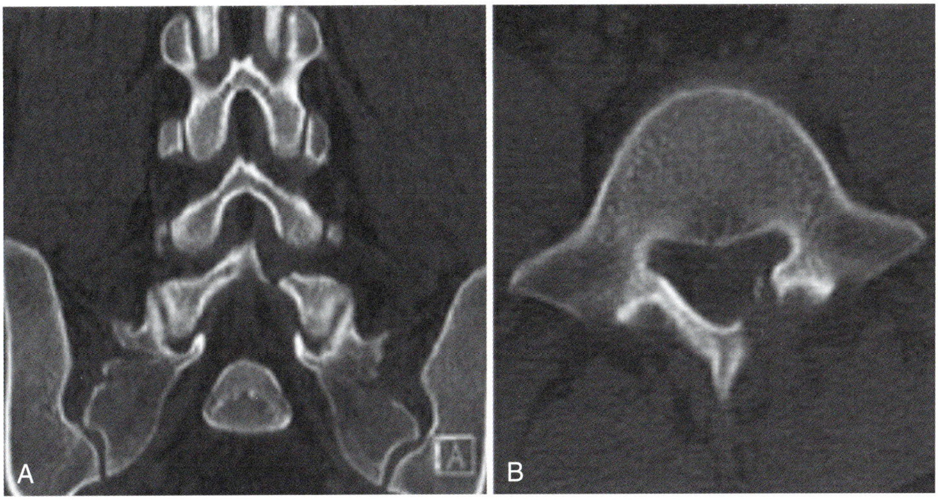

FIG. 17.8 (A) Coronal section. (B) Axial section of the Post-operative CT scan. Postoperative CT scan demonstrating the minimal but targeted robotic-assisted interlaminar laminotomy defect that permitted enough of a working window in which to complete the endoscopic discectomy of a large extruded fragment.

Procedural Advantages

The interlaminar endoscopic approach is distinct from the transforaminal approach in that it utilizes a slightly paramedian incision and approach, and requires drilling (except in some situations at L5–S1) and flavectomy in order to reach the neural elements. Drilling through an endoscopic portal allows the surgeon to visualize pathology directly, similar to other minimally invasive (e.g., tubular) techniques. However, there are limitations of this approach, which must be appreciated compared to traditional MIS and open approaches. First, apart from what is seen through the endoscopic lens, there is no easy way to orient yourself precisely by comparison to the neighboring anatomic structures. Excessive wanding of the rigid endoscope is limited by superficial structures; therefore, only structures within millimeters of the working portal can be visualized. Second, despite continuous irrigation, drilling is often performed in an "on/off" pattern in order to clear away the bone particles that obstruct endoscopic visualization. The weight of the drill in the operating hand plus balancing the working portal and endoscope itself with the other hand can lead to inadvertent movements and fatigue. Third, for novice users, the tactile and audible feedback from the drill may not alert the surgeon as to when they are about to break through the inner cortical surface and on to the neural elements.

Robotic assistance, in this type of case, helps to circumvent these concerns.[15] Preoperative planning of the target bone to be drilled is precise and provides real-time feedback of the exact location that is being resected; therefore, orientating yourself to neighboring structures which cannot be visualized is not required. The custom-made adapter used in this case provides rigid support and serves to hold the weight of the drill and eliminate inadvertent micromotions of the surgeon, as well as to prevent plunging through the inner cortical layer of the lamina. Collectively, the advantages of robotic-assisted endoscopic laminotomy allow for a smaller surgical footprint, a risk-reduced and ergonomically superior experience for the surgeon, and mitigation of potential iatrogenic instability through targeted bony resection, which all ultimately benefit the patient's outcomes.

FUTURE DIRECTIONS

Leveraging robotic technology to synergize and augment other areas of spine surgery continues to evolve. Among the other exciting technological advancements in current spine surgery practice has been the development of augmented and virtual reality systems. These technologies leverage heads-up displays, allowing the incorporation of intraoperative CT imaging with three-dimensional navigation capabilities that allow for precise anatomic localization and instrumentation placement. Another advantage is overlaying and color-coding of the relevant anatomy (such as nerve roots, pars, facet joints, and dura). Burström et al.[13] from the Karolinska Institute recently described their initial experience with a custom robotic arm that was integrated into a hybrid operating room (OR) equipped with an augmented reality surgical navigation system (ARSN). The robot was mounted on the OR table and used to assist in placing Jamshidi needles in 113 pedicles in multiple cadavers, while the ARSN system was used for planning screw paths and directing the robot. A ceiling-mounted C-arm was used for initial image capture, which was registered in three-dimensional space with four optical cameras placed around the hybrid OR. The robotic arm autonomously aligned with the planned screw trajectory, and the surgeon's only role was the insertion of the Jamshidi needle into the pedicle. This semi-autonomous system used the ARSN system to incorporate the data from the optical tracking cameras with the C-arm intraoperative images, and therefore the robotic arm itself was not being tracked, but rather entirely directed by the feedback fed into it by the ARSN. The authors found a clinical accuracy rate of 100% for projected pedicle screw placement and found statistically significant improvements compared with the ARSN systems used for screw placement without robotic assistance.

Another exciting area of current research is leveraging artificial intelligence with robotic surgical technologies. In this sense, the goal is to move away from the fully controlled model of human-controlled robotic assistance to one where the robotic can use input from multiple feedback vectors to make informed decisions for itself or at least to relay potential sources of error or complications to the surgeon. For example, as previously described, using the robot for spinal decompression allows for precise bony removal without violation of the inner cortical surface. However, what happens if a portion of the cortex is fractured during more superficial drilling? Since the robot is only registered with presurgical inputs and planning that the surgeon has devised, an unnoticed crack in the cortex can potentially shift the bone fragment and create an unprotected path to the dura that the robot or surgeon will not recognize immediately intraoperatively. To this end, researchers, such as Sun et al.,[14] have described using multimodal methods of informing the surgical robot to deviations from the original plan. They described the use of force and sound sensors that have been programmed into the robot based on artificially obtained intelligence from ex vivo dynamic experimentation and allow for a robotic-assisted mode that allows the robot to stop drilling autonomously if a breach in the cortex is detected within 30 milliseconds, far faster than a human could response to the same tactile feedback. This type of technology is now further opening avenues for the exploration of tele-surgery, where the spine surgeon may not even be in the same city as the operation; this is only augmented by the recent implementation of 5 G technology for faster and secure remote information transmission.

CONCLUSION

Robotics is just one of many exciting technological advancements in spine surgery over the past two decades. The incorporation of robotics with endoscopic surgery is an area where precision and minimal invasiveness intersect to create an even safer and more efficient experience for the patient and surgeon. Moving past just accuracy for pedicle screw insertion, the robot will be increasingly utilized with endoscopic technologies, three-dimensional navigation, and robotic-controlled instrumentation to allow the expansion of its utility in various spinal procedures, including trajectory planning, bony decompressions, and potentially osteotomy localization for complex deformities. Future research is well underway in incorporating robotics into "smart", hybrid ORs for spine surgery which can take up less footprint than the current systems and allow for a more ergonomically friendly operation for the surgeon. Moreover, leveraging artificial intelligence and spinal robotics will facilitate further evolution and autonomy that will allow this technology to respond faster and more precisely than a surgeon's hand ever could, as has already been witnessed in other industries such as avionics, transportation, and manufacturing.

ACKNOWLEDGMENTS

Disclosures: IH: Nothing to disclose. **MYW:** Royalty payments from DePuy-Synthes Spine, Inc, Children's Hospital of Los Angeles, Springer Publishing, and Quality Medical Publishing; consultant for DePuy-Synthes Spine, Inc, Stryker Spine, K2M, and Spineology; advisory board member for Vallum; stock in Spinicity and Innovative Surgical Devices; and grants from the Department of Defense.

Funding: N/A

REFERENCES

1. Wallace DJ, Vardiman AB, Booher GA, et al. Navigated robotic assistance improves pedicle screw accuracy in minimally invasive surgery of the lumbosacral spine: 600 pedicle screws in a single institution. *Int J Med Robot.* 2020;16(1):e2054. https://doi.org/10.1002/rcs.2054.
2. Pechlivanis I, Kiriyanthan G, Engelhardt M, et al. Percutaneous placement of pedicle screws in the lumbar spine using a bone mounted miniature robotic system: first experiences and accuracy of screw placement. *Spine (Phila Pa 1976).* 2009;34(4):392–398. https://doi.org/10.1097/BRS.0b013e318191ed32.
3. Peng YN, Tsai LC, Hsu HC, Kao CH. Accuracy of robot-assisted versus conventional freehand pedicle screw placement in spine surgery: a systematic review and meta-analysis of randomized controlled trials. *Ann Transl Med.* 2020; 8(13):824. https://doi.org/10.21037/atm-20-1106.
4. Tarawneh AM, Salem KM. A systematic review and meta-analysis of randomized controlled trials comparing the accuracy and clinical outcome of pedicle screw placement using robot-assisted technology and conventional freehand technique. *Glob Spine J.* 2021;11(4):575–586. https://doi.org/10.1177/2192568220927713.
5. Jiang B, Pennington Z, Zhu A, et al. Three-dimensional assessment of robot-assisted pedicle screw placement accuracy and instrumentation reliability based on a preplanned trajectory. *J Neurosurg Spine.* 2020:1–10.
6. Vardiman AB, Wallace DJ, Booher GA, et al. Does the accuracy of pedicle screw placement differ between the attending surgeon and resident in navigated robotic-assisted minimally invasive spine surgery? *J Robot Surg.* 2020;14(4):567–572. https://doi.org/10.1007/s11701-019-01019-9.
7. Zhang JN, Fan Y, He X, Liu TJ, Hao DJ. Comparison of robot-assisted and freehand pedicle screw placement for lumbar revision surgery. *Int Orthop.* 2021;45(6):1531–1538. https://doi.org/10.1007/s00264-020-04825-1.
8. Liounakos JI, Kumar V, Jamshidi A, et al. Reduction in complication and revision rates for robotic-guided short-segment lumbar fusion surgery: results of a prospective, multi-center study. *J Robot Surg.* 2021;15(5):793–802. https://doi.org/10.1007/s11701-020-01165-5.
9. Li J, Fang Y, Jin Z, Wang Y, Yu M. The impact of robot-assisted spine surgeries on clinical outcomes: A systemic review and meta-analysis. *Int J Med Robot.* 2020;16(6):1–14. https://doi.org/10.1002/rcs.2143.
10. Zhang Q, Xu YF, Tian W, et al. Comparison of superior-level facet joint violations between robot-assisted percutaneous pedicle screw placement and conventional open fluoroscopic-guided pedicle screw placement. *Orthop Surg.* 2019;11(5):850–856. https://doi.org/10.1111/os.12534.
11. Zhou LP, Zhang RJ, Sun YW, Zhang L, Shen CL. Accuracy of pedicle screw placement and four other clinical outcomes of robotic guidance technique versus computer-assisted navigation in thoracolumbar surgery: a meta-analysis. *World Neurosurg.* 2021;146:e139–e150. https://doi.org/10.1016/j.wneu.2020.10.055.
12. Liounakos JI, Wang MY. Lumbar 3-lumbar 5 robotic-assisted endoscopic transforaminal lumbar interbody fusion: 2-dimensional operative video. *Oper Neurosurg (Hagerstown).* 2020;19(1):E73–E74. https://doi.org/10.1093/ons/opz385.
13. Burstrom G, Balicki M, Patriciu A, et al. Feasibility and accuracy of a robotic guidance system for navigated spine surgery in a hybrid operating room: a cadaver study. *Sci Rep.* 2020;10(1):7522. doi:10.1038/s41598-020-64462-x.
14. Sun Y, Wang L, Jiang Z, Li B, Hu Y, Tian W. State recognition of decompressive laminectomy with multiple information in robot-assisted surgery. *Artif Intell Med.* 2020;102:101763. https://doi.org/10.1016/j.artmed.2019.101763.
15. Li Y, Wang MY. Robotic-assisted endoscopic laminotomy: 2-dimensional operative video. *Oper Neurosurg (Hagerstown).* 2021;20(5):E361. https://doi.org/10.1093/ons/opaa441.
16. Kolcun JPG, Brusko GD, Basil GW, Epstein R, Wang MY. Endoscopic transforaminal lumbar interbody fusion without general anesthesia: operative and clinical outcomes in 100 consecutive patients with a minimum 1-year follow-up. *Neurosurg Focus.* 2019;46(4):E14. https://doi.org/10.3171/2018.12.FOCUS18701.
17. Fanous AA, Tumialán LM, Wang MY. Kambin's triangle: definition and new classification schema. *J Neurosurg Spine.* 2019;32(3):390–398. https://doi.org/10.3171/2019.8.SPINE181475.

INDEX

Page numbers followed by "*f*" indicate figures, "*t*" indicate tables, "*b*" indicate boxes.